MEDICAL RADIOLOGY
Diagnostic Imaging

Editors:
A. L. Baert, Leuven
K. Sartor, Heidelberg

P. Lefere · S. Gryspeerdt (Eds.)

Virtual Colonoscopy

A Practical Guide

With Contributions by

F. Booya · D. Burling · A. H. Dachman · A. H. de Vries · H. Fenlon · J. T. Ferrucci
J. G. Fletcher · S. Gryspeerdt · S. Halligan · A. Laghi · P. Lefere · A. Maier · T. Mang
B. G. McFarland · K. J. Mortelé · A. S. Odulate · A. O'Hare · P. Paolantonio · P. Pokieser
W. Schima · J. Stoker · S. Taylor · R. E. van Gelder · J. Yee · H. Yoshida · M. E. Zalis

Foreword by

A. L. Baert

With 173 Figures in 407 Separate Illustrations, 115 in Color and 11 Tables

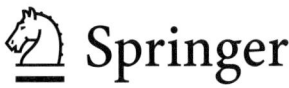

Philippe Lefere, MD
Stedelijk Ziekenhuis
Department of Radiology
Bruggesteenweg 90
8800 Roeselare
Belgium

Stefaan Gryspeerdt, MD
Stedelijk Ziekenhuis
Department of Radiology
Bruggesteenweg 90
8800 Roeselare
Belgium

Medical Radiology · Diagnostic Imaging and Radiation Oncology
Series Editors: A. L. Baert · L. W. Brady · H.-P. Heilmann · M. Molls · K. Sartor

Continuation of Handbuch der medizinischen Radiologie
Encyclopedia of Medical Radiology

Library of Congress Control Number: 2005928418

ISBN 3-540-22865-9 Springer Berlin Heidelberg New York
ISBN 978-3-540-22865-3 Springer Berlin Heidelberg New York

This work is subject to copyright. All rights are reserved, whether the whole or part of the material is concerned, specifically the rights of translation, reprinting, reuse of illustrations, recitations, broadcasting, reproduction on microfilm or in any other way, and storage in data banks. Duplication of this publication or parts thereof is permitted only under the provisions of the German Copyright Law of September 9, 1965, in its current version, and permission for use must always be obtained from Springer-Verlag. Violations are liable for prosecution under the German Copyright Law.

Springer is part of Springer Science+Business Media

http//www.springeronline.com
© Springer-Verlag Berlin Heidelberg 2006
Printed in Germany

The use of general descriptive names, trademarks, etc. in this publication does not imply, even in the absence of a specific statement, that such names are exempt from the relevant protective laws and regulations and therefore free for general use.

Product liability: The publishers cannot guarantee the accuracy of any information about dosage and application contained in this book. In every case the user must check such information by consulting the relevant literature.

Medical Editor: Dr. Ute Heilmann, Heidelberg
Desk Editor: Ursula N. Davis, Heidelberg
Production Editor: Kurt Teichmann, Mauer
Cover-Design and Typesetting: Verlagsservice Teichmann, Mauer

Printed on acid-free paper – 21/3151xq – 5 4 3 2 1 0

Foreword

Modern spiral multidetector computed tomography enables isotropic voxel data acquisition and has opened up the way for superb multiplanar reconstruction, resulting in exquisite pathologic radiological correlation. CT angiography and CT colonography are examples of the clinical applications of this new technology. Both new radiological procedures have already secured their specific role in everyday radiological practice.

During the previous decade, radiologists made fundamental contributions to the study and diagnosis of colon diseases with the introduction of single and double contrast barium examinations of the colon. Due to progress in endoscopic techniques both classical radiological procedures have rapidly lost their importance.

With CT colonography begins yet a new era for radiology of the colon and offers very attractive possibilities for non-invasive detection and diagnosis of colon tumors.

As for many other radiological procedure, meticulous methodology and appropriate training in the interpretation of the imaging features are needed in order to obtain optimal results with this new method.

This volume explains in the most comprehensive way all practical details to be observed by those starting virtual coloscopy in their practice. These include: patient preparation, correct CT scanning parameters and imaging interpretation.

Both editors are pioneers in the field and have long-standing clinical experience with virtual coloscopy. In addition, they have been able to secure the collaboration of several other internationally recognised experts who have contributed individual chapters.

I congratulate the editors and the contributing authors for this outstanding, well researched, well structured and superbly illustrated book.

I am convinced that this volume on a hot clinical topic will be of great interest for both radiologists in training and certified radiologists wishing to become familiar with virtual coloscopy, as well as for gastroenterologists and abdominal surgeons.

I sincerely hope that this volume will enjoy the same success as so many other volumes previously published in the series: Medical Radiology – Diagnostic Imaging.

Leuven ALBERT L. BAERT

Preface

Virtual colonoscopy or computed tomographic (CT) colonography is a recent radiological technique enabling detection of tumoral lesions in the colon. As in the past two decades its radiological predecessor, double-contrast barium enema (DCBE), has lost most of its adherents, CT colonography constitutes a real opportunity for gastrointestinal radiologists to play a preponderant role in the diagnosis and treatment of colorectal cancer and the adenoma. Since its introduction by David Vining in 1994, CT colonography has very rapidly shown its virtues as a possible substitute for DCBE. The first important study on CT colonography by Helen Fenlon from the Boston Medical Center, published in 1999 in the New England Journal of Medicine, reporting very good lesion detection, underscored this aspiration. Since then CT colonography has dramatically evolved by the refinement of existing techniques and the introduction of new ones: faecal tagging with the option of reducing the cathartic or laxative part of the preparation, the use of carbon dioxide to inflate the colon, the introduction of multi-detector CT scanners producing spectacular images with isotropic resolution and reducing the examination time for the patient, the use of ultra-low-dose scan protocols reducing the radiation burden, improvement of the image post-processing with fast three-dimensional functions, and computer-aided diagnosis (CAD). These technical improvements help both the radiologist and the patient. For the former there is an improvement of the reading conditions, possibly improving diagnostic accuracy; for the latter the preparation and examination are more comfortable.

Despite these improvements in technique, however, CT colonography has not yet been able to break through as an acceptable tool for colorectal cancer screening. This is because of the disappointing results in some recent large multi-centre trials. Most probably sub-optimal technique in preparation, colonic distension, scanning parameters and image post-processing was the main cause of this failure. In fact, each of these stages needs rigorous attention if one is to achieve optimal results like those obtained in another momentous study, performed by Perry Pickhardt and published in the New England Journal of Medicine in 2003. Based upon a meticulous technique of preparation with faecal tagging, colonic inflation, scanning parameters and reading conditions, CT colonography obtained better scores than optical colonoscopy in this study. Furthermore, the examinations were interpreted by a team of radiologists experienced in CT colonography. This brings us to another important aspect of CT colonography. As was the case with DCBE, the degree of experience needed to adequately read and interpret CT colonography should not be underestimated.

In experienced hands CT colonography seems to be ripe for prime-time colorectal cancer screening. However it is not yet ready for widespread application of screening for the aforementioned reasons. CT colonography is now at an important crossroads, and serious efforts should be undertaken to take it to the level of being a widely accepted screening method for colorectal cancer. To fulfil this goal tremendous efforts are being undertaken in both Europe and the United States to educate radiologists with workshops, data banks and numerous scientific publications.

With contributions from several leaders in the field, this book, entirely dedicated to this exciting technique, sets out to be a guide for both the beginner and the experienced CT colonographer. It provides the reader with a wealth of information on all the prerequisites to perform state-of-the-art CT colonography.

We want to express our sincere gratitude and appreciation to all the renowned radiologists experienced in CT colonography who have contributed to this volume. We also thank Professor Albert L. Baert, who gave us the unique opportunity to edit this book and to bring it to a successful conclusion.

We hope that the reader will enjoy this work and will find it a help when performing CT colonography.

Roeselare, Belgium   PHILIPPE LEFERE and STEFAAN GRYSPEERDT

Contents

CTC: Why We Do It
JOSEPH T. FERRUCCI 1

1 Starting CT Colonography in Your Department
ALAN O'HARE and HELEN FENLON. 7

2 The Eligible Patient: Indications and Contraindications
AYODALE S. ODULATE and KOENRAAD J. MORTELE 13

3 Patient Preparation for CT Colonography
JUDY YEE 23

4 The Alternative: Faecal Tagging
PHILIPPE LEFERE and STEFAAN GRYSPEERDT. 35

5 How to Get the Colon Distended?
DAVID BURLING, STUART TAYLOR, and STEVE HALLIGAN 51

6 The Right Scanner Parameters to Use
ANDREA LAGHI and PASQUALE PAOLANTONIO 61

7 How to Interpret the Data Sets?
BETH G. MCFARLAND 73

8 How to Avoid Pitfalls in Imaging. Causes and Solutions
to Overcome False Negatives and False Positives
STEFAAN GRYSPEERDT and PHILIPPE LEFERE. 87

9 3D Imaging: Invaluable for the Correct Diagnosis?
AYSO H. DE VRIES, ROGIER E. VAN GELDER, and JAAP STOKER 117

10 Extracolonic Findings in CT Colonography
STEFAAN GRYSPEERDT and PHILIPPE LEFERE. 129

11 The Future: Computer-Aided Detection
HIROYUKI YOSHIDA 137

12 Quality and Consistency in Reporting CT Colonography
ABRAHAM H. DACHMAN and MICHAEL ZALIS 153

13 Virtual Colonoscopy Beyond Polyp Detection?
   Thomas Mang, Wolfgang Schima, Andrea Maier, and Peter Pokieser 161

14 Pictorial Overview of Normal Anatomy, Mimics of Disease,
   and Neoplasia at CT Colonography
   Joel G. Fletcher and Fargol Booya. 175

Subject Index 193

List of Contributors. 199

CTC: Why We Do It

JOSEPH T. FERRUCCI

Question: Why do we climb Mt. Everest?
Answer: Because it is there.
                                        Anonymous

CONTENTS

1 Introduction *1*
2 Colorectal Cancer Screening (CRCS): Rationale *2*
3 Colon Polyp: Natural History/Target of Screening *2*
4 Clinical Results *4*
5 Acceptance of CTC *4*
6 Conclusion *5*
   References *5*

1
Introduction

Computed tomographic colonography (CTC), commonly known as Virtual Colonoscopy (VC) has recently emerged as a fundamentally new technique for radiologic imaging of the colon with the unique potential for broad application in population screening for colorectal cancer. Yet, when framed in the philosophic question of "why do we do CTC?", the analogy to Mt. Everest becomes clear. We do CTC because the technology exists.

In the early 1990s, the introduction of spiral CT scanners, and powerful new computer workstations for image processing prompted individual pioneers to exploit the new technology at least in part, because they could. Coin obtained a United States patent for CT reconstruction of the colon (COIN et al. 1995), while Vining is credited with the first clinical demonstration of what he termed 'virtual colonoscopy' (VINING and GELFAND 1994). Hara at the Mayo Clinic (HARA et al. 1996) and Royster at Boston University (ROYSTER et al. 1997) confirmed clinical feasibility for polyp detection. Fenlon then showed that the sensitivity of CTC equaled that of conventional colonoscopy for detection of large polyps and cancers in a landmark 100 patient Boston University study published in the New England Journal of Medicine (FENLON et al. 1999). As they say, the rest is history.

As CTC enters its second decade, it is no longer new, but retains many compelling features. Technologically it maintains its sophisticated, innovative appeal and still exhibits great potential to evolve further. Scientifically, CTC is reframing strategies for colorectal cancer screening and now challenges the primacy of colonoscopy and the specialty of gastroenterology for the diagnosis of colon disorders. At the same time, CTC has been a dominant focus of research in abdominal and gastrointestinal radiology for several years, stimulating an enormous volume of original scientific investigation as well as media and industry attention. Impressive clinical results continue to appear from investigators throughout the world, including North America, Europe, and Australia (YEE et al. 2001; MACARI et al. 2002; IANNACONE et al. 2003; EDWARDS et al. 2004). Even more important is the totally non-invasive aspect of CTC (no drugs, no contrast media and no injections) which has won the favor of many physicians and their patients, especially when compared to optical colonoscopy. In preference studies comparing the two tests, patients usually prefer CTC despite the unavoidable biases of pre-endoscopy sedation (SVENSSON 2002). It is this patient friendly, 'compliance enhancer' nature of CTC which has been able to attract otherwise reluctant patients to undergo colorectal cancer screening. A recent U.S. hospital think tank reported that some 60% of patients having virtual colonoscopy had never had any prior form of colorectal cancer screening (ADVISORY BOARD 2004) (Fig. 1). In the United States, several HMOs have begun to reimburse for colorectal cancer screening using CTC, and wider reimbursement coverage is expected in 2006 which should lead to rapid wide dissemination into clinical practice.

J. T. FERRUCCI, MD
Chair Emeritus and Professor of Radiology, Boston University School of Medicine, Boston Medical Center, 88 East Newton Street, Boston, MA 02118

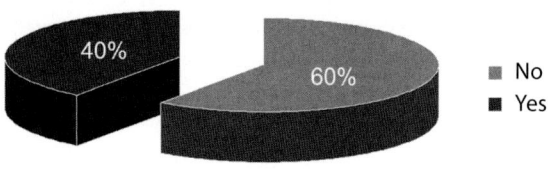

Fig. 1. CTC as a 'compliance enhancer'. Pie chart from a US hospital think tank study showing that among patients having virtual colonoscopy 60% had never had any prior colon cancer screening

2
Colorectal Cancer Screening (CRCS): Rationale

Across the developed world, colorectal cancer is the second or third leading cause of cancer deaths. While a small percentage (10–20%) of colorectal cancers occur in high risk genetically predisposed patients, the majority, i.e., ca. 80% of colorectal cancers occur sporadically in otherwise low risk individuals. In the vast majority of such cases, the cancers are believed to arise from pre-existing adenomatous polyp pre-cursors in series of events that have a well characterized origin in genetic mutations with a consequent histopathologic sequence of degeneration into frank invasive cancer. However, this process is rather leisurely, requiring some 10–15 years or more and interruption of this progression by detection and removal of threatening pre-cursor adenomas by endoscopic polypectomy results in a decline of cancer related mortality by as much as 30%.

Guidelines for colorectal screening in asymptomatic populations have been developed on the basis of scientific medical evidence, by professional organizations and government agencies throughout Europe and North America. Most recommend that screening begin in asymptomatic individuals at low or average risk at age 50 years and permit several different testing strategies. These include annual screening with fecal occult blood tests, flexible sigmoidoscopy every five years, the combination of fecal occult blood and flexible sigmoidoscopy every five years, double contrast barium enema every five years or colonoscopy every ten years. However, none of these test strategies is ideal and proponents of the various strategies continue to engage in contentious debate. For example, the specific limitations of FOBT and flexible sigmoidoscopy have led to the concept of the desirability of an anatomic or structural examination of the whole colon. This has led to the emergence of colonoscopy as the de facto gold standard for colorectal screening as well as colon diagnosis generally. The more focused debate has revolved around whether colonoscopy should be offered as a universal once in a lifetime test, e.g., at age 60 or reserved for selective application when results of other preliminary screening tests are positive. In the latter case, the broader goal of colorectal cancer screening becomes the use of less invasive, less expensive tests for triage selection of patients to undergo therapeutic optical colonoscopy. (Parenthetically, the double contrast barium enema is rapidly falling out of favor in the U.S. for primary colorectal cancer screening.)

Yet, despite wide medical, public health and lay media airing as to the importance of colorectal cancer screening, the public has remained generally reluctant to undergo these tests which are perceived as unpleasant and embarrassing such that overall compliance with colorectal cancer screening rarely exceeds 30–40%. Recently in the specific instance of colonoscopy in the United States, compliance rate have increased slightly to ca.40–50%, but only in selected well insured patient groups. Moreover, manpower resources of colonoscopists are strained, at least in the United States, with long 6–12 month waiting lists for elective appointments. Thus, new alternative tests for colorectal cancer screening are needed and awaited and, along with fecal DNA testing, CTC appears a procedure whose time has come.

3
Colon Polyp: Natural History/Target of Screening

The progressive transformation of adenomatous polyps to invasive adenocarcinoma has been characterized as "the adenoma carcinoma sequence" (MUTO 1975). However, because the prevalence of undetected cancer in an asymptomatic screening population is very low at ca.1%, colon polyp size is widely accepted as a surrogate end point for outcomes assessment in colorectal cancer screening programs. Thus, the concept of the "advanced adenoma" has been developed which is defined as an adenomatous polyp measuring 10 mm or greater or one containing villous or dysplastic components at histologic examination (WINAWER and ZAUBER 2002). However, in the context of CRC screening, the actual prevalence of advanced adenomas or at least polyps 10 mm or greater is rather low at approximately 5–10%. By the same token, approximately 50% of adults age 50 years will harbor some form of a polyp at colonoscopy with the prevalence of polyps increasing linearly in the 6th and 7th decades thereafter. Thus, as Bartrum has stated, it is "normal to have a polyp at age 50 years" (BARTRUM 2000).

Herein, the emergence of CTC creates a new conundrum for those assessing colorectal cancer screening strategies. Because colon polyps are so common, while advanced adenomas are relatively rare and frank cancers even rarer still, there is a sudden new focus of interest in better characterizing the natural history of polyps detected by radiologic CTC colon screening. When using optical colonoscopy for screening, every polyp detected is simply removed and it is more or less academic to deliberate further on their histopathology or malignant potential. However, many if not most small polyps are either not adenomas and are merely hyperplasic or non-specific inflammatory response on histology. Further, even if they are in fact adenomas, they are so small that their potential for malignant degeneration will never be expressed in the patient's life (BOND 2001). In studies of colonoscopic screening of average risk populations, approximately 60% of patients had no evidence of neoplasia while another 20–25% of patients had only one or two subcentimeter polyps (LEIBERMAN et al. 2000; PICKHARDT et al. 2003). Thus, in terms of colon cancer prevention, the detection and removal of such diminutive polyps will convey little or no direct benefit to the individual patient in terms of cancer prevention.

Considerations such as the above contain epidemiologic and public health policy implications as they highlight the distinction in benefits from colorectal screening that may apply to a single individual patient vs the strategic allocation of resources for colon cancer prevention in a population at large. In this context, the benefit harms ratio of screening asymptomatic populations is a critical concern. In colon screening, unlike screening for breast or lung cancer, the target lesion for detection is merely a benign precursor, rather than an actual frank histological malignancy and the intervention becomes cancer prevention rather than cancer detection. Thus, it is even more critical to obtain a careful balance of variables such as risk, resource cost and testing interval (Fig. 2).

As suggested in the foregoing, the new issue for CRC screening will become the proper management of polypoid lesions detected at CTC in terms of follow up surveillance or referral to colonoscopy for polypectomy. Guidelines currently recommended by the Working Group for Virtual Colonscopy (a informal federation of VC researchers) is shown in Fig. 3. Of note, is the relative unimportance of polyps less than 5 mm in diameter and the recommendation that lesions 10 mm or larger be referred for polypectomy. Much of the future debate, therefore, will be reserved for management of intermediate sized polyps 6–9 mm in size. For this group of patients, multiple factors (age, co-morbidities) will require consideration leading to individualized patient decisions.

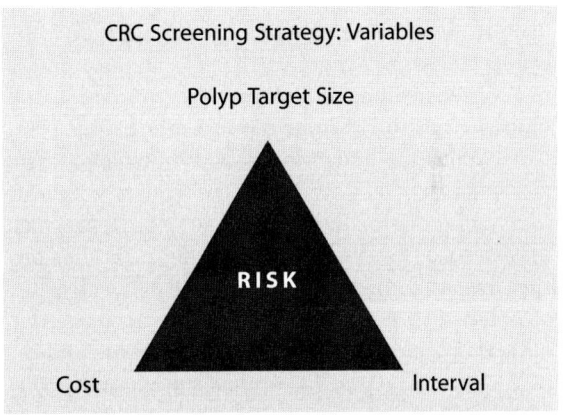

Fig. 2. Balancing variables in strategies for CRC screening

RECOMMENDATIONS

Colonoscopy?

	% of Patients	Recomendations
No polyps	(c. 40%)	NO ACTION (Routine surveillance)
Polyp 5 mm or <	(c. 30%)	NO ACTION (Routine surveillance)
Polyp 6–9 mm	(c. 20%)	INDIVIDUALIZE pt age, co-morbidities ? Multiple polyps esp > 3
Polyp 10 mm or >	(c. 10%)	COLONOSCOPY

Fig. 3. Recommendations for management of CTC detected polyps developed by the Working Group for Virtual Colonoscopy (WGVC), at the 5th International Symposium for Virtual Colonoscopy, Boston Oct 2004

4
Clinical Results

CTC researchers have developed several conventions for standardizing result reporting (FENLON et al. 1999; DACHMAN and ZALIS 2004). Results are reported on a per polyp as well as a per patient basis. Results based on per poly analysis are the most rigorous as they imply direct comparison to colonoscopy. Per patient analysis, however, is the more clinically relevant parameter in terms of referral of the patient for therapeutic optical colonoscopy. Polyp detection rates are usually grouped according to size as under 6 mm in diameter, 6–9 mm and 10 mm or greater. Polyp location is given either by anatomical colon segment (six or eight segments) or by recording the linear colon center line distance from the anal verge from workstation software. Polyp measurements are usually given as the longest linear dimension either by 2D or 3D viewing and there is also an emerging consensus that some form of a confidence limit modifier may be of some clinical merit.

To date, the most important published result has been that of a multi-center trial of screening in asymptomatic adults from the U.S. Department of Defense. (PICKHARDT et al. 2003). In that prospective study of 1233 patients, CTC detected 96% of polyps 8 mm or greater, was more accurate than optical colonoscopy, and found 55 polyps and one of 2 cancers missed by optical colonoscopy. CTC also gave a negative predictive value of 98% for any polyp greater than 10 mm in size, and showed that over 50% of patients had no polyps whatsoever present in their colon. The excellent results in that study were considered to be multi-factorial in nature and included the use of primary endoluminal 3D viewing, aggressive double dose phosphosoda bowel preparation, knowledgeable radiologist readers, and the use of a novel segmental unblinding technique which produced a new consensus 'ground truth' by direct virtual and optical colonoscopic correlation. As a result of that study, gastroenterologists in the U.S. and their national professional organizations conceded that CTC was a technique that was likely to be of wide value and encouraged its "use" by gastroenterologists. However, a subsequent smaller study conducted by U.S. gastroenterologists several months later gave much poorer results (COTTON et al. 2004). However, that study was widely discredited by CTC radiologist researchers because of outmoded techniques and flawed study execution (FERRUCCI et al. 2004; PICKHARDT 2004; HALLIGAN et al. 2004). Nevertheless, some doubt as to the generalizability of CTC performance was raised and the issue was left open as to whether or not additional studies of CTC in screening populations were really required. Two such large multi-center trials are underway as of this writing, one in the U.S conducted by the American College of Radiology Imaging Network (ACRIN) and another in the U.K. carried out for the National Health Service by the Special Interest Group for Gastrointestinal and Abdominal Radiology (SIGGAR). However, the results of these two trials are not likely to be widely available before 2006–2007. In the meantime, rapid further technical advances in CTC including the use of newer 16–64 slice multi-row detector scanners, laxative free colon cleansing schemes, and computer aided detection will become more widespread. Thus even these studies now well underway are destined to be characterized as outdated by the time their results are eventually published.

5
Acceptance of CTC

Several factors will likely converge in the very near future to precipitate wide-spread acceptance of CTC for colorectal screening.
- Continued excellent results from single center trials will add to existing cumulative data of its efficacy.
- Evidence-based comparisons with existing approved screening tests (FOBT, flexible sigmoidoscopy, double contrast barium enema, colonoscopy) will show that none is perfect and that CTC has a sufficient number of benefits and unique attractions to make it a legitimate addition.
- Continued deployment of modern CT scanner capability will make it apparent to community hospitals and private practitioners that there is a very low entry cost to introduce this new imaging product and hospital administrators will persuade radiologists, referring clinicians and gastroenterologists to adopt the procedure.
- Radiology professional organizations will develop and promulgate appropriate practice standards, guidelines, reporting schema, training curricula and accreditation programs to insure that the technique and the reading radiologists have credibility with the public and insurance carriers, as well as other physicians and governmental policy makers. The precedent of mammography in the U.S. where quality standards have been developed

- by the American College of Radiology has been invaluable to the public and radiologists alike. Similar programs are necessary and in fact inevitable for CTC.
- Gastroenterologists performing colonoscopy will increasingly understand that CTC is not so much a competitive threat, as it is in fact a case multiplier in that it will detect and deliver patients to them with truly actionable large polyps for beneficial polypectomy.
- Practical models for integration of virtual and optical colonoscopy into practice will evolve, especially those involving single day one stop shopping cross referral between radiologists and colonoscopists for positive findings at CTC and by the same token for failed colonoscopies allowing an immediate follow-up same day virtual exam with only a single colon prep.

6
Conclusion

It can be predicted that final certifying examinations for young radiologists completing residency training will soon contain examples of CTC studies. This is especially likely in as much as the current generation of trainees is no longer able to perform an adequate number of barium enemas to become proficient. Even though most diagnostic radiologists already consider themselves significantly overworked, it is now inevitable that CTC will be incorporated into daily radiologic practice in the very near future. Also predictable is that the clinical techniques for performing CTC will evolve even further with acquisitions faster, computer aided detection ubiquitous, small polyps ignored and recommendations for further management conveyed in a structured and illustrated computer generated report. Indeed, in leading academic CT research departments, the future is already here.

References

Advisory Board (2004) www.advisoryboardcompany.com. The Advisory Board, Washington, DC

Bartrum C (2000) Personal communication

Bond JH (2001) Clinical relevance of the small colorectal polyp. Endoscopy 33:454–457

Coin CG, Bond WC, Stafford TO (1995) Computed tomographic colonoscopy. United States Patent 5,458,111. Oct 17, 1995

Cotton PB, Durkalski VL, Pineau BC et al. (2004) Computed tomographic colonography (virtual colonoscopy): a multicenter comparison with standard colonoscopy for detection of colorectal neoplasia. JAMA 291:1713–1719

Dachman AH, Zalis ME (2004) Quality and consistency in CT colonography and research reporting. Radiology 230:319–323

Edwards JT, Mendelson RM, Fritschi L, Foster NM, Wood C, Murray D, Forbes GM (2004) Colorectal neoplasia screening with CT colonography in average-risk asymptomatic patients: community-based study. Radiology 230:459–464

Fenlon HM, Nunes DP, Schroy PC et al. (1999) A comparison of virtual colonoscopy and conventional colonoscopy for the detection of colorectal polyps. N Engl J Med 341:1496–1503

Ferrucci JT et al. (2004) Virtual colonoscopy. Letter to the Editor. JAMA 292:431–432

Halligan S et al. (2004) Virtual colonoscopy Letter to the Editor. JAMA 292:431–432

Hara AK, Johnson CD, Reed JE et al. (1996) Detection of colorectal polyps by computed tomographic colography: feasibility of a novel technique. Gastroenterology 110:284–290

Iannacone R, Laghi A, Catalano C et al. (2003) Performance of lower dose multi-detector row helical CT colonography compared with conventional colonoscopy in the detection of colorectal lesions. Radiology 229:775–781

Leiberman DA, Weiss DG, Bond JH et al. (2000) Use of colonoscopy to screen asymptomatic adults for colorectal cancer. N Engl J Med 343:162–174

Macari M, Bini EJ, Xue X, Milano A, Katx SS, Resnick D, Chandarana H, Krinsky G, Klingenbeck K, Marshall CH, Megibow AJ (2002) Colorectal neoplasms: prospective comparison of thin-section low-dose multidetector row CT colonography and conventional colonoscopy for detection. Radiology 224:383–392

Muto T, Bussey HJR, Morson BC (1975) The evolution of cancer of the colon and rectum. Cancer 36:2251–2270

Pickhardt P (2004) Virtual colonoscopy. Letter to the Editor. JAMA 292:431

Pickhardt PJ, Choi JR, Hwang I et al. (2003) CT virtual colonoscopy to screen for colorectal neoplasia in asymptomatic adults. N Engl J Med 349:2189–2198

Royster AP, Fenlon HM, Clarke PD et al. (1997) CT colonoscopy of colorectal neoplasms; two-dimensional and three-dimensional virtual-reality techniques with colonoscopic coreelation. AJR 169:1237–1242

Svensson MH, Svensson E, Lasson A et al. (2002) Patient acceptance of CT colonography and conventional colonoscopy: prospective comparative study in patients with or suspected of having colorectal disease. Radiology 222:337–345

Vining DJ, Gelfand DW (1994) Non-invasive colonoscopy using helical CT scanning. 3D reconstruction and virtual reality. Syllabus. 23rd Annual Meeting Society of Gastrointestinal Radiologists, Maui, Hawaii

Winawer SJ, Zauber AG (2002) The advanced adenoma as the primary target of screening. Gastrointestinal Endoscopy Clinics of North America, vol 12, pp 1–9

Yee J, Akerkar GA, Hung RK, Steinauer-Gebauer AM, Wall SD, McQuaid KR (2001) Colorectal neoplasia: performance characteristics of CT colonography for detection in 300 patients. Radiology 219:685–692

1 Starting CT Colonography in Your Department

Alan O'Hare and Helen Fenlon

CONTENTS

1.1 Introduction 7
1.1.1 Technical Requirements 7
1.1.2 CT Colonography Protocols 8
1.1.3 Reading and Training 9
1.2 Reading Conditions 10
1.2.1 Patient Information, Referral and Follow-Up 11
1.2.2 Cost and Financial Implications 12
1.3 Quality Assurance 12
References 12

1.1
Introduction

CT colonography (Virtual Colonoscopy) has rapidly evolved since its initial description just over a decade ago. It has gradually moved from being a research tool that was largely confined to academic teaching hospitals to a clinical test that is now widely available in many community-based hospitals. With its potential to become a credible tool for colon cancer screening many radiologists are interested in establishing CT colonography in their departments, physicians are requesting the test more frequently and, increasingly, patients are demanding it. The following chapter examines the essential components, minimum requirements and potential hurdles in establishing an effective CT colonography service in a busy diagnostic radiology department.

1.1.1
Technical Requirements

Progress made in the clinical implementation of CT colonography would not have been possible without significant advances that have been made in CT imaging technology over the past 10 years. Availability and ease of access to this technology is crucial for any CT colonography service to allow rapid acquisition, processing and reading of CT colonography datasets.

Technologically, there are three basic components to a CT colonography examination: 1) multislice CT hardware for image acquisition, 2) software and associated platforms for post processing and reading of data sets and 3) adequate transfer networks between the hardware and software components with appropriate image data storage facilities.

While techniques for image post processing and rendering have a major impact on how the final image is viewed, the spatial quality of the dataset will fundamentally be determined by the initial CT acquisition parameters. Although much of the early work on CT colonography was performed on single row helical scanners (Fenlon et al. 1999), multidetector CT (MDCT) is now the accepted standard for current CT colonography research protocols and for performing clinical examinations in everyday practice. MDCT allows acquisition of a single breathhold thin section CT examination of the entire colon in relatively short scan times. A typical acquisition takes 12–15 s using a 16-slice MDCT with a decrease in both respiratory artefacts and improved colonic distension compared with single slice acquisition (Hara et al. 2001). Image artefacts and misregistration secondary to motion and breathing at single slice CT scanning have been shown to increase both diagnostic errors and evaluation times (Fletcher et al. 1999). These artefacts are virtually eliminated using MDCT acquisition. Any department purchasing a new CT scanner to include an expansion of their service to include CT colonography should choose an MDCT.

Once the CT data is acquired, images should be reconstructed according to a standard protocol and automatically transferred to a reading workstation for review. There are numerous options available with regard to CT colonography workstations. Appropriate software is available from both the leading CT manufacturers and specific CT colonography

A. O'Hare, MD; H. Fenlon, MD
Department of Radiology, Mater Misericordiae University Hospital, Eccles Street, Dublin 7, Ireland

software vendors. Such workstations allow datasets to be read in a variety of formats, most commonly 2D images with multiplanar reconstructions (MPR) and 3D endoluminal views for problem solving. Furthermore, software programmes are now capable of generating automated 3D reconstructions of the colonic mucosa from the acquired datasets with an average time for reconstruction in the order of 5–8 min for a complete 3D fly-through. The relative merits of each method will be discussed in a subsequent chapter.

Consideration must also be given as to how CTC datasets will be archived and how datasets may be retrieved to facilitate comparison with previous CT colonography studies. The volume of data generated for each CT colonography examination precludes hardcopy printing of all acquired images. Using a 16-slice MDCT with 3-mm slice acquisition and 1.5- mm slice overlap, a standard study with 40 cm of Z-axis coverage in both supine and prone positions will typically comprise over 600 slices. At the standard 512 512 bits of resolution each study will require over 500 MB of memory for storage. A single patient's examination, therefore, will occupy almost an entire conventional compact disc (CD) which has a memory capacity of 700 MB. An alternative to CD for archiving is DVD. While relatively inexpensive, use of DVD requires purchase of a DVD reader as most commercially available workstations come with only an integrated CD reader. The actual hard drive memory capacities of workstations vary (14,000 MB in our department) which if used for CT colonography alone can accommodate only 20 cases. In reality, these workstations are also used for 3D reconstruction of other studies including vascular and orthopaedic examinations, resulting in a real need for external storage.

Without an integrated PACS system effective high volume CT colonography that allows rapid image retrieval and comparison with previous studies is extremely difficult. Many issues relating to memory storage and networking infrastructure are simply resolved with the implementation of PACS. PACS offers numerous potential advantages including the viewing of studies in remote locations, a decrease in the number of lost datasets, and the large capacity image storage. Its greatest advantage is that it facilitates the rapid retrieval of previous studies which is a significant advantage in the setting of a screening program. Until recent years many CT workstations did not have a PACS compatible interface. Furthermore many radiology departments do not yet have PACS. When choosing a workstation for CT colonography interpretation, careful consideration should be given to its PACS compatibility.

The network interface between the CT workstation and reading workstations must be seamless, transfer of datasets must be fast and automatic, and datasets must be available for reading without any loss of diagnostic information. Transferring datasets of this size places a considerable demand on any network whether it involves transmission from CT workstations to reading workstations or from the primary reading stations to remote reader locations. The connecting network cable must be at least a category 5 UTP connection with switches producing speeds up to 100 Mb/s. Speed of transfer will be compromised if the network is of insufficient size and if high volumes of data are being transferred simultaneously.

1.1.2
CT Colonography Protocols

Specific CT colonography protocols should be established at a local level and should be based on the currently available published evidence. Protocols should address the method of bowel preparation (clean colon vs fluid or faecal tagging), use or not of intravenous contrast, use or not of spasmolytics, method of colon distension, scanning parameters, and methods of interpretation. The specifics of many of these options are discussed in subsequent chapters.

The basic equipment required for the CT colonography examination is little more than a red rubber catheter with a hand held insufflation bulb similar to that used for barium enema examinations. There are a variety of rectal catheters available of varying size, typically 5–15 mm in diameter. Although we routinely use a balloon-tipped enema catheter, many researchers now avoid balloon insufflation. Traditionally room air has been the gas of choice for colonic insufflation at CT colonography due to its availability and lack of additional expense. However, there is a growing body of evidence advocating the use of carbon dioxide (CO_2) which is associated with less abdominal cramps and is more rapidly reabsorbed (YEE and GALINDO 2002). CO_2 is supplied from a refillable cylinder via a disposable administration set which allows constant gas pressure influx with the facility to record both gas pressures and the volume of CO_2 administered.

In our practice, the radiologist is responsible for the practicalities of rectal tube insertion and subsequent colonic insufflation. Depending on departmental time constraints, radiology staffing and volume of CT colonography examinations, consideration may be given to training a dedicated CT colonography technician or nurse and this has been successfully established in some institutions. Furthermore, some centres allow patients to 'self-inflate' in order to improve patient acceptance of the technique.

Much research has been published from both in vivo and phantom studies on the effect of different scan parameters (particularly slice collimation, pitch and mAs) on the quality of CT colonography studies, the associated artefacts and patient radiation doses. As with any radiologic study there will be a trade off between image quality (the diagnostic value of the study) and radiation dose. Typical parameters for CT colonography will be specifically discussed in a later chapter. In establishing a CT colonography service it is important to agree on a standard scan protocol so that patients are imaged and the data set acquired in a consistent and reproducible manner. This creates a uniformity among studies, which facilitates interpretation and comparison with previous studies. Published literature advocates that all patients be scanned in both supine and prone positions as dual positioning allows redistribution of air, stool and fluid and is associated with an increased sensitivity for polyp detection. In one particular study, the reported sensitivity of CT colonography for detection of polyps greater than 10 mm in size was 92.7% for dual positioning compared with 58.5 and 51% for supine and prone scanning alone (YEE et al. 2003).

1.1.3
Reading and Training

After image acquisition and transfer of datasets, studies should be read and reported in a timely fashion. The following discussion will address aspects of image interpretation including who should read the datasets, how much training is required, how many readers are required and when and where studies should be read.

The primary aim of CT colonography is accurate identification of significant colorectal polyps and cancers in a minimally invasive manner. For CT colonography to be a safe, accurate and attractive alternative to colonoscopy, radiologists reading these studies must confidently recognise polyps and cancers, identify pitfalls and therefore reduce the number of false positive findings, and report significant extracolonic findings in a consistent and reliable manner. It is increasingly clear that to achieve this, radiologists must have specific CT colonography training. The effect of training and experience on reader performance has been the subject of a number of studies to date and has been a topic of intense discussion at many scientific meetings including the annual International Symposia on Virtual Colonoscopy in Boston. Training and its relationship to an individual's ability to report accurately CT colonography studies is a complex issue and is currently the subject of investigation of an ESGAR-funded research study. It appears that radiologists with a specific interest in CT colonography who have read many hundreds of cases perform better than abdominal radiologists who have been trained on 50 cases alone, who, in turn, perform better than those with little or no specific CT colonography training. This is as one might expect – however what is not clear is just how steep the learning curve is and when, or if, one reaches a plateau in reader performance.

Current recommendations are that radiologists should be specifically trained in a supervised manner on cases that have either endoscopic verification or have been read by an 'expert' reader. The datasets should include an appropriate mix of normal studies, cancers of various morphology, polyps (pedunculated and flat), and extracolonic findings as well as studies limited by underdistension and poor bowel preparation. Emphasis should also be placed on familiarity with CT colonography software applications and recognition of the various pathologies in both 2D and 3D formats. While supervised training on 50 proven cases has been regarded as a minimum initial requirement, it would be wrong to assume that this is adequate for every radiologist or that it provides a level of 'expertise' as performance clearly improves with increasing experience.

Differences in reader experience has been identified as one of the factors contributing to the wide range of reported accuracies of CT colonography. In recent studies the reported sensitivities for detection of polyps >1 cm varied from 52 to 92% (JOHNSON et al. 2003A; COTTON et al. 2004; PICKHARDT et al. 2003). Although there were some differences in the study populations and the methods used for bowel preparation, image acquisition, and interpretation, it is widely believed that differences in performance were due, at least in part, to variability in reader experience. Adequate and widespread access to reader training will be required before acceptance of CT colonography as a screening tool.

Clearly, if a radiology department is to offer a CT colonography service, at least one 'experienced' radiologist will be required to read studies, and likely more depending on workload. Experience as a general radiologist does not automatically qualify one to reading datasets as even the most experienced radiologists can miss large lesions on CT colonography (Halligan et al. 2004). Experience as an abdominal radiologist confers some advantage compared with a general radiologist but it by no means qualifies as adequate training.

Further evidence that reader experience impacts on the diagnostic performance of CT colonography comes from the ACRIN 1 trial (American college of Radiology Imaging Network). This study examined the ability of radiologists of various experience to detect clinically important neoplasia (lesions >1 cm). The results suggest that readers could achieve high accuracies only with extensive experience (Johnson et al. 2003b). Reader inexperience not only impacted on the ability of the reader to detect polyps but also increased inter- and intraobserver errors with regard to polyp size measurement. In another study Belloni et al. examined the performance of novice readers after every 25 patients for almost 100 CT colonography examinations. They found that the sensitivity achieved by readers for polyps of all sizes increased from 32% after the first 25 cases to 92% for the final 25 cases (Spinzi et al. 2001). Although controversy remains as to what qualifies as 'adequate experience' a minimum of 40–50 proven datasets was proposed based on a questionnaire sent to 18 international experts and presented by Dr J.A. Soto at the RSNA in 2004.

Even with suitable training errors of judgment will continue to be made by even the most experienced of radiologists. Potential 'pitfalls' leading to both false positive and negative results must be highlighted. These pitfalls typically relate to retained stool, complex fold and polyp morphology, and the relationship of polyps to folds and flexures. A number of publications have addressed these pitfalls (Fenlon 2002; Macari and Megibow 2001; Gleucker et al. 2004), and training courses should include examples. Training courses should also include formal lectures on image acquisition parameters, non-interpretive matters and a review of the data supporting virtual colongraphy for screening.

Training courses are available that meet these criteria in many centres in both North America and Europe. These courses are typically held over a two-day period. Although there is currently no obligation on radiologists to receive specific training prior to reporting CT colonography studies it may become mandatory in the future if screening with CT colonography becomes a reality. Ferrucci has compared such a colonic screening program with the template that already exists for mammographic screening (Ferruci 2000). He correctly predicts that in the setting of a colon screening program there will be a demand by certain third parties such as insurance companies or the American college of Radiologists that radiologists reporting CT colonography studies reach certain levels of competence and maintain those standards. The impact of such a step is to be welcomed as it would establish pre-requisites that every reporting radiologist should meet in terms of their training and level of experience.

In our practice and most others, radiologists perform the study and interpret the scans. However, some believe that CT colonography studies could be performed and read by trained radiographers in the same way as barium enema examinations are provided in some institutions. The data supporting the use of non-radiologists is limited – at the 5th International Symposium on Virtual Colonoscopy in Boston 2004 results were presented from a multicentre trial, suggesting that there is no significant difference in reader performance or the time taken to read studies between radiology trainees and radiographic technicians. However in a recent consensus on training from 18 leading radiologists in the field of CT colonography, 78% of those questioned felt that radiologists alone should report datasets and, currently, it is the view held by ourselves.

1.2
Reading Conditions

Reading conditions also impact on reader performance. CT colonography studies should ideally be batch-read in a quiet environment with each batch consisting of no more than five or six cases. This helps to reduce the impact of reader fatigue which adversely effects reader concentration and performance in terms of polyp detection. Although an experienced radiologist may take as little as 5 min to read a study in 2D format, interpretation requires a high level of concentration to maintain ones focus on the lumen while scrolling back and forth through the colon. In the setting of a busy department with many conflicting demands on radiologists, CT colonography readers should be careful to avoid the impulse to read rapidly studies or the latter stages of studies as this may result in a significant decrease in polyp detection rates (TAYLOR et al. 2004). The time allocated to reading these studies should be protected in a manner similar to the reading of screening mammograms.

Using the mammography analogy, it is likely that the sensitivity for polyp detection increases when studies are double read compared with single read examinations. A second reader does not necessarily have to be a trained radiologist – this role could potentially be filled by computer aided detection (CAD). CAD is an automated computer software mechanism used to highlight abnormalities within a colon that may be missed by the radiologist. CAD could act as the first reader with a trained radiologist acting as the second. The benefits of CAD have been shown in other radiological applications such as mammography and lung nodule detection. There is considerable interest among academic radiologists and commercial companies in this tool and, although not yet fully FDA approved or verified in multicentre trials, CAD is a rapidly developing tool that may become standard in CT colonography reading in the future.

A standard report format should also be agreed upon at a local level. If used by all reporting radiologists a standard printed report would help improve communication with the referring clinician or patient and help direct appropriate patient follow-up and management. Such a report would stratify patients into specified groups depending on the CT colonography findings. The factors which decide group designation would include polyp size, morphology, location and attenuation. A system has been proposed similar to the B-RADS system used in mammography that is called C-RADS. Patients would be classified into groups C1 to C5 and the report would also include an E1 to E5 categorisation based on the presence or absence of significant extracolonic findings. Development of such a system is currently underway and is based on the coordinated efforts of the American College of Radiology and the Working Group on Virtual Colonoscopy.

The successful implementation of any new practice requires that there be adequate and proper utilization of that resource that justifies the expense of providing the equipment, training the staff, performing the studies and reading the datasets. This requires close collaboration and communication between radiologists and many different staff, including radiographers, secretarial and nursing staff in radiology, primary care physicians, endoscopy staff and gastroenterologists. The success of any CT colonography service is close liaison between the radiology and gastroenterology departments. A good working relationship between the two groups allows free exchange of information and ideas, promotes patient referrals and, most importantly of all, provides a clear mechanism for follow-up of any abnormal cases. It is up to the radiologist to promote the technique within their hospital by meeting local physician groups, particularly the gastroenterologists, and explaining the advantages and disadvantages, indications and contraindications of this new procedure. Easy same-day access to CT colonography following failed colonoscopy is appealing to both patients and gastroenterologists and is an effective way of introducing and promoting this technique at a local level. Gastroenterologists as a group are only too aware of the potential significance of CT colonography as a screening tool for colon cancer and its implications for both their future practice and ours. It is vital that we gain their confidence from the outset and that we are sufficiently familiar with current literature on colon cancer screening and CT colongraphy to address any issues or questions that may arise.

1.2.1
Patient Information, Referral and Follow-Up

For patients and the population in general, particularly those considering a screening test, easy access to information regarding the procedure and clear communication with the providers are also important. There should exist within a department a means by which patients can be informed of the procedure, the necessary preparation, potential risks and complications, implications of a normal and abnormal result and what mechanism for follow-up exists. The most practical way of achieving this would be through printed literature on the test and access to a liaison staff member such as a nurse or radiographer who has been specifically trained.

We agree with Mark. E. Klein, Washington Radiology Associates who recently spoke at the 5th International Virtual Colonoscopy Conference that a department introducing a CT colonography service would be well advised to perform a 'mini study' on the first 40 patients with conventional colonoscopy correlation in each case. This gives the radiologist a valuable opportunity to become familiar with all aspects of the technique and to address organisational issues including the process of patient referrals, timing of appointments, the staffing and infrastructure required, optimal bowel preparation and distension, to become familiar with the reading software and issues related to interpretation and to consider mechanism for follow-up when required.

1.2.2
Cost and Financial Implications

The economic implications of setting up a CT colonography service must also be considered. Each department must consider whether or not it is financially viable for them to provide this service. Estimates suggest that, when all factors are considered, the real cost of providing a CT colonography examination is in the order of 250 Euro. Balanced against this is the ongoing difficulty with reimbursement, which varies widely from country to country and even from state to state in North America. Apart from a handful of health care providers there is currently no reimbursement for screening CT colonography and limited and inconsistent reimbursement when the test is performed in symptomatic patients. Although many patients are willing to pay for CT colonography this is clearly not sustainable nor appropriate. Radiologists must be able to address and discuss these issues with their local health insurance companies to ensure that the interests of their patients are protected and that they are appropriately reimbursed for capital costs and their professional time.

1.3
Quality Assurance

Establishing a CT colonography service requires a major investment in time, cost and personal commitment. However maintaining a quality service and insuring high quality clinical standards is equally important, particularly when considering screening populations. This will involve setting standards, measuring competence, continuous medical education, clinical audit and quality control. Appropriate audit and quality control will assess the various systems involved in a CT colonography service from the time an appointment is made right through to patient follow-up so that potential deficiencies can be identified and appropriate changes implemented as required.

References

Cotton PB, Durkalski VL, Pineau BC, Palesch YY, Mauldin PD, Hoffman B, Vining DJ, Small WC, Affronti J, Rex D, Kopecky KK, Ackerman S, Burdrick JS, Brewington C, Turner MA, Zfass A, Wright AR, Iyer RB, Lynch P, Sivak MV, Butler H (2004) Computed tomographic colonography (virtual coloscopy): a multicentre comparison with standard colonoscopy for detection of colorectal neoplasia. JAMA 291:1713–1719

Fenlon HM (2002) CT colonography:pitfalls and interpretation. Abdominal Imaging 27(3):284–291

Fenlon HM, Nunes DP, Schroy PC et al. (1999) Comparison of virtual and conventional colonoscopy for the detection of colorectal polyps. N Engl J Med 341(20):1496–1503

Ferruci JT (2000) CT colonography for colorectal cancer: lessons from mammography. Am J Roentgenol 174(6):1539–1541

Fletcher JG, Johnson CD, MacCarty RL, Welch TJ, Hara AK (1999) CT colonography: potential pitfalls and problem solving techniques. AJR Am J Roentgenol 172(5):1271–1278

Gleucker TM, Fletcher JG, Welch TJ, MacCarty RL, Harmsen WS, Harrington JR, Ilstrup D, Wilson LA, Corcoran KE, Johnson CD (2004) Characterisation of lesions missed on interpretation of CT colonography using a 2D search method. Am J Roentgenol 182(4):881–889

Halligan S, Taylor S, Burling D (2004) Letter. JAMA 292:432

Hara AK, Johnson DC, MacCarty RL et al. (2001) CT colonography: single-versus multi-detector row imaging. Radiology 219:461–465

Johnson DC, Harmsen WS, Wilson LA, MacCarty RL, Welch TJ, Ilstrup DM, Ahlquist DA (2003a) Prospective blinded evaluation of computed tomographic colonography for screen detection of colorectal polyps. Gastroenterology 125(a):311–319

Johnson DC, Toledano AY, Herman BA, Dachman AH, McFarlend EG, Barish MA, Brink JA et al. (2003b) Computerised tomographic colonography: performance evaluation in a retrospective multicentre setting. Gastroenterology 125(3):688–695

Macari M, Megibow AJ (2001) Pitfalls of using three dimensional CT colonography with two dimensional imaging correlation. Am J Roentgenol 176(1):137–143

Pickhardt PJ, Choi JR, Hwang l, Butler JA, Puckett ML, Hildebrandt HA, Wong RK, Nugent PA, Mysliwiec PA, Schindler WR (2003) Computed tomographic virtual colonoscopy to screen for colorectal neoplasia in asymptomatic adults. N Engl J Med 349:2191–2200

Spinzi G, Belloni G, Martegani A, Sangiovanni A, Del Favero C, Minoli G (2001) Computed tomographic colonography and conventional colonoscopy for colon disease: a prospective blinded study. Am J Gastroenterol 96:394–400

Taylor SA, Halligan S, Burling D, Morley S, Bassett P, Atkin W, Bartram CI (2004) CT colonography: effect of experience and training on reader performance. Eur Radiol 14:1025–1033

Yee J (2002) CT colonography: examination prerequisites. Abdom Imaging. 27(3):244–252

Yee J, Kumar NN, Hung RK, Akerkar GA, Kumar PR, Wall SD (2003) Comparison of supine, prone scanning separately and in combination at CT colonography. Radiology 226:653–661

2 The Eligible Patient: Indications and Contraindications

AYODALE S. ODULATE and KOENRAAD J. MORTELE

CONTENTS

2.1 History 13
2.2 Indications 14
2.2.1 Screening CT Colonography 14
2.2.2 Diagnostic CT Colonography 16
2.2.3 Pre-operative Assessment 18
2.2.4 Post-operative Colorectal Cancer Surveillance 18
2.2.5 Incomplete Conventional Colonoscopy 18
2.2.6 Inflammatory Bowel Disease Surveillance 19
2.3 Contraindications 19
2.3.1 Absolute Contraindications 20
2.3.2 Relative Contraindications 20
2.4 Current Reimbursable Indications 21
2.5 Future Indications 21
2.6 Summary 21
References 21

2.1 History

The development of computed tomography (CT) independently by both Godfrey N Hounsfield and Allan M Cormack in 1972 has forever changed the practice of medicine in the detection, surveillance and treatment of disease. In the past three decades, we have seen an explosion in technological innovation, particularly in the field of CT. As CT has become more sophisticated, so has the radiologist in the detection and diagnosis of disease.

In 1994, Vining and Gelfand introduced computed tomographic colonography (CTC), also referred to as virtual colonoscopy (VC), as a tool to evaluate the insufflated colon (VINING et al. 1994). Early work in CT colonography involved patient populations with an increased risk of colon cancer with the goal of detecting colorectal cancer. Also, early studies were performed with single detector CT scanners with thick collimated slices and were primarily read in the 2D axial plane. We have advanced significantly from the days of single detector scanners with 4, 8, 16, and 64 multidetector-row scanners now available. Total volume imaging in a single breath-hold, as a result of multidetector-row scanning, has been shown to improve accuracy of polyp detection by decreasing breathing artifacts (GRYSPEERDT et al. 2004). Also, due to significant software improvements, post-processing reformations are currently reconstructed in any plane in a manner of seconds (BRUZZI et al. 2001) and continued advancement in 3-D software development has made virtual endoscopic flythrough of the colon feasible (SIEMENS 2002).

The practical execution of CT colonography is still somewhat variable: patient bowel preparation, method of insufflating the colon, scanning acquisition parameters and post-processing software vary. Methods of interpretation also vary with some proponents advocating a primary 3D read with 2D images for problem solving versus a primary 2D read with 3D flythrough for problem solving (DACHMAN et al. 1998). No technique has yet been proven to be superior to any other consistently and differences are seen regionally. Overall, however, the CT colonography literature has shown consistent improvement in the sensitivity and specificity of polyp and colorectal cancer detection as the technology has improved.

CT colonography as a screening tool for colon cancer continues to improve and a credible alternate and non-invasive tool to evaluate the colon now exists. Initial studies in the mid- to late 1990s demonstrated sensitivities of polyp detection ranging from 50 to 90% for polyps larger than 1 cm with specificities ranging from 70 to 90% (VAN DAM et al. 2004). As the technology and application of

A. S. ODULATE, MD
Resident in Radiology, Department of Radiology, Brigham and Women's Hospital, 75 Francis Street Boston, Massachusetts 02115 USA

K. J. MORTELE, MD
Associate Professor of Radiology, Harvard Medical School; Director, Abdominal and Pelvic MRI; Associate Director, Division of Abdominal Imaging and Intervention, Department of Radiology, Brigham and Women's Hospital, 75 Francis Street Boston, Massachusetts 02115 USA

CTC developed over time, the detection of colon cancer and polyps, even those smaller than 10 mm, improved (YEE et al. 2001). In certain patient populations, CTC may in fact be the examination of choice for evaluating the colon, compared to available current alternatives, such as double-contrast barium enema (DCBE), flexible sigmoidoscopy and conventional colonoscopy. Studies have proven that CTC is better at detecting colon cancers and polyps compared to DCBE, and arguably is as good as conventional colonoscopy for the same purposes. CT colonography has yet to be adopted and integrated into the screening algorithm.

This chapter explores the current indications and contraindications of CTC, and provides recommendations regarding which patients are eligible to undergo CTC. Current reimbursable indications in the US by major third party payers are briefly described. Lastly, the current technologies under development with possible future indications are discussed.

2.2
Indications

The indications for CTC closely follow the indications for conventional optical colonoscopy with few exceptions. These indications include screening asymptomatic high- and average-risk patient populations, pre-operative assessment of the colon proximal to an obstructing mass, evaluation of patients with change in bowel habits, surveillance of patients post colorectal cancer surgery, and incomplete or failed colonoscopy. Patients with bleeding diathesis, contraindications to sedation, and frail and elderly patients may also be better suited for CTC than conventional colonoscopy.

2.2.1
Screening CT Colonography

In the United States, 1 in 17 people will develop colorectal cancer. According to reports from the National Cancer Institute, colorectal cancer is the third most common cancer in US men and women. The overall incidence of colorectal cancer increased until 1985 and then began decreasing at an average rate of 1.6% per year. Approximately 75% of all colorectal cancers occur among persons of average risk, i.e., those without predisposing conditions, such as inflammatory bowel disease, familial adenomatous polyposis, hereditary nonpolyposis colorectal cancer, or a first degree relative with a history of colorectal adenoma or colorectal cancer (WINAWER et al. 1991; AHSAN et al. 1998). The age range for development of colon cancer is late 40s to 70s in average-risk patients. The high-risk patient population accounts for approximately 25% of the colorectal cancer incidence in the United States. Deaths from colorectal cancer rank third after lung and prostate cancer in men and third after lung and breast cancer in women.

The proposed natural history of colon cancer in the average-risk patient, as described in the National Polyp Study in 1990, confirmed the expected developmental course of colorectal cancer beginning with an adenomatous polyp, progressing to high-grade dysplasia, and then, frank carcinoma. However, the majority of polyps resected less than 10 mm in size represent hyperplastic polyps and other benign findings. Therefore, the goal of polypectomy should be adenoma resection. Research suggests that there is about a five-year development interval between the stages of adenomatous polyp and adenoma with high-grade dysplasia, and another five-year interval to develop frank cancer (O'BRIEN et al. 1990). The majority of adenomas that will develop into cancer are polypoid or villous in shape (Fig. 2.1). A small proportion of adenomas are so called flat or depressed and have been shown to be difficult to identify on conventional colonoscopy and other colonic imaging modalities. Positive predictive characteristics of an adenoma with increased propensity to develop into cancer are its size and total number of adenomas. Polyps greater than 10 mm in diameter and more that three in number, regardless of their size, have been reported as risk factors for transformation into colorectal cancer through the "adenoma-carcinoma sequence", as described above. Despite prior reports, flat or depressed adenomas do not have an increased risk of developing cancer when compared to the polypoid or villous configurations (WINAWER and ZAUBER 2002). Overall, the literature suggests that the risk of an adenoma, 5 mm or less in greatest dimension, to develop into cancer is significantly low, approximating 0.9% (O'BRIEN et al. 1990).

The goal of colorectal cancer screening is to reduce the morbidity and mortality of colon cancer by early detection and resection of adenomas and cancer (FRAZIER et al. 2000). The screening guidelines from the National Cancer Institute, and adopted by the American Gastroenterological Association, currently call for screening of the average-risk

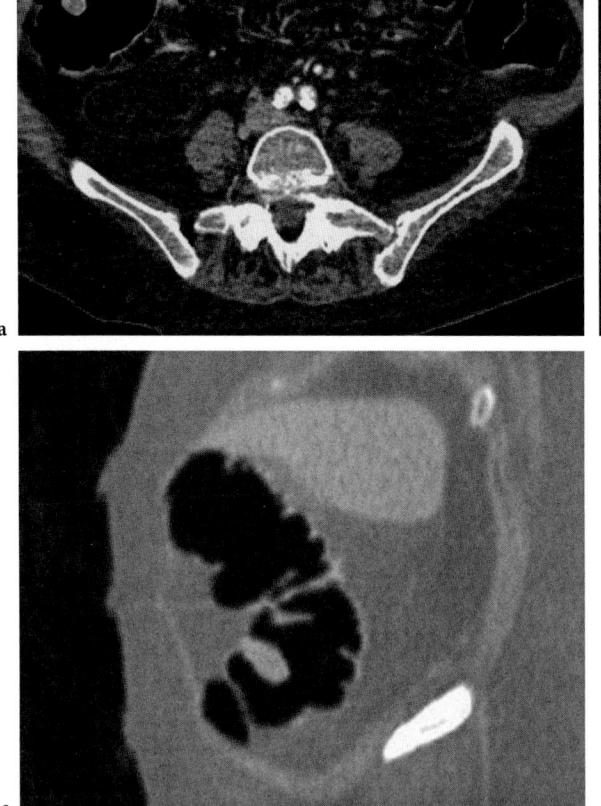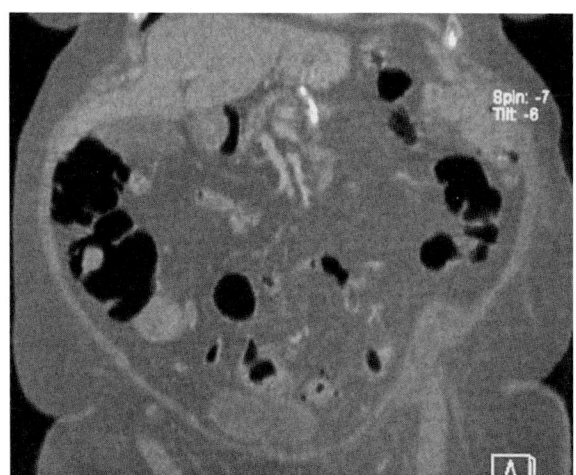

Fig. 2.1a–c. Colonic adenoma: a axial CT image demonstrates a soft tissue polypoid lesion located off of the anterior aspect of the ascending colon. CT images (lung window settings) show a discrete polypoid lesion in the ascending colon identified on the reformatted coronal and sagittal images; b reformatted coronal image; c reformatted sagittal image

asymptomatic patient with an annual digital rectal examination, annual fecal occult blood testing, and flexible sigmoidoscopy every 5 years beginning at age 50. In addition, double contrast barium enema is recommended every 5 years or optical colonoscopy every 10 years beginning at age 50 (ANDERSON et al. 2002; WINAWER et al. 1997). Patients classified as high-risk for developing colorectal cancer undergo screening at a much younger age, as specified by their personal risk factors.

Albeit imperfect with a documented adenoma miss rate ranging from 6 to 27% (depending on the size of the lesion), conventional colonoscopy is still the gold standard for colon cancer screening (REX et al. 1997). Cancers have also been missed by conventional colonoscopy. A study performed in Canada reported a cancer miss rate of 4% in cancers originating in the right colon (BRESSLER et al. 2004). Several reasons exist why cancers are missed on conventional colonoscopy: poor bowel prep, slippage of the endoscope around flexures, redundant colon, misinterpretation of findings and failure to biopsy (LEAPER et al. 2004). A false negative conventional colonoscopy may have serious implications, as patients may not have another colon screening test for a decade.

Conventional colonoscopy is also not without risk to the patient and significant morbidity and mortality has been reported (GARBAY et al. 1996). The most common adverse outcome associated with conventional colonoscopy includes hemorrhage and perforation. The rate of perforation of the colon ranges from 0.2 to 0.4% after diagnostic colonoscopy, increases with polypectomy, and approximates 5% with hydrostatic balloon dilatation of colonic strictures (ZUBARIK et al. 1999).

A landmark multicenter study published by Pickhardt et al. compared CT colonography and conventional colonoscopy in asymptomatic average-risk patient population. As a screening study, comparable adenoma and colorectal cancer detection rates were reported (PICKHARDT et al. 2003). In fact, the sensitivity and specificity per patient and per polyp were similar and not statistically different between CTC and conventional colonoscopy for adenomas greater than 10 mm. The sensitivity of CTC for adenomatous polyps was 93.8% for polyps at least 10 mm in diameter, 93.9% for polyps at least 8 mm in diameter, and 88.7% for polyps at least 6 mm in diameter. The sensitivity of conventional colonoscopy for adenomatous polyps was 87.5, 91.5, and 92.3% for the three sizes of polyps, respectively. The specificity of CTC for adenomatous polyps was 96.0% for polyps at least 10 mm in diameter, 92.2% for polyps at least 8 mm in diameter, and 79.6% for polyps at least 6 mm in diameter (PICKHARDT et al. 2003).

Detection rates for polyps less than or equal to 5 mm in size are lower and the debate over the significance of these smaller lesions continues. Again, the aim of colorectal cancer screening is to detect cancer and adenomas. With respect to adenomas, the term "advanced adenoma" has been used to describe clinically significant adenomas that have the greatest likelihood to develop into cancer. Current understanding is that adenomas larger or equal to 10 mm reside in this category and should undergo resection. Polyps ranging in size from 5 mm to 9 mm should undergo short-term interval follow-up (VAN DAM et al. 2004).

The most recent guidelines presented at the 5th Annual International Symposium on Virtual Colonoscopy in Boston, MA for reporting CTC findings are the following: mass lesion, direct referral to surgery; single or multiple polyps ≥10 mm, direct referral for colonoscopy and polypectomy; single polyp <10 mm but greater than or equal to 6 mm, three year follow up; ≥3 polyps, each 6 mm -9 mm, referral to colonoscopy and polypectomy; polyps "5 mm, seven year follow up study (ZALIS 2004).

CT colonography as a screening tool has the potential to have wider public acceptance compared to conventional colonoscopy. Acceptance of a screening study by a population is multi-factorial. Many physical and psychological barriers to colorectal cancer screening have been described. Surveys have reported patients' reluctance to undergo colorectal cancer screening because of time commitment for the conventional colonoscopy, use of colon cathartics, sedation requirements, prior painful experience and even embarrassment (ROZEN and PIGNONE 2003). CT colonography is relatively fast without the need for sedation or a driver post procedure. Patients have described the post procedure discomfort less for CTC than conventional colonoscopy.

Several studies have shown that patients' acceptance of CTC is greater than conventional colonoscopy or double contrast barium enema (TAYLOR et al. 2003). Development of minimal bowel prep or prep-less CTC through fecal tagging and electronic cleansing appears to be within reach, thus making a truly prep-less colorectal screening test an attractive possibility (LEFERE et al. 2002).

A subset of patients, including the elderly, those with cardiovascular disease, bleeding diathesis and a history of failed colonoscopies, are better suited to undergo CTC for colorectal cancer screening compared to colonoscopy or DCBE.

2.2.2
Diagnostic CT Colonography

Patients with positive bowel symptoms, such as change in bowel habits, lower gastrointestinal bleeding, iron deficiency anemia and abdominal pain are eligible to undergo a diagnostic CTC. The patient is scanned in both the supine and prone position, but unlike a screening CTC, the patient is injected with intravenous iodinated contrast material during the supine acquisition (CHEN et al. 1999). Injection of contrast aids in the differentiation of polyps versus adherent stool. Studies have also demonstrated increased accuracy of polyp detection with the use of intravenous contrast (MORRIN 2000). A contrast-enhanced scan may aid in the detection of extra-colonic causes of the patient's symptoms. Finally, diagnostic CTC has the ability to detect and stage colorectal cancer, unlike the other two alternatives, conventional colonoscopy and double contrast barium enema.

The indications for diagnostic CTC closely follow those for conventional colonoscopy (RANKIN 1987). Rectal bleeding, heme positive stool, anemia and constipation are just a few examples. Indications for screening and diagnostic CTC are summarized in Table 2.1.

Diagnostic CTC may be used to further evaluate findings on conventional colonoscopy. Not infrequently, diagnostic CTC is performed in patients with suspicious intramural or extra-mural masses detected on optical colonoscopy (Fig. 2.2).

Occasionally, patients are unable to undergo conventional colonoscopy due to presence of a colonic stricture, redundant sigmoid, or contraindications to intravenous conscious sedation. Flexible sigmoidoscopy can be performed without sedation; however, the majority of the colon is not evaluated.

The Eligible Patient: Indications and Contraindications

Table 2.1. Indications and contra-indications for CT colonography

Indications for CTC		Contra-indications for CTC
Screening	Diagnostic	
Age ≥ 50 years[a]	Colorectal cancer detection in patients with:	Acute abdomen
Bleeding diathesis	Lower gastrointestinal bleeding	Recent pelvic or abdominal surgery
Failed colonoscopy	Change in bowel habits	Acute diverticulitis
Polyp detection	Lower abdominal pain	Toxic megacolon
Elderly	Iron deficiency anemia	Colonic hernia
Contraindication to sedation	Obstructing colon mass	Scanner weight limitations
	Post-operative colorectal cancer surveillance	Pregnancy[c]
	High risk patients[b]	Hip joint replacement[c]
		Incompetent ileocecal valve[c]
		Claustrophobia[c]

[a] Average risk patient
[b] Patients with inflammatory bowel disease, familial adenomatous polyposis, hereditary nonpolyposis colorectal cancer, first degree relative with colorectal cancer or patients with prior history of colorectal cancer.
[c] Relative contraindication

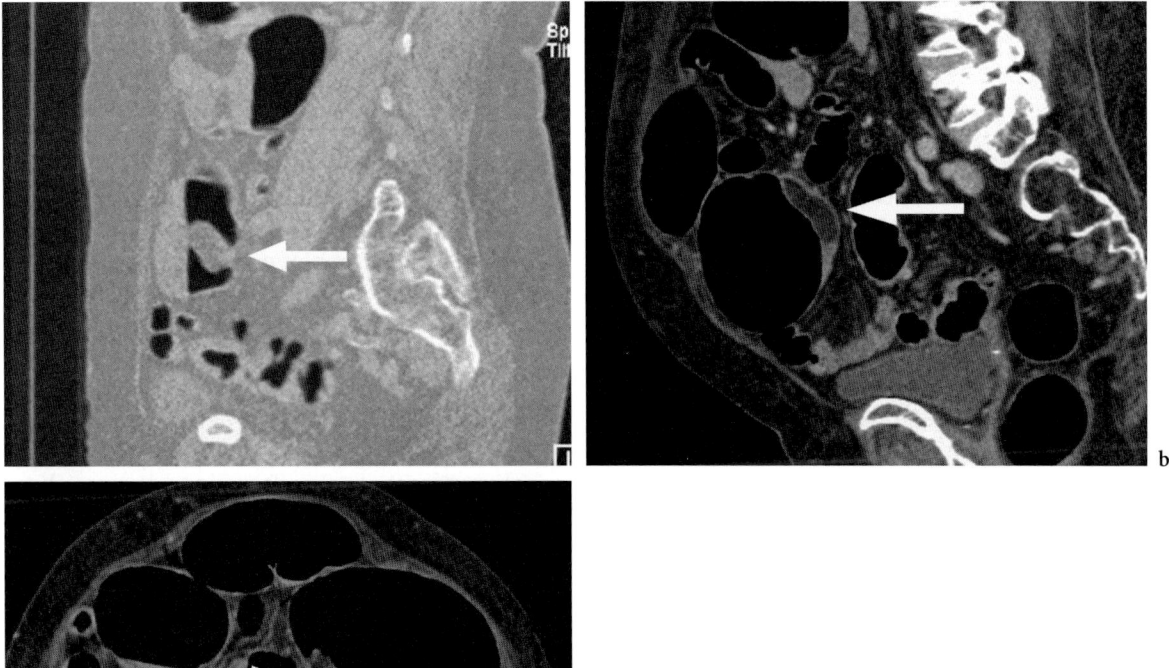

Fig. 2.2a–c. Submucosal colonic lipoma: **a** sagittal reformatted CT image (lung window settings) acquired in prone position shows a 1.8-cm intramural lesion within the cecum (*arrow*); **b** sagittal reformatted CT image in supine position (soft tissue settings) demonstrates a fatty mass (*arrow*) along the posterior border of the cecum in the same location as seen on the prone image; **c** supine axial CT image (soft tissue settings) demonstrates again the fatty mass consistent with a submucosal lipoma

Although double contrast barium enema evaluates the entire colon, many proponents of the new technology believe that CTC should be the study of choice for patients whom are unable to undergo conventional colonoscopy. Several studies reveal that the sensitivity and specificity of polyp detection is higher for CTC compared to DCBE (JOHNSON et al. 2004; FENLON et al. 1999b).

2.2.3
Pre-operative Assessment

The assessment of colon proximal to an obstructing colonic mass has been a shortcoming of conventional colonoscopy. In the past, inter-operative palpation or post-operative colonoscopy was performed with the possibility of a second surgery required for a missed synchronous cancer or adenoma. The sensitivity of hand palpation is fairly low and intraoperative insufflation of the colon increases the risk of peritoneal contamination.

Double contrast barium enema remains in the algorithm for work-up of colorectal cancer in evaluation of the proximal bowel in cases of an obstructing mass. This examination is not preferred, as the proximal colon often does not drain all of the barium by the time of surgery. Patients are also at increased risk for post-operative morbidity if a reactive peritonitis develops secondary to barium contamination intra-operatively.

The incidence of synchronous neoplasia in the colon has been described at a rate of 1.5–9%. Adenomas harboring in the colon in patients with colon cancer have been reported at an incidence of 27–55%. Fenlon et al. compared CTC to pre-operative double contrast barium enema in the evaluation of patients with an obstructing carcinoma (FENLON et al. 1999a). CTC identified all of the cancers including 2 synchronous cancers proximal to the obstructing mass that were missed by barium enema (FENLON et al. 1999a). In addition, CTC demonstrated 16 of 18 polyps in the proximal colon.

2.2.4
Post-operative Colorectal Cancer Surveillance

The American Society of Clinical Oncology developed in 1999 a set of guidelines for the surveillance of the post-operative patient with colorectal cancer after thorough review of the literature of common surveillance protocols. Protocols were reviewed on the basis of reduction in morbidity and five-year disease free survival. Monitoring carcino-embryonic antigen (CEA) levels and colonoscopy were found to be the most effective in many protocols, with liver function evaluation, fecal occult blood testing, liver ultrasound and chest X-ray being less effective in overall outcome (DESCH et al. 1999). Colonoscopy appears to have the best predictive value for morbidity. A pre-operative or peri-operative evaluation of the entire colon is essential in the surveillance algorithm with a polyp free colon a must. Metachronous adenomas and neoplasms have been reported on surveillance colonoscopy at a fairly high rate (FUKUTOMI et al. 2002). Surveillance colonoscopy can be performed in three to five years if polyp free after surgery. However, colorectal surgeons surveyed stated they typically use a more frequent algorithm, such as 6–12 months intervals for the first 5 years.

The role of CT colonography has been evaluated specifically in this patient population. Incomplete colonoscopies secondary to post-operative strictures and rigid mesentery have been reported. In 2002, Gollub et al. reported a conventional colonoscopy failure rate of 4%-29% in post-operative or post-radiotherapy patients (GOLLUB et al. 2002). These patients would undergo a double contrast barium enema for complete evaluation of the colon. As discussed, CTC sensitivity for polyp detection is greater than DCBE and thus makes it a superior surveillance tool in this subset of patients.

The additional benefit of CTC for surveillance includes evaluation of the abdominal and pelvic viscera. The anastomosis can be specifically evaluated. In some surveillance algorithms, patients undergo colonoscopy and liver ultrasound. Laghi et al. reported on a group of patients undergoing surveillance with CEA, liver ultrasound, colonoscopy and chest X-ray (LAGHI et al. 2003). In his study, the patients underwent contrast-enhanced CTC and findings were directly compared to conventional colonoscopy findings. CTC detected all polyps seen with conventional colonoscopy with two false positives. The study was also able to diagnose liver metastases and basal lung nodules. Therefore, contrast-enhanced CTC appears to be a valuable alternative surveillance tool in post-operative patients at increased risk for adenomas and cancer.

2.2.5
Incomplete Conventional Colonoscopy

CTC has been shown to be superior to double contrast barium enema following incomplete conventional colonoscopy and, in fact, failed colonoscopy was the first established indication for CTC. An incomplete colonoscopy is defined as failure to intubate up to the cecum. The reported rate of failed colonoscopy ranges from 8% to as high as 35%. Patients with a history of an incomplete colonoscopy have a significantly increased risk of failing a second attempt. A multitude of reasons contribute to a failed conventional colonoscopy: poor bowel preparation, redundant colon, strictures, history of failed colonoscopies and patient discomfort. Double contrast barium enema was usually the next step in the algorithm of colon evaluation and in most cases performed the same day. On some occasions, however, DCBE is suboptimal as well, sometimes due to poor bowel prep, patient's inability to move on the table or inadequate barium coating of the colonic mucosa secondary to an air block from the previous incomplete colonoscopy (Macari et al. 1999).

In patients with failed colonoscopy, Macari et al. reported CTC sensitivities of polyp detection of 87%, compared with 45% for DCBE. The specificity was also better for CTC than DCBE; 98 vs 89%, respectively (Macari et al. 1999). Therefore, in this subset of patients who have failed conventional colonoscopy, CTC rather than a second attempt of conventional colonoscopy or DCBE may be prudent.

2.2.6
Inflammatory Bowel Disease Surveillance

The cancer surveillance algorithm is augmented for high-risk patients. Patients with pancolitis for more than 7–10 years and patients with left-sided ulcerative colitis for more than 15 years are at increased risk of developing colon cancer. The current recommendation for screening colonoscopy for these groups is every 1–2 year with random biopsies of the colon (American Society of Gastrointestinal Endoscopy 1998). Patients with ulcerative colitis and Crohn's disease have an increased risk of cancer the longer the disease progresses and an approximate overall 3% risk of colon cancer has been reported (Mpofu et al. 2004). For this reason, surveillance usually begins eight years after initial diagnosis and patients are usually screened by conventional colonoscopy with polypectomy and occasionally colectomy. However, no clear evidence exists that surveillance improves colon cancer survival in this patient population (Mpofu et al. 2004).

In this patient population with history of colitis and possible prior segmental colonic resections, fistulas and strictures often develop at the anastomosis and make passage of the colonoscopy device impossible. Scarring of the mesentery may also cause rigidity and may lead to failed colonoscopies. Historically, patients would then go on to double contrast barium enema for complete evaluation of the colon.

Ota et al. reported a study of 33 patients with Crohn's disease and compared CTC with conventional colonoscopy and DCBE in the detection of lesions in the colon proximal to a stenosis (Ota et al. 2003). CT colonography was found to be superior to both DCBE and conventional colonoscopy in the evaluation of the proximal colon. Although conventional colonoscopy was limited in the evaluation of the mucosa, CTC had the added advantage of being able to evaluate the entire bowel wall as well as extra-luminal tissues.

Patients with Crohn's disease primarily in the region of the ileocecal valve have an increased risk of colon cancer similar to patients with ulcerative colitis. In this subset of Crohn's patients who often have a history of multiple abdominal surgeries for fistulas, a described failed colonoscopy rate exists. Biancone et al. described a beneficial use for CTC in this particular subset of patient with strictures and failed colonoscopies (Biancone et al. 2003). His study was performed in 16 patients who had undergone partial colectomy, including ileo-colonic anastomosis, for Crohn's colitis and his study was conducted to evaluate for recurrence at the anastomosis. Patients underwent both conventional colonoscopy and CTC. CT colonography was found to be just as accurate in the detection of recurrence at the site of anastomosis with the added evaluation of small bowel dilatation proximal to the stricture and degree of bowel wall thickening. A significant limitation of CTC was its inability to perform biopsies. In patients with inflammatory bowel diseases, CTC is a good tool for further subdividing the patient populations into those who have positive findings and need to go on to conventional colonoscopy and biopsy and those who have negative findings and can continue to be screened at regular intervals.

2.3
Contraindications

The contraindications to CTC are few and, in general, different than these encountered with conventional colonoscopy (Rex et al. 1987). Weight and girth limitations of the scanner, artifacts from metal prosthesis and claustrophobia are examples of contraindications unique to CT. Absolute contraindications to instrumentation of the colon include presence of an acute abdomen, recent abdominal or pelvic surgery, colonic hernia, and acute diverticulitis (Fig. 2.3). Relative contra-indications include pregnant patients, patients with hip replacements, claustrophobia and an incompetent ileocecal valve (Fig. 2.4).

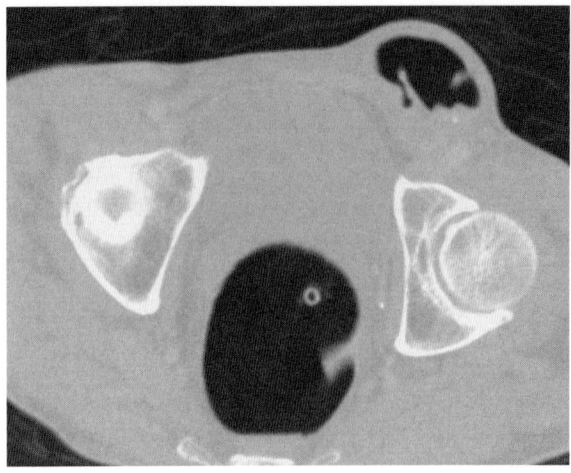 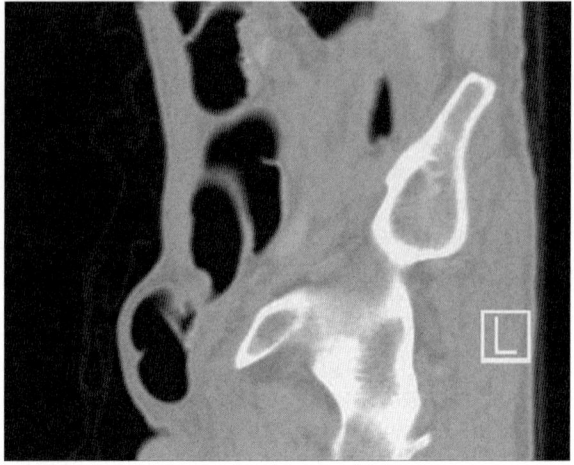

Fig. 2.3a,b. Left inguinal colonic hernia: a supine CT image (lung window setting) shows loops of bowel presumed to represent colon in a left inguinal hernia; b sagittal reformatted CT image shows distended colon within a left inguinal hernia

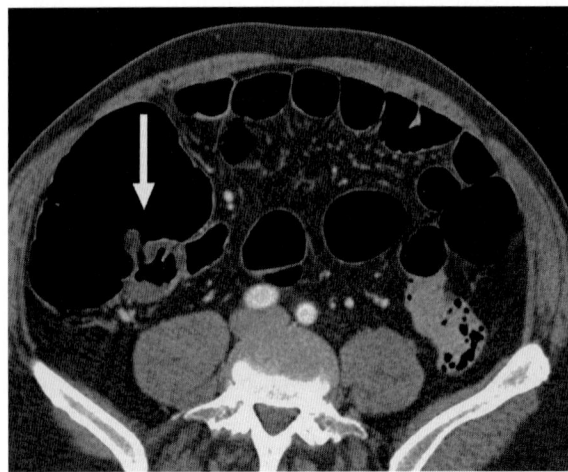 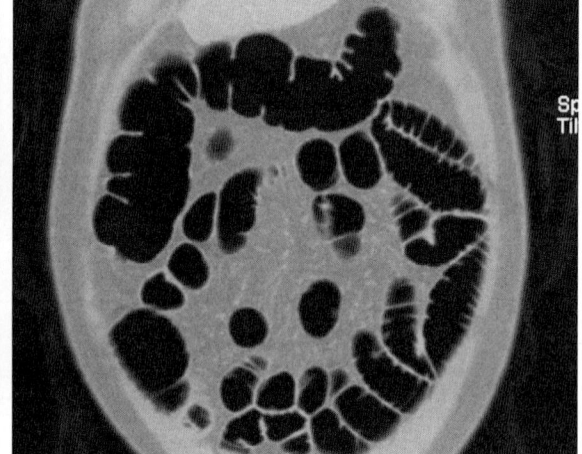

Fig. 2.4a,b. Incompetent ileocecal valve: a axial CT image (soft tissue window) demonstrates a gaping ileocecal valve (*arrow*); b coronal reformatted CT image lung window settings shows gas filled and distended loops of small bowel and colon

2.3.1
Absolute Contraindications

Many CT scanners have a weight limit of 300 to 400 pounds and a circumferential girth limit of 60 cm.

A patient with an acute abdomen should not be inflated with room air or CO_2, and a consultation with a surgeon is most appropriate. Patients with active diverticulitis should not be referred to CT colonography. If an abscess or free air is suspected, a CT of the abdomen and pelvis can be performed with oral and IV contrast. Insufflation of the colon is contraindicated and may cause perforation and widespread peritonitis. Similarly, if a patient has recently undergone pelvic or abdominal surgery, in the past four months, insufflation of the colon is contraindicated. Patients with a known history of colonic hernia or toxic megacolon should also not undergo colonoscopy or CTC.

2.3.2
Relative Contraindications

Pregnancy is a relative contraindication to CTC. The radiation dose and absorbed dose to the fetus during the dual scan is the major issue. In these rare instances that a pregnant patient is suspected to have a colorectal cancer, there is a real risk of perforation with conventional colonoscopy and CTC may be the safer alternative. The gestational age of the fetus is an important factor when contemplating risk. The relative risk of childhood cancers is 1.4 with an exposure of 10 mGy in utero (KUSAMA and OTA 2002). Radiation doses are heavily regulated and the effective dose limit to the fetus is 0.5 rem (5 mSv) (HUDA and STONE 2003). The effective dose of thin-section low dose CTC is 5.0 mSv for men and 7.8 mSv for women. The effective dose to the fetus in utero, however, is less than the stated dose of 7.8 mSv (IANNACCONE et al. 2003 and MACARI et al. 2002).

Patients with metallic hip joint replacements will have significant artifacts in the pelvis with limited evaluation of colonic segments in this region. This is a relative contraindication depending on the clinical question asked. Intravenous iodinated contrast allergy is also a relative contraindication as any patient with a history of a mild contrast allergy can be premedicated for the exam or not receive the injection. Claustrophobia is also a relative contra-indication to the study. Patients can take an oral sedative prior to the study. An incompetent ileocecal valve is another relative contra-indication for CTC as distention of the colon may be suboptimal.

2.4
Current Reimbursable Indications

The first reimbursable indication for CT colonography was studying the colon following a failed colonoscopy. Currently, CT colonography is coded under the CPT category III code 0066T for screening and 0067T for diagnostic CT colonography. Reimbursement of CTC exams by Medicare and many third party payers is approved for diagnostic CTC only and only with specified ICD-9 codes. Medicare does not currently cover colon cancer screening and, therefore, patients have to pay out of pocket in the US. To date, Wisconsin is the lone state that has successfully lobbied the local major third party payers and secured reimbursement for screening CTC. This is likely just the beginning of trends to come in the near future (BARISH 2004).

2.5
Future Indications

The need for colon cleansing with bowel cathartics may be a technique of the past with further development of electronic bowel cleansing software and prep-less fecal tagging protocols. This promises to significantly increase the overall percentage of patients willing to participate in colorectal cancer screening and, therefore, reduce morbidity and ultimately mortality related to colorectal cancer.

Polyp surveillance with CTC may be further refined and some patients ultimately spared from unnecessary polypectomy. Concerns raised regarding radiation dose may be further reduced with continued dose reduction software development.

2.6
Summary

Virtual colonoscopy, now ten years old, has made substantial progress in the detection of adenomas and colorectal cancer. Recent studies report comparable sensitivities and specificities to conventional colonoscopy for polyps 10 mm or larger on a per polyp basis. CTC is currently approved by Medicare as a diagnostic study in patients with positive symptoms and after failed colonoscopy. Work continues to approve CTC as a colorectal cancer screening exam. Many experts believe CTC is also ready to be adopted into the colorectal screening algorithm.

References

Ahsan H, Neugut A, Garbowshi G et al. (1998) Family history of colorectal adenomatous polyps and increased risk for colorectal cancer. Ann Intern Med 128:900–905

American Society for Gastrointestinal Endoscopy (1998) The role of colonoscopy in the management of patients with inflammatory bowel disease. Gastrointest Endosc 48:689–690

Anderson W, Guyton K, Hiatt R et al. (2002) Colorectal cancer screening for persons at average risk. J Natl Cancer Inst 94:1126–1133

Barish M (2004) Billing and reimbursement of virtual colonoscopy. Fifth Annual Symposium on Virtual Colonoscopy, Boston, USA

Biancone L, Fiori R, Tosti C et al. (2003) Virtual colonoscopy compared with conventional colonoscopy for stricturing postoperative recurrences in Crohn's disease. Inflammatory Bowel Dis 9:343–350

Bressler B, Paszat LF, Vinden C et al. (2004) Colonoscopic miss rates for right-sided colon cancer: a population-based analysis. Gastroenterology 127:452–456

Bruzzi J, Moss A, Fenlon H.(2001) Clinical results of CT colonoscopy. Eur Radiol 11:2188–2194

Chen S, Lu D, Hecht J, et al. (1999) CT colonography: value of scanning in both the supine and prone positions. Am J Roentgenol 172:595–599

Dachman A, Kuniyoshi J, Boyle C et al. (1998) CT colonography with three-dimensional problem solving for detection of colonic polyps. Am J Roentgenol 171:989–995

Desch C, Benson A, Smith T et al. (1999) Recommended colorectal cancer surveillance guidelines by the American Society of Clinical Oncology. J Clin Oncol 17:1312

Fenlon H, McAneny D, Nunes D et al. (1999a) Occlusive colon carcinoma: virtual colonoscopy in the preoperative evaluation of the proximal colon. Radiology 210:423–428

Fenlon H, Nunes D, Schroy P et al. (1999b) A comparison of virtual and conventional colonoscopy for the detection of colorectal polyps. N Engl J Med 341:1496–1503

Frazier A, Lindsay M, Graham A et al. (2000) Cost-effectiveness of screening for colorectal cancer in the general population. JAMA 284:1954–1961

Fukutomi Y, Moriwaki H, Nagase S et al. (2002) Metachronous colon tumors: risk factor and rationale for the surveillance colonoscopy after initial polypectomy. J Cancer Res Clin Oncol 128:569–574

Garbay J, Suc B, Rotman N et al. (1996) Multicentre study of surgical complications of colonoscopy. Br J Surg 83:42–44

Gollub M, Ginsberg M, Cooper C et al. (2002) Quality of virtual colonoscopy in patients who have undergone radiation therapy or surgery: how successful are we? Am J Roentgenol 178:1109–1116

Gryspeerdt S, Herman M, Baekelandt M, et al. (2004) Supine/left decubitus scanning: a valuable alternative to supine/prone scanning in CT colonography. Eur Radiol 14:768–777

Huda W, Stone RM (2003) Review of radiologic physics, 2nd edn. Lippincott Williams and Wilkins, Philadelphia

Iannaccone R, Laghi A, Catalano C et al. (2003) Detection of colorectal lesions: lower-dose multi-detector row helical CT colonography compared with conventional colonoscopy. Radiology 229:775–781

Johnson C, MacCarty R, Welch T et al. (2004) Comparison of the relative sensitivity of CT colonography and double-contrast barium enema for the screen detection of colorectal polyps. Clin Gastroenterol Hepatol 2:314–321

Kusama T, Ota K (2002) Radiological protection for diagnostic examination of pregnant women. Congenital Anomalies 42:10–14

Laghi A, Iannaccone R, Bria E et al. (2003) Contrast-enhanced computed tomographic colonography in the follow-up of colorectal cancer patients: a feasibility study. Eur Radiol 13:883–889

Leaper M, Johnston MJ, Barclar M et al. (2004) Reasons for failure to diagnose colorectal carcinoma at colonoscopy. Endoscopy 36:499–503

Lefere P, Gryspeerdt S, Dewyspelaere J et al. (2002) Dietary fecal tagging as a cleansing method before CT colonography: initial results polyp detection and patient acceptance. Radiology 224:393–403

Macari M, Berman P, Dicker M et al. (1999) Usefulness of CT colography in patients with incomplete colonoscopy. AJR 173:561–564

Macari M, Bini E, Xue X et al. (2002) Colorectal neoplasms: prospective comparison of thin-section low-dose multi-detector row CT colonography and conventional colonoscopy for detection. Radiology 224:383–392

Morrin M, Farrell R, Kruskal J et al. (2000) Utility of intravenously administered contrast material at CT colonography. Radiology 217:765–771

Mpofu C, Watson A, Rhodes J (2004) Strategies for detecting colon cancer and/or dysplasia in patients with inflammatory bowel disease. Cochrane Database Syst Rev 2:CD000279

O'Brien M, Winawer S, Zauber A et al. (1990) The national polyp study. patient and polyp characteristics associated with high grade dysplasia in colorectal adenomas. Gastroenterology 88:371–379

Ota Y, Matsui T, Ono H et al. (2003) Value of virtual computed tomographic colonography for Crohn's colitis: comparison with endoscopy and barium enema. Abdom Imaging 28:778–783

Pickhardt P, Choi J, Hwang I et al. (2003) Computed tomographic virtual colonoscopy to screen for colorectal neoplasia in asymptomatic adults. N Engl J Med 349:2191–2200

Rankin GB. (1987) Indications, contraindications, and complications of colonoscopy. In: Sivak MV (ed). Gastrointestinal endoscopy. WB Saunders, Philadelphia, pp 873–878

Rex D, Cutler C, Lemmel G et al. (1997) Colonoscopic miss rates of adenomas determined by back-to-back colonoscopies. Gastroenterology 112:24–28

Rozen P, Pignone M (2003) Implementing colon cancer screening. Recommendations from an international workshop. Oncology 9:17–22

Siemens AG (2002) Medical solutions. Computed tomography; its history and technology. Brochure. Siemensstr. 1, D-91301 Forcheim, Germany. Telephone ++49913184-0. www. SiemensMedical.com

Taylor S, Halligan S, Saunders B et al. (2003) Acceptance by patients of multidetector CT colonography compared with barium enema examinations, flexible sigmoidoscopy, and colonoscopy. Am J Roentgenol 181:913–921

Van Dam J, Cotton P, Johnson D et al. (2004) AGA Future Trends Report: CT colonography. Gastroenterology 127:970–984

Vining D, Gelfand D, Bechtold R et al. (1994) Technical feasibility of colon imaging with helical CT and virtual reality. Am J Rotenography 162(suppl):104

Winawer S, Schottenfeld D, Flehinger B (1991) Colorectal cancer screening. J Natl Cancer Inst 83:243–253

Winawer S, Fletcher R, Miller L et al. (1997) Colorectal cancer screening: clinical guidelines and rationale. Gastroenterology 112:594–642

Winawer S, Zauber A (2002) The advanced adenoma as the primary target of screening. Gastrointest Endosc Clin North Am 1212:1–9

Yee J, Akerkar G, Hung R et al. (2001) Colorectal neoplasia: performance characteristics of CT colonography for detection in 300 patients. Radiology 219:685–692

Zalis M (2004) Presentation 5th Annual Symposium on Virtual Colonoscopy, Boston, MA, USA

Zubarik R, Fleischer DE, Mastropietro C et al. (1999) Prospective analysis of complications 30 days after outpatient colonoscopy. Gastrointest Endosc 50:322–328

3 Patient Preparation for CT Colonography

Judy Yee

CONTENTS

3.1 Colonic Preparation 24
3.1.1 Polyethylene Glycol 25
3.1.2 Sodium Phosphate 26
3.1.3 Magnesium Citrate 27
3.2 Colonic Distension 27
3.2.1 Room Air 29
3.2.2 Carbon Dioxide 29
3.3 Anti-Spasmodic Agents 30
3.3.1 Glucagon 30
3.3.2 Hyoscine *n*-Butylbromide 31
References 32

CT colonography or virtual colonoscopy has increasing support as a screening tool for colorectal polyps and carcinoma. This radiologic examination uses the patient data acquired from a helical CT scanner and combines it with computer software that post-processes the data to generate both two- and three-dimensional images of the colon for analysis. However, before the patient undergoes the CT scan, there are initial steps that must be taken to help obtain images of the colon that are of high diagnostic quality. The key element for a high-quality CT colonography examination is a well-cleansed and well-distended colon (Figs. 3.1, 3.2). When the colon contains residual fluid and/or stool, this can cause false negative and false positive results. If the colon is poorly distended, this too can lead to lesions being missed, and an area of collapse may simulate the apple-core appearance of a carcinoma. Patients are typically scanned in two opposing positions (supine and prone) so that portions of the colon that have residual material or poor distension in one position may be re-evaluated in the opposing view.

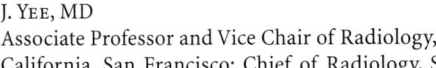

J. Yee, MD
Associate Professor and Vice Chair of Radiology, University of California, San Francisco; Chief of Radiology, San Francisco VA Medical Center, 4150 Clement Street, San Francisco, CA 94121, USA

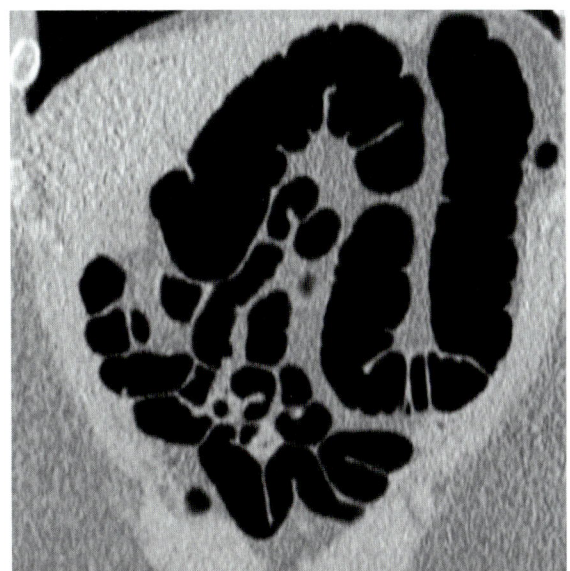
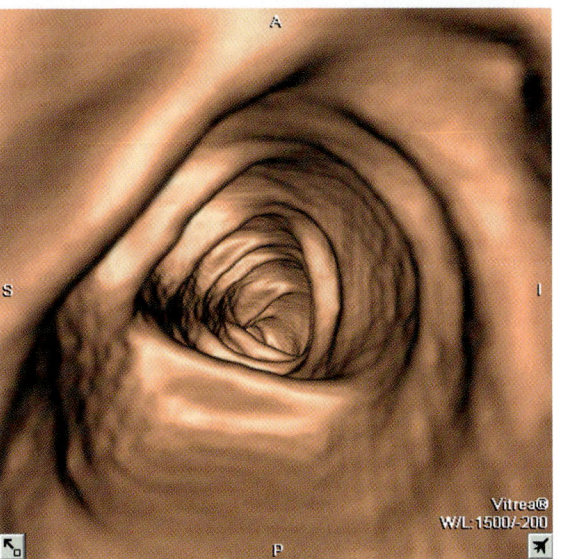

Fig. 3.1. a Coronal multiplanar reformat demonstrates a well-cleansed transverse colon with no layering fluid or residual solid stool. **b** Three-dimensional endoluminal view from the same patient showing normal haustral folds which are easily evaluated because of the absence of residual material

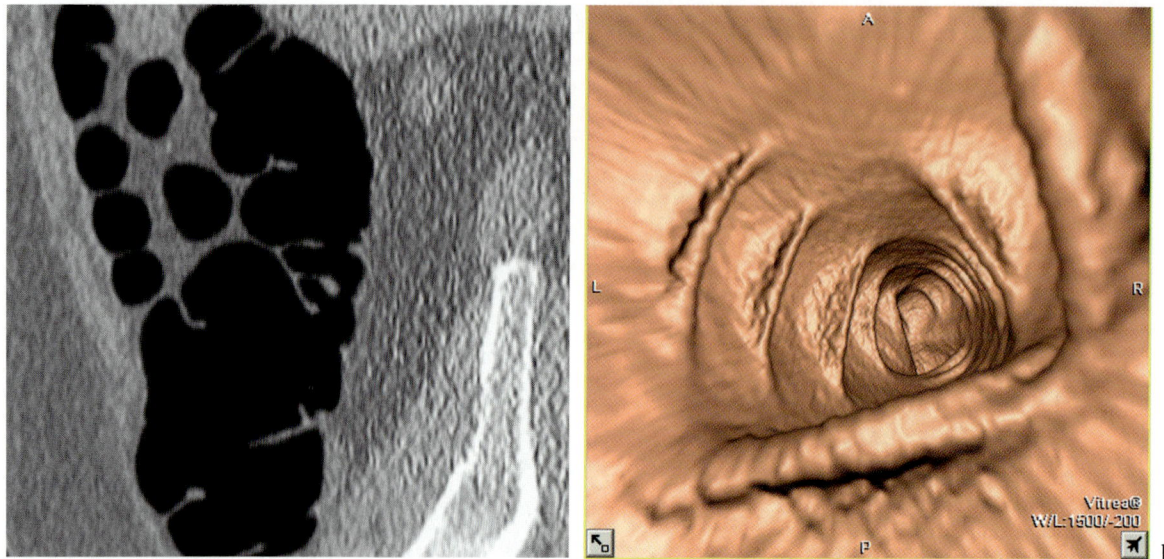

Fig. 3.2. a Excellent distension of the ascending colon and cecum on a sagittal multiplanar reformat optimizes diagnostic ability. **b** A well-distended segment in the same patient on the endoluminal view allows easy navigation

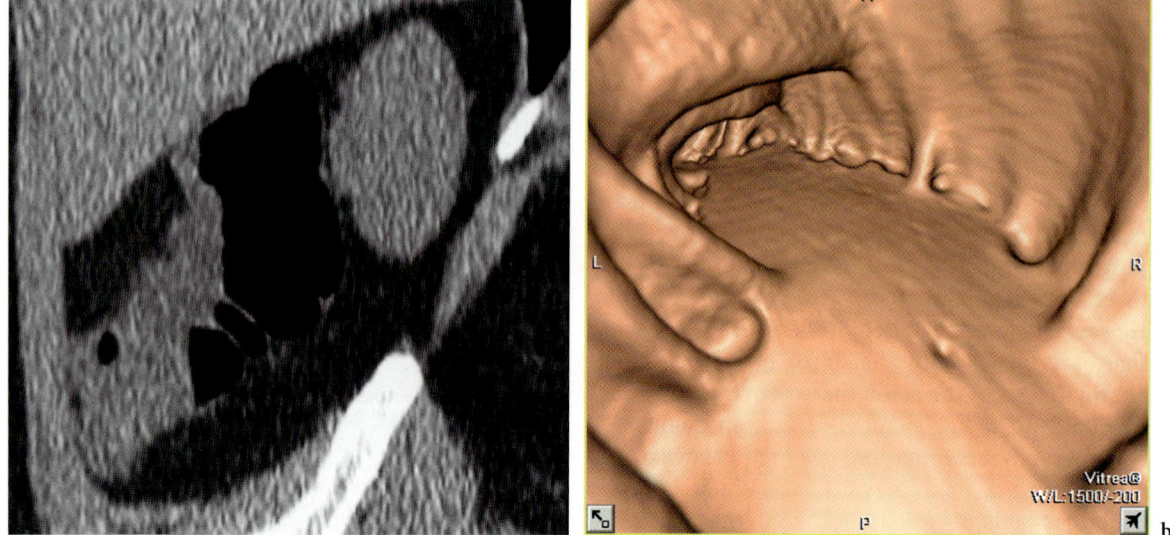

Fig. 3.3. a Suboptimal bowel preparation due to a large amount of residual fluid layering along the dependent wall of the colon as seen on this sagittal multiplanar reformatted view. **b** Poor cleansing with a large amount of layering fluid that obscures the colonic wall beneath it on this endoluminal view in the same patient

3.1
Colonic Preparation

Proper cleansing of the colon is essential if the radiologist is to identify colonic lesions accurately on CT colonography. Remaining pools of fluid in the colon can hide polyps and cancer both on two-dimensional axial and reformatted images and on the three-dimensional endoluminal views (Figs. 3.3, 3.4). Residual solid stool may be misdiagnosed as a polyp, particularly if homogeneous and non-mobile. Large amounts of residual stool can obscure true colorectal polyps and even cancer. Bowel cleansing for CT colonography is currently similar to that used for other colon tests such as the barium enema and standard colonoscopy. There are two main strategies, the first consisting of maintaining a clear liquid diet starting about 24 h before the CT scan. The

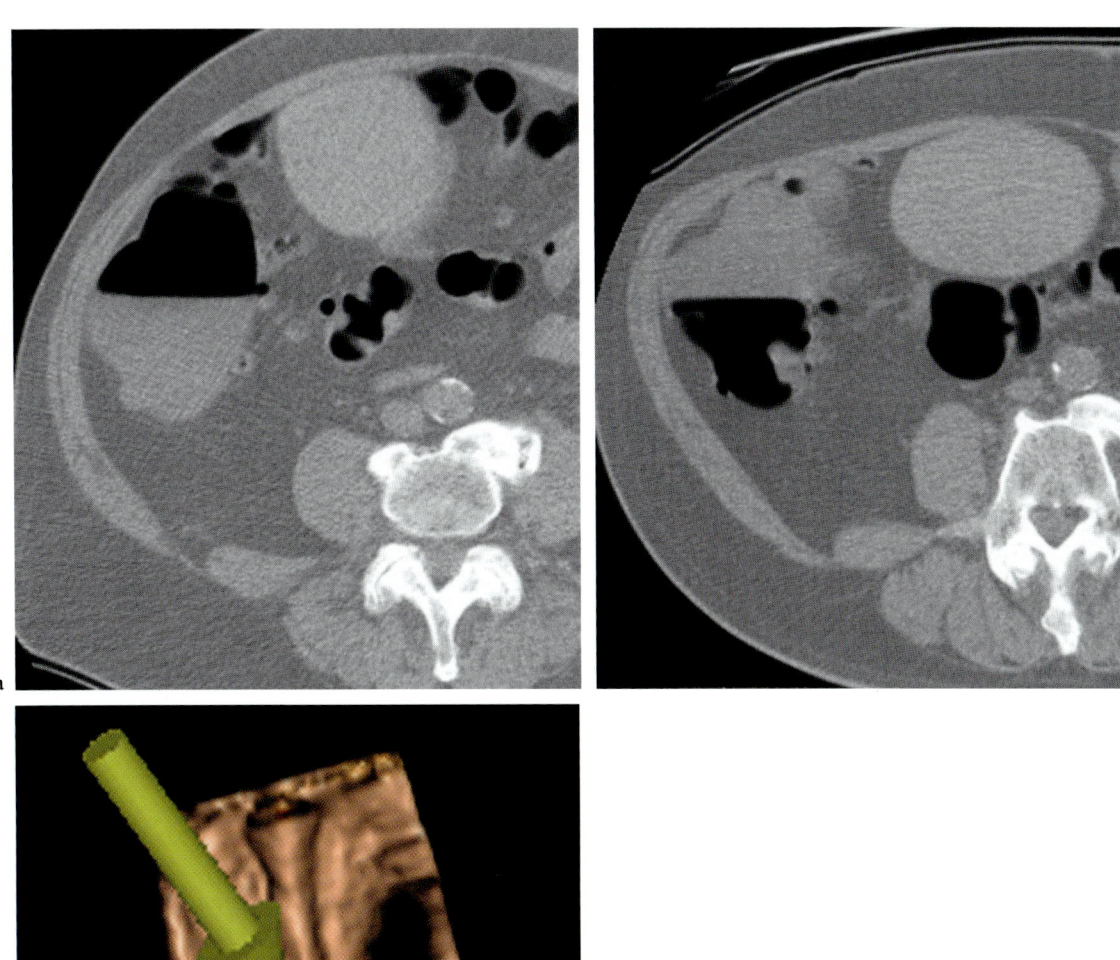

Fig. 3.4. a Supine axial view of the ascending colon demonstrates greater than 50% of the lumen filled with fluid. **b** Prone axial view in the same patient demonstrates the large adenomatous polyp that would have been missed if dual-position imaging had not been performed. **c** Prone three-dimensional cube view shows the same large irregular adenomatous polyp

second strategy is to clean the colon by having the patient ingest a cathartic or laxative that promotes emptying of the colon. Polyethylene glycol is an electrolyte lavage solution in a nonabsorbable medium that patients drink in large volumes to bring about colonic evacuation. Sodium phosphate and magnesium citrate are saline cathartics which are highly osmotic agents containing inorganic ions that draw fluid into the bowel lumen to induce peristalsis and elimination of bowel contents.

3.1.1
Polyethylene Glycol

Polyethylene glycol electrolyte lavage solution is often the agent preferred by gastroenterologists for colonic cleansing in patients prior to fiberoptic colonoscopy. One unit of the solution is composed of 236 g of polyethylene glycol as well as electrolytes such as sodium and potassium and is administered orally in a large volume to empty the colon.

The product typically comes in powder form in a large container and is mixed with about 4 l of water. Patients are instructed to drink the 4 l of polyethylene glycol solution within a 3-h period during the afternoon or early evening before the day of the procedure. Polyethylene glycol is not contraindicated in patients with renal failure or congestive heart failure. However, many patients, especially the elderly, have a difficult time ingesting this large volume during the limited period, and patient compliance may be a problem. Additionally, patients may experience abdominal discomfort, nausea and bloating. In a study of patients being prepared for surgery, 100 patients underwent bowel cleansing with polyethylene glycol and 100 patients received sodium phosphate. Although the quality of the colonic cleansing was similar in both groups, it was found that patients tolerated the sodium phosphate (65% stated they would take the same agent again, 95% completed the preparation) significantly better than the polyethylene glycol (25% would take the same preparation again, 37% ingested the entire amount) (Oliviera et al. 1997).

Polyethylene glycol is not an optimal bowel cleansing agent for CT colonography because it is a "wet preparation". Although it is very effective in clearing solid material, polyethylene glycol often leaves a large amount of residual fluid which may compromise the diagnostic ability of the CT. Excess fluid in the colon does not often hinder the colonoscopy evaluation, since the gastroenterologist is able to aspirate or remove the extra fluid at the time of the procedure to reveal the underlying mucosa. Many of the studies that have been published evaluating the accuracy of CT colonography have used standard colonoscopy as the reference standard, which is typically performed on the same day. In these studies, patients have usually received polyethylene glycol for colonic cleansing.

In a study evaluating the effect of different bowel preparations on residual fluid at CT colonography, 11 patients undergoing same-day CT colonography and screening colonoscopy received polyethylene glycol. Thirty-one patients undergoing CT colonoscopy within 1 week after incomplete colonoscopy received sodium phosphate preparation. Three readers who were blinded to the preparation used in the patients independently evaluated the quantity of residual fluid in six segments of the colon using a four-point scale: 1 = no residual fluid; 2 = less than 25% of the lumen filled with fluid; 3 = 25%-50% of the lumen filled with fluid; and 4 = greater than 50% of the lumen filled with fluid. A statistically significant difference was found between the two groups, with the mean summed residual fluid score equal to 16.3 for the sodium phosphate group and a mean summed score of 26.9 for the polyethylene glycol group (Macari et al. 2001). In a prospective randomized study evaluating bowel cleansing methods prior to CT colonography in 50 patients, the overall quality of bowel cleansing was found to be better for sodium phosphate than with polyethylene glycol and the sodium phosphate preparation was better tolerated with significantly less nausea and less fecal incontinence (Ginnerup Pedersen et al. 2002).

3.1.2 Sodium Phosphate

Sodium phosphate (also known as phospho-soda) is a saline cathartic that is familiar to radiologists since it is often used as a cleansing agent prior to double-contrast barium enema. The laxative effect of sodium phosphate results from its osmotic properties which causes large outflow from the colon. A kit is commercially available containing a 1.5-oz or 45-ml bottle of monobasic and dibasic sodium phosphate, four bisacodyl tablets (5 mg each) and one bisacodyl suppository (10 mg). Bisacodyl is a contact laxative that stimulates parasympathetic reflexes to induce evacuation (Gelfand et al. 1991). Patients are instructed to mix the 45 ml of sodium phosphate with 4 oz (ca. 125 ml) of water and to ingest this with an additional 8 oz (ca. 250 ml) of water at about 6 PM the evening before the procedure. The time to onset of the laxative effect is about 1 h in general, and patients are instructed to remain close to a restroom. The four bisacodyl tablets are taken at about 9 p.m. the same evening and the bisacodyl suppository is administered the morning of the procedure.

Reported complications from the use of sodium phosphate are rare and may result from induced hypovolemia, or patients can develop significant electrolyte disturbances, such as hypernatremia, hyperphosphatemia, hypocalcemia, and hypokalemia (Ehrenpreis et al. 1996; Vukasin et al. 1997). Sodium phosphate is contraindicated in patients with known renal failure, pre-existing electrolyte abnormalities, congestive heart failure (particularly if on diuretic therapy), ascites, and ileus (Fass et al. 1993). Although some gastroenterologists and radiologists prescribe a "double dose" (3 oz or 90 ml) of sodium phosphate for colonic cleansing, this must be administered with caution, especially in older patients, given the increased potential for serious blood electrolyte abnormalities. The first dose of 45 ml is given the evening before and the second dose is administered the morning of the procedure, the two doses separated by about 10--12 h (Pickhardt et al. 2003). The US Food and Drug Administration (FDA) has released a warning about the potential toxicity of oral sodium phosphate as a colonic cleansing agent for colonoscopy (FDA 2002). To avoid serious adverse events, it has been advised that oral sodium phosphate be administered as recommended to patients without major comorbid conditions (Hookey et al. 2002).

In contrast to polyethylene glycol lavage solution, sodium phosphate is known as a "dry preparation" since little fluid typically remains in the colon. In the setting of a dry colon, even small amounts of residual solid material may be seen as pseudo-polypoid lesions on CT colonography. There are multiple published studies evaluating the adequacy of bowel cleansing in patients using sodium phosphate versus polyethylene glycol. Whereas some colonoscopy studies have found similar quality of bowel cleansing irrespective of the purgative agent used (Afridi et al. 1995; Golub et al. 1995; Marshall et al. 1993), other studies have found sodium phosphate to be more effective at cleansing the bowel than polyethylene glycol (Cohen et al. 1994; Kolts et al. 1993; Vanner et al. 1990). A meta-analysis including 1,286 patients from eight colonoscopist-blinded trials comparing sodium phosphate and polyethylene glycol lavage solution found that overall sodium phosphate is as effective as polyethylene glycol and is a more easily completed preparation. A cost saving of approximately $40 per colonoscopy was also identified with the use of sodium phosphate (Hsu and Imperiale 1998). A study evaluating the quantity of fluid retention and adequacy of bowel wall coating in patients receiving sodium phosphate versus polyethylene glycol prior to having a barium enema found that there was no significant difference(O'Donovan et al. 1997).

3.1.3
Magnesium Citrate

Magnesium citrate is a saline cathartic that may also be used as a bowel cleansing agent prior to CT colonography. It prevents water resorption and also stimulates cholecystokinin, which causes increased fluid secretion into the small bowel (Bartram 1994). Magnesium citrate comes in either a powder form which is reconstituted with 8 oz (ca. 250 ml) of water or as a premixed solution in a 10-oz (ca. 310 ml) bottle. This is ingested in the late afternoon on the day prior to the procedure with an additional 8 oz (ca. 250 ml) of water. Bisacodyl tablets and suppository are typically used in conjunction with magnesium citrate similar to sodium phosphate.

An advantage of using magnesium citrate is that it is known as a low-sodium preparation. It contains 12 mg of sodium in its mixed form, compared with 5,004 mg of sodium for sodium phosphate. Although in rare instances sodium phosphate has been associated with clinically significant electrolyte disturbances, the use of magnesium citrate has not been found to cause any similar abnormalities. A study found that all patients receiving sodium phosphate had significant elevations in phosphorus levels followed by a decline in serum calcium levels compared with patients receiving magnesium citrate (Oliviera et al. 1998).

Magnesium citrate has been used with a reduced total volume of polyethylene glycol lavage solution prior to colonoscopy as a strategy to improve patient compliance and tolerance. This has also been found to improve the quality of colonic cleansing and to decrease preparation times (Sharma et al. 1998).

3.2
Colonic Distension

Proper distension of the colon is necessary to allow the radiologist the ability to visualize polyps and cancers that may impinge upon the lumen on CT colonography (Figs. 3.5, 3.6). A segment of colon that is poorly distended or collapsed can simulate a malignant narrowing such as that caused by an annular carcinoma (Fig. 3.7). A well-trained technologist or nurse can assist in placing the rectal tube with care and performing the colonic insufflation, depending upon local guidelines. With the patient in a right-side-down decubitus position on the CT table, the rectal tube is placed. Various types of administration sets are available when performing manual insufflation, including a rectal tip attached to tubing and an insufflation bulb or a Foley catheter attached to an insufflation bulb. Preliminary insufflation in this position is suggested, allowing for filling of the rectosigmoid and the descending colon. The patient is then turned to a supine position and insufflation continues to fill the transverse colon and then the right colon. In general it will take

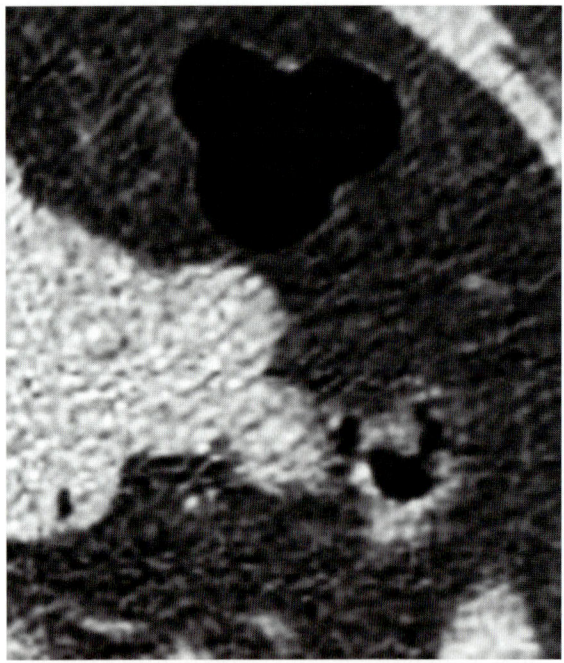
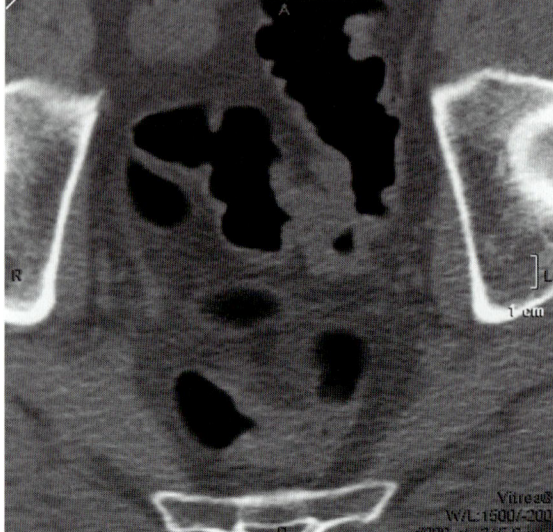
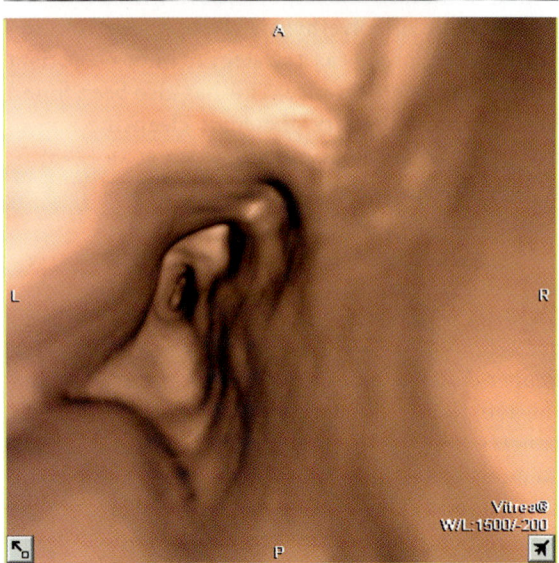
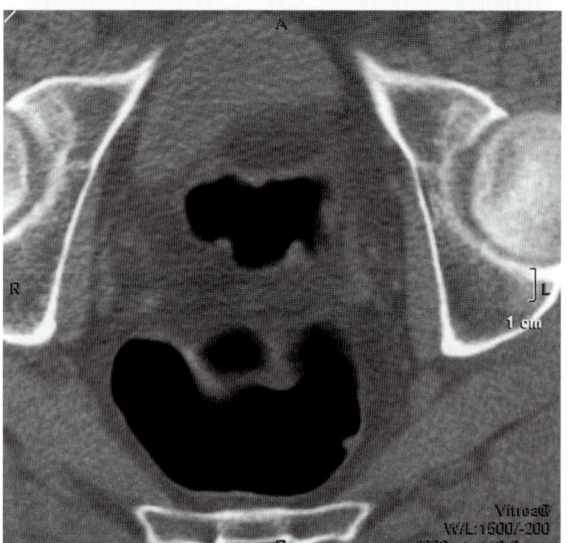

Fig. 3.5. a Poor distension of the descending colon limits the diagnostic ability for lesions on this axial image. **b** Endoluminal view in the same patient showing suboptimal distension which inhibits navigation through this segment

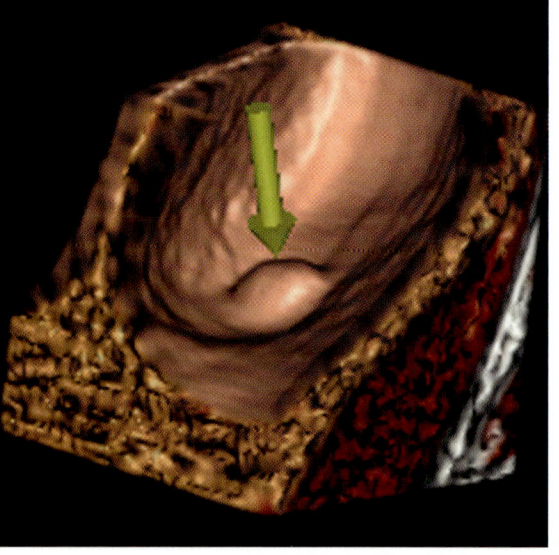

Fig. 3.6. a Collapse of a portion of the rectum in the supine position on an axial image. **b** Excellent distension of the rectum with the same patient in a prone position, demonstrating a small polyp along the left posterolateral colonic wall. **c** Three-dimensional cube view of the same polyp seen in the prone position

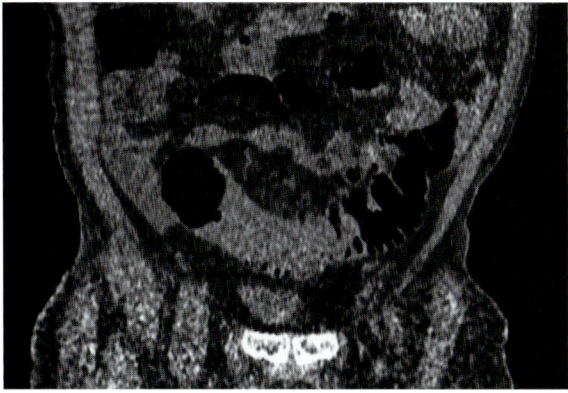
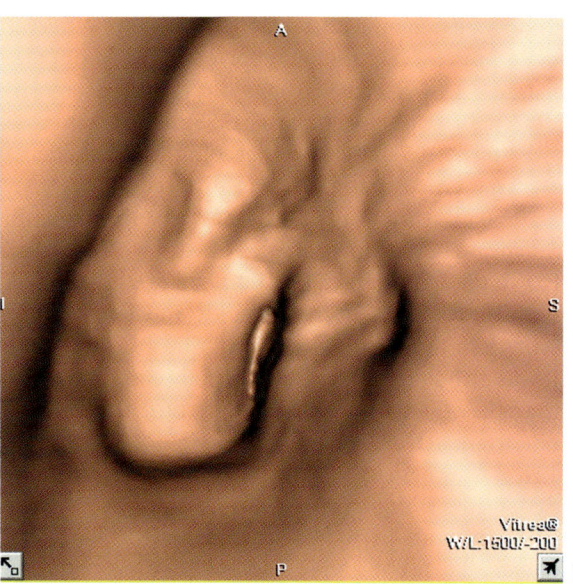

Fig. 3.7. a Collapse of a long length of the sigmoid on coronal multiplanar reformatted view simulating annular carcinoma. b Occlusion of the lumen on endoluminal view due to collapse of the sigmoid in the same patient. This appearance may also be caused by an occluding carcinoma, and proper colonic distension is essential for differentiation

at least 2–3 l of gas to adequately distend the colon. A CT scout view is obtained of the abdomen and pelvis. If the entire colon, particularly the sigmoid, is not well distended then repeat administration of gas is performed according to maximum patient tolerance. Following supine axial image acquisition, the patient is turned prone and another CT scout image is obtained with additional gaseous insufflation given if segments of colon with suboptimal distension are noted on the scout view.

3.2.1
Room Air

Currently room air is used most frequently to manually insufflate the colon for CT colonography. Its ease of use and familiarity to radiologists and technologists because of a similar route of administration per rectum for double-contrast barium enema examinations have made it easily adaptable for CT colonography. It is also readily available at no additional cost. A large component of room air is nitrogen, which is inert, so that there is no active diffusion across the bowel wall when the colon is distended with air. Thus, following retrograde insufflation of the colon with room air, the colon will remain filled until the air is passed distally. Occasionally patients may experience severe pain and distension up to several hours after the CT colonography examination because of excess residual air within the colon. In an evaluation of symptom rates, 7% of subjects experienced significant pain and 13% had severe distension following air insufflation of the colon for barium enema (SKOVGAARD et al. 1995).

3.2.2
Carbon Dioxide

Carbon dioxide (CO_2) has been used instead of atmospheric air for insufflation of the colon for colonoscopy as well as for barium enema examination because it has been found to decrease patient discomfort. CO_2 is readily resorbed through the colonic wall because of a steep diffusion gradient and it is then exhaled from the lungs. One hundred patients were randomized to undergo colonoscopy with insufflation with either air or CO_2. Post-procedural pain was reported in 45% and 31% of patients receiving air at 1 h and 6 h, respectively, after colonoscopy compared with 7% and 9%, respectively in subjects insufflated with CO_2 (SUMANAC et al. 2002). In a study of 142 subjects, approximately half of the patients received room air and the other half received CO_2 to distend the colon for barium enema. Patients who received CO_2 were found to have a reduced incidence of both immediate and delayed pain, from 31% to 12.5% and from 12.9% to 4.2% respectively (ROBSON et al. 1993). In another study of 151 patients undergoing barium enema, 86 received room air and 65 received CO_2 for colonic insufflation. Almost one-third of patients who received room air experienced pain versus only 11% of patients who underwent colonic distension with CO_2. Whereas none of the CO_2 patients reported severe pain, five patients who received room air reported significant pain (COBLENTZ et al. 1985). In a comparative study, 105 patients undergoing barium enema received either manually administered air, CO_2, or a 50/50 mixture of the two gases. No difference in mucosal coating was found. Patients who received CO_2 had significantly less immediate and delayed pain than those who received air and less delayed pain than those insufflated with the 50/50 mixture. It was also found that air provided better distension than the other two gases although the difference did not attain statistical significance (HOLEMANS et al. 1998). Another study identified less optimal colonic distension with manually administered CO_2 than with room air in 100 patients referred for barium enema. It was concluded that poor distension could lead to diagnostic errors and thus outweigh any advantages in patient acceptability when using CO_2 as an insufflation agent (SCULLION et al. 1995).

More recently, CO_2 has also been used to distend the colon for CT colonography. The retrograde administration of CO_2 may be performed either manually, similar to retrograde air insufflation, or electronically using a specific commercially available mechanical device developed for CT colonography. Although manual administration of CO_2 may lead to suboptimal bowel distension as described above, our experience shows more reliable and consistent optimal bowel distension with the use of electronic CO_2 insufflation for CT colonography, which maintains a constant infusion of CO_2 into the colon up to a certain preset pressure. For colonoscopy, a pressure maintained at 35 mmHg with a CO_2 flow rate of 1 l/min has been proven safe (PHAOSAWASDI et al. 1986). For CO_2 administration during CT colonography, the maximum pressure setting allowed using the mechanical device is 25 mmHg. With a fixed flow rate of 3 l/min, the pressure is set at about 15 mmHg to start with and then slowly increased to a maximum of 25 mmHg depending upon patient tolerance. CO_2 instillation is continued in the supine and prone positions until completion of the scan. The total amount of CO_2 insufflated during CT colonography is typically about 4 l due to the relatively short procedural time. This amount is far less than during an average laparoscopic procedure of approximately 2 h using CO_2 flow rates of 5--15 l/min with a total CO_2 consumption of approximately 40 l (TASKIN et al. 1998). No complications have been reported in the literature to date for intracolonic CO_2 insufflation.

3.3
Anti-Spasmodic Agents

Anti-spasmodic agents are used to relax the bowel wall and to minimize peristalsis. Glucagon has been employed for CT colonography in the USA, although its usefulness has not been substantiated. Butyl scopolamine is used in Europe for CT and MR colonography, where it has been found to be cheaper than glucagon and more effective than glucagon as a spasmolytic agent. However, the utility of butyl scopolamine for CT and MR colonography is also controversial.

3.3.1
Glucagon

Glucagon is a polypeptide hormone normally produced by the pancreatic islets of Langerhans. It causes an increase in blood glucose, but is perhaps better known for its clinical use as a hypotonic agent for the stomach, small bowel, and colon. Glucagon relaxes the smooth muscle of the gastrointestinal tract and is thought to improve bowel distension and decrease patient discomfort due to spasm. The effectiveness of glucagon is dependent upon location, and it has been found to be most effective on the duodenum and least effective on the colon (CHERNISH and MAGLINTE 1990). Although uncommon, the most frequently encountered side effects of glucagon are nausea, vomiting and headache. One study found that 4% of patients experienced nausea following the intravenous administration of glucagon prior to CT colonography.(MORRIN et al. 2002). Rarely, generalized allergic-type reactions such as urticaria, respiratory distress and hypotension may occur. Glucagon is contraindicated in patients with pheochromocytoma, insulinoma, poorly controlled diabetes or a known hypersensitivity to glucagon.

Glucagon was used in the past, and is still being used at some sites, as a spasmolytic agent for CT colonography. Many of the older published trials evaluating the performance of CT colonography for polyp detection were performed on subjects who had received 1 mg of glucagon intravenously. The routine use of glucagon for colonic evaluation had been adopted from barium enema practice. Some studies have found decreased discomfort during and after barium enema when glucagon is given prior to the procedure (BOVA et al. 1993; MEEROFF et al. 1975). However, it has also been reported that there was no improvement in colonic distension on double-contrast barium enema after the administration of glucagon [33] and that there was also no improvement in colon polyp detection rates on double-contrast barium enema with glucagon administration (THOENI et al. 1984). Important differences exist between the barium enema examination and CT colonography when considering the usefulness of glucagon for these studies. Liquid barium may cause colonic spasm during the barium enema examination, but this does not occur during CT colonography. Additionally CT colonography is a much more rapid study than barium enema. Colonic insufflation with air is important during the scan phase of the CT, which is very short and occupies less than 15 s in each position, whereas a distended colon is needed for at least 15 min after glucagon is administered for the barium enema examination.

Trials specifically evaluating the value of intravenous glucagon for CT colonography have been conducted. CT colonography was performed in 60 patients following manual air insufflation of the colon up to maximum patient tolerance. Thirty-three patients received 1 mg of glucagon immediately prior to the CT scan and the remaining patients did not (YEE et al. 1999a). Segmental as well as overall colonic distension was evaluated. The colon was divided into eight segments in both supine and prone positions for a total of 16 segments per patient. It was found that glucagon administration did not significantly improve colonic distension in supine or prone positions. In patients receiving glucagon, 222 segments (84.1%) were considered adequately distended. In patients not receiving glucagon, 187 segments (86.6%) were adequately distended. No statistically significant differences were identified between the glucagon group and the non-glucagon group for overall colonic distension scores in the prone, supine, or combined positions.

Another study also found that colonic distension at CT colonography is improved by dual positioning but not by the administration of intravenous glucagon (MORRIN et al. 2002). In a study of 96 patients, 74 subjects received 1 mg of glucagon intravenously immediately prior to CT scanning and 22 patients did not. A five-point scale was used to score adequacy of distension, with 1 = collapsed and 5 = excellent distension. There was no statistically significant difference between the glucagon and non-glucagon groups (mean distension scores 3.6 and 3.9, respectively). We do not administer glucagon routinely for CT colonography at our institution, but we use it in specific cases where there is significant patient discomfort or evidence of colonic spasm on the scout CT view. Initial investigation has also found that glucagon does not appear to improve the sensitivity of CT colonography for detection of colorectal polyps (YEE et al. 1999b).

3.3.2
Hyoscine *n*-Butylbromide

Hyoscine *n*-butylbromide (Buscopan) is an anticholinergic agent that has been used as a muscle relaxant for the barium enema examination as well as for CT and MR colonography in Europe. It has not received approval for use in the USA. Buscopan has a different mechanism of action than glucagon and is less expensive. Hypotonia of the colon is induced by its action on the postganglionic parasympathetic receptors in smooth muscle. Contraindications to the use of anticholinergic agents include glaucoma, severe prostatic hyperplasia, unstable heart disease, bowel obstruction or ileus, and myasthenia gravis. Anticholinergics can cause side effects such as tachycardia, dry mouth, acute urinary retention, and acute gastric dilatation.

In a study comparing various antispasmodic agents for barium enema, 106 patients received a placebo, 109 patients received 1 mg intravenous glucagon, and 109 patients received 20 mg intravenous Buscopan prior to the enema (GOEI et al. 1995). Results showed that Buscopan performed better than glucagon for colonic distension, although about 5% of patients who received Buscopan experienced blurry vision. The routine use of Buscopan for CT colonography is controversial. In a study of 73 patients undergoing CT colonography, 36 patients received 20 mg of Buscopan intravenously and 37 subjects received no muscle relaxant immediately prior to scanning. Intravenous Buscopan was not found to improve the adequacy of colonic distension, and there was no significant improvement in the accuracy of polyp detection (ROGALLA et al. 2005). It was concluded that the routine use of intravenous Buscopan for CT colonography was not supported. Another study performed on 136 patients randomized subjects to receive either 20 mg or 40 mg of Buscopan or no muscle relaxant prior to CT colonography (BRUZZI et al. 2003). Significantly improved distension was found in the cecum and in the ascending and transverse colon in the supine position and in the ascending and descending colon in the prone position. No incremental advantage was found with the larger dose of 40 mg. This study also found that the use of a rectal balloon catheter did not improve distension. A recently published study compared patients not receiving an anti-spasmodic agent with patients receiving 1 mg of glucagon intravenously and subjects receiving 20 mg of Buscopan intravenously immediately prior to supine-only CT colonography.(TAYLOR et al. 2003). Mean colon volumes and radial distensibility were significantly better with Buscopan only when comparing patients who received Buscopan with patients who did not receive any muscle relaxant. The value of Buscopan for CT colonography using dual positioning remains controversial.

References

Afridi SA, Barthel JS, King PD, Pineda JJ, Marshall JB (1995) Prospective, randomized trial comparing a new sodium phosophate-bisacodyl regimen with conventional PEG-ES lavage for outpatient colonoscopy preparation. Gastrointest Endosc 41:485–489

Bartram CI (1994) Bowel preparation -- principles and practice. Clin Radiol 49:365–367

Bova JG, Jurdi RA, Bennett WF (1993) Antispasmodic drugs to reduce discomfort and colonic spasm during barium enemas: comparison of oral hyoscyamine, iv glucagon, and no drug. AJR 161:965–968

Bruzzi JF, Moss AC, Brennan DD, MacMathuna P, Fenlon HM (2003) Efficacy of IV buscopan as a muscle relaxant in CT colonography. Eur Radiol 13:2264–2270

Chernish SM, Maglinte DDT (1990) Glucagon: common untoward reactions -- review and recommendations. Radiology 177:145–146

Coblentz CL, Frost RA, Molinaro V, Stevenson GW (1985) Pain after barium enema: effect of CO2 and air on double-contrast study. Radiology 157:35–36

Cohen SM, Wexner SD, Binderow SR, Nogueras JJ, Daniel N, Ehrenpreis ED, Jensen J, Bonner GF, Ruderman WB (1994) Prospective, randomized, endoscopic-blinded trial comparing precolonoscopy bowel cleansing methods. Dis Colon Rectum 37:689–696

Ehrenpreis ED, Nogueras JJ, Botoman VA, Bonner GF, Zaitman D, Secrest KM (1996) Serum electrolyte abnormalities secondary to Fleet's phospho-soda colonoscopy prep. Surg Endosc 10:1022–1024

Fass R, Do S, Hixson LJ (1993) Fatal hyperphosphatemia following Fleet phospho-soda in a patient with colonic ileus. Am J Gastroenterol 88:929–932

Food and Drug Administration (2002) Science background: safety of sodium phosphates oral solution. Center for Drug Evaluation and Research. Food and Drug Administration, Washington, DC

Gelfand DW, Chen MYM, Ott DJ (1991) Preparing the colon for the barium enema examination. Radiology 178:609–613

Ginnerup Pedersen B, Christiansen TE, Mortensen FV, Christensen H, Laurberg S (2002) Bowel cleansing methods prior to CT colonography: a prospective, comparative, randomized blinded study. Acta Radiol 43:306–311

Goei R, Nix M, Kessels AH, Tentusscher MPM (1995) Use of antispasmodic drugs in double contrast barium enema examination: glucagon or buscopan? Clin Radiol 50:553–557

Golub RW, Kerner BA, Wise WE, Meesig DM, Hartmann RF, Khanduja KS, Aguilar PS (1995) Colonoscopic bowel preparations -- which one? A blinded, prospective, randomized trial. Dis Colon Rectum 38:594–599

Holemans JA, Matson MB, Hughes JA, Seed P, Rankin SC (1998) A comparison of air, CO2 and and air/CO2 mixture as insufflation agents for double contrast barium enema. Eur Radiol 8:274–276

Hookey LC, Depew WT, Vanner S (2002) The safety profile of oral sodium phosphate for colonic cleansing before colonoscopy in adults. Gastrointest Endosc 56:895–902

Hsu CW, Imperiale TF (1998) Meta-analysis and cost comparison of polyethylene glycol lavage versus sodium phosphate for colonoscopy preparation. Gastrointest Endosc 48:276–82

Kolts BE, Lyles WE, Achem SR, Burton L, Geller AJ, MacMath T (1993) A comparison of the effectiveness and patient tolerance of oral sodium phosphate, castor oil, and standard electrolyte lavage for colonoscopy or sigmoidoscopy preparation. Am J Gastroenterol 88:1218–1223

Macari M, Lavelle M, Pedrosa I, Milano A, Dicker M, Megibow AJ, Xue X (2001) Effect of different bowel preparations on residual fluid at CT colonography. Radiology 218:274–277

Marshall JB, Pineda JJ, Barthel JS, King PD (1993) Prospective, randomized trail comparing sodium phosphate solution with polyethylene glycol-electrolyte lavage for colonoscopy preparation. Gastrointest Endosc 39:631–634

Meeroff JC, Jorgens J, Isenberg JI (1975) The effect of glucagon on barium enema examinations. Radiology 115:5–7

Morrin MM, Farrell RJ, Keogan MT, Kruskal JB, Yam CS, Raptopoulos V (2002) CT colonography: colonic distention improved by dual positioning but not intravenous glucagon. Eur Radiol 12:525–530

O'Donovan AN, Somers S, Farrow R, Mernagh J, Rawlinson J, Stevenson GW (1997) A prospective blinded randomized trial comparing oral sodium phosphate and polyethylene glycol solutions for bowel preparation prior to barium enema. Clin Radiol 52:791–793

Oliviera L, Wexner SD, Daniel N, DeMarta D, Weiss EG, Nogueras JJ, Bernstein M (1997) Mechanical bowel preparation for elective colorectal surgery -- a prospective, randomized, surgeon-blinded trial comparing sodium phosphate and polyethylene glycol-based oral lavage solutions. Dis Colon Rectum 40:585–591

Phaosawasdi K, Cooley W, Wheeler J, Rice P (1986) Carbon dioxide-insufflated colonoscopy: an ignored superior technique. Gastrointest Endosc 32:330–333

Pickhardt P, Choi JR, Hwang I, Butler J, Puckett M, Hildebrandt H, et al (2003) Computed tomographic virtual colonoscopy to screen for colorectal neoplasia in asymptomatic adults. Radiology 349: 2191–2200

Robson NK, Lloyd M, Regan F (1993) The use of carbon dioxide as an insufflation agent in barium enema -- does it have a role? Br J Radiol 66:197–198

Sharma VK, Chockalingham SK, Ugheoke EA, Kapur A, Ling PH, Vasudevaa R, Howden CW (1998) Prospective, randomized, controlled comparison of the use of polyethylene glycol electrolyte lavage solution in four-liter versus two-liter volumes and pretreatment with either magnesium citrate or bisacodyl for colonoscopy preparation. Gastrointest Endosc 47:167–171

Skovgaard N, Sloth C, Von Benzon E, Jensen GS (1995) The role of carbon dioxide and atmospheric air in double-contrast barium enema. Abdom Imaging 20:436–439

Sumanac K, Zealley I, Fox BM, Rawlinson J, Salena B, Marshall JK, Stevenson GW, Hunt RH (2002) Minimizing postcolonoscopy abdominal pain by using CO2 insufflation: a prospective, randomized, double-blind, controlled trial evaluating a new commercially available CO2 delivery system. Gastrointest Endosc 56:190–194

Scullion DA, Wetton CWN, Davies C, Whitaker L, Shorvorn PJ (1995) The use of air or CO2 as insufflation agents for double contrast barium enema: is there a qualitative difference? Clin Radiol 50:558–561

Taskin O, Buhur A, Birincioglu M, et al (1998) The effects of duration of CO2 insufflation and irrigation on peritoneal microcirculation assessed by free radical scavengers and total glutathione levels during operative laparoscopy. J Am Assoc Gynecol Laparosc 5:129–133

Rogalla P, Lembcke A, Ruckert JC, Hein E, Bollow M, Rogalla NE, Hamm B (2005) Spasmolysis at CT colonography: butyl scopolamine versus glucagon. Radiology 236:184–188

Taylor SA, Halligan S, Goh V, Morley S, Bassett P, Atkin W, Bartram CI (2003) Optimizing colonic distention for multidetector row CT colonography: effect of hyoscine butylbromide and rectal balloon catheter. Radiology 229:99–108

Thoeni RF, Vandeman F, Wall SD (1984) Effect of glucagon on the diagnostic accuracy of double-contrast barium enema examinations. AJR 142:111–114

Vanner SJ, MacDonald PH, Paterson WG, Prentice RS, DaCosta LR, Beck IT (1990) A randomized prospective trial comparing oral sodium phosphate with standard polyethylene glycol-based lavage solution (Golytely) in the preparation of patients for colonoscopy. Am J Gastroenterol 4:422–427

Vukasin P, Weston LA, Beart RW (1997) Oral Fleet phosphosoda laxative-induced hyperphosphatemia and hypocalcemic tetany in an adult. Dis Colon Rectum 40:497–499

Yee J, Hung RK, Akerkar GA, Wall SD (1999a) The usefulness of glucagon hydrochloride for colonic distention in CT colonography. AJR 173:1–4

Yee J, Hung RK, Steinauer-Gebauer AM, Akerkar GA, Wall SD, McQuaid KM (1999b) Colonic distention and prospective evaluation of colorectal polyp detection with and without glucagon during CT colonography [Abstract]. Radiology 213 [Suppl]:256

4 The Alternative: Faecal Tagging

Philippe Lefere and Stefaan Gryspeerdt

CONTENTS

4.1 Introduction 35
4.2 What is Faecal Tagging? 35
4.3 The Rationale of Performing Faecal Tagging 36
4.3.1 Improving Diagnosis 36
4.3.2 Improving Patient Compliance 36
4.4 How We Do It! 36
4.4.1 The Preparation 36
4.4.1.1 A Low Residue Diet 37
4.4.1.2 Faecal Tagging with Barium 37
4.4.1.3 Mild Cathartic Cleansing 37
4.4.1.4 Instruction Folder 37
4.4.2 The Examination 38
4.4.3 Indications 38
4.5 Imaging Findings 39
4.5.1 Reading the Data Sets 39
4.5.2 Stool Tagging 39
4.5.2.1 Tagged Stool 39
4.5.2.2 Non-Tagged Stool 41
4.5.3 Fluid Tagging 43
4.5.4 Miscellaneous Findings 45
4.5.4.1 Mucous Filaments 45
4.5.4.2 Foam 45
4.6 Results 47
4.7 The Future: Laxative-Free CT Colonography 48
4.7.1 Principles 48
4.7.2 Results 48
4.8 Conclusion 48
References 48

4.1
Introduction

As described in the previous chapter, preparing the colon is one of the prerequisites to perform CT colonography adequately. The option of an intensive preparation to obtain a colon as clean and dry as possible has been approved in a consensus statement developed by several experts in CT colonography (Barish et al. 2005). However, although recently published, this consensus statement was already developed back in 2003 shortly before the publication of the study by Pickhardt et al. (2003) in the *New England Journal of Medicine*. Since then opinion might have changed. Theoretically an intensive preparation should produce the best performance of polyp detection. Indeed, in a well distended, clean and dry colon, conspicuity of tumoral lesions should be at its best. However, this expectation has not been accomplished in some recent multi-centre trials. Two recently published large multi-centre studies obtained very disappointing results of polyp detection using a regular preparation (Cotton et al. 2004; Rockey et al. 2005). Of the many drawbacks these trials have been afflicted with, the lack of faecal tagging, was considered a major shortcoming (Ferrucci 2005a and author reply Ferrucci 2005b). Furthermore, to date the best results of polyp detection have been obtained in a large average-risk population of 1233 patients, using a preparation based on faecal tagging by Pickhardt et al. (2003). In this way, faecal tagging is an appealing technique and is becoming the preparation of choice to perform CT colonography (van Dam et al. 2004; Ferrucci 2005a,b).

The purpose of this chapter is: 1) to explain what faecal tagging is; 2) to demonstrate why this particular type of preparation is important; 3) to explain how faecal tagging is performed at our institution; 4) to show imaging findings.

4.2
What is Faecal Tagging?

Faecal tagging means labelling of faecal residue in the colon. Stool tagging refers to labelling of residual stool, while fluid tagging refers to labelling of residual fluid. The technique is based on the oral ingestion of positive contrast material (barium and/or iodine) as part of the preparation prior to CT colonography. The orally ingested contrast material impregnates the residual stool and mixes with the

P. Lefere, MD; S. Gryspeerdt, MD
Stedelijk Ziekenhuis, Department of Radiology, Bruggesteenweg 90, 8800 Roeselare, Belgium

residual fluid in the colon. By doing so the residual stool and fluid, remaining in the colon after the preparation, have a hyperdense or white aspect on the two-dimensional CT images.

4.3
The Rationale of Performing Faecal Tagging

The rationale of developing a preparation with faecal tagging was twofold: 1) improving diagnosis; 2) improving patient compliance.

4.3.1
Improving Diagnosis

Despite an intensive cleansing of the colon using regular preparations without faecal tagging, both residual stool and fluid in the colon not infrequently cause diagnostic difficulties (Johnson and Dachman 2000) (see also Chap. 8). Residual stool may appear isodense to the colonic wall and cause pseudopolypoid images, mimicking lesions and possibly resulting in false positive findings (Fenlon 2002; Macari and Megibow 2001a). Residual fluid is also isodense to the colonic wall and tumoral lesions. Hence, when present in a large amount, some parts of the colon can be obscured in both supine and prone position, resulting in incomplete visualization of the colonic wall. This may of course result in false negative findings. Occasionally, a polyp mimics residual stool and even fluid, possibly resulting in false negative findings. By labelling both residual stool and fluid in the colon with positive contrast material, both these false positives and negatives could be avoided and consequently facilitate and improve diagnosis (Fig. 4.1) (see also imaging findings).

4.3.2
Improving Patient Compliance

Intensively cleansing the colon mostly causes interruption of the normal daily activity. In fact preparations for full structural examinations of the colon are based on the intensive use of cathartics and produce more or less heavy diarrhoea. Besides this major inconvenience, side effects such as nausea, vomiting, and dizziness frequently occur. This important discomfort is known as a major barrier to complying with standard screening recommendations (Morrin et al. 1999) resulting in less than one half of the population participating in a colorectal cancer screening programme (van Dam et al. 2004; Bromer and Weinberg 2005). To avoid preparation related side effects and to increase patient compliance, a reduced cathartic cleansing in combination with faecal tagging has been developed. In fact as the faecal residue is labelled in the colon, more residue can be left over in the colon without compromising the diagnostic performance of CT colonography. This offers the opportunity of reducing the cathartic cleansing part of the preparation and should enable improvement of patient compliance. This improved patient compliance was confirmed by Lefere et al. (2002). They compared the patient discomfort experienced the day before CT colonography in 2 groups of 50 patients. The former group was prepared with an intensive cathartic cleansing, while the latter was prepared with a combination of a reduced cathartic cleansing and faecal tagging. There were significantly less side effects (such as nausea, vomiting, and abdominal cramps) in the group prepared with the reduced cathartic cleansing and faecal tagging. This resulted in an improved final opinion.

4.4
How We Do It!

4.4.1
The Preparation

The preparation takes one day and is performed the day before CT colonography. It consists of three

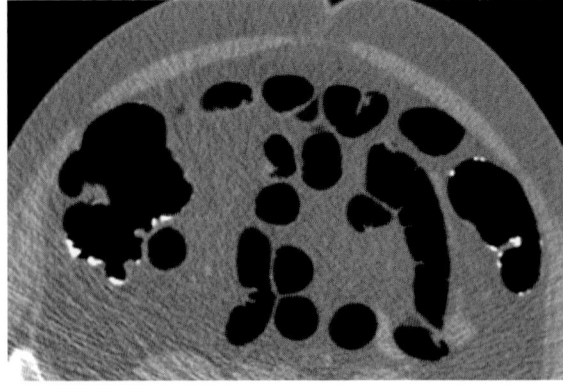

Fig. 4.1. The residual stool in the ascending and descending colon is tagged and appears *white* on the two-dimensional images, facilitating diagnosis

main parts: 1) a low residue diet; 2) faecal tagging with barium; 3) mild cathartic cleansing (LEFERE et al. 2005a). The preparation can be performed in an ambulatory manner without interrupting the normal daily activity and is routinely used at our department.

4.4.1.1
A Low Residue Diet

The patients receive a dedicated low residue diet (Nutra Prep®, E-Z-EM, Lake Success, NY, USA). This diet is provided in a box and supplies the patient with all the meals and drinks for the entire day before CT colonography (Fig. 4.2). This box contains powdered drinks with vanilla flavour, fruit drinks, soups, chips and nutrition bars. The diet reduces the fat intake and the faecal output. Patients are allowed to have breakfast (8 a.m.), lunch (noon) and dinner (5 p.m.). Breakfast consists of a tropical fruit juice, one vanilla drink and tea or coffee. At lunch patients drink another tropical fruit juice and vanilla drink and/or apple sauce, a soup and tea or coffee. At dinner they can have another soup and/or vanilla drink. Between the meals they can eat the chips and nutrition bars. The patients are allowed to drink as much additional water as they want to.

4.4.1.2
Faecal Tagging with Barium

Faecal tagging is performed with a 40% weight/volume barium suspension (Tagitol V®, E-Z-EM). The patients only have to drink a total of 60 ml: 20 ml at breakfast, lunch and dinner respectively. The patients are instructed to drink the barium at once after the meal.

We use barium as sole tagging agent. Several authors advocate the use of iodine or a combination of barium and iodine to achieve fluid tagging (ZALIS and HAHN 2001; ZALIS et al. 2003; PICKHARDT 2003; IANNACCONE et al. 2004). Although its efficacy in fluid tagging is well established, we are not in favour of using iodine. Why not ? In our experience of performing dietary faecal tagging with barium as sole tagging agent, only a few segments presented with a considerable amount of non-tagged fluid. The taste of the barium suspension is improved by adding a flavour (for instance apple flavour) whereas iodine has a bad taste. Furthermore, using iodine, adverse effects such as nausea, vomiting and diarrhoea quite

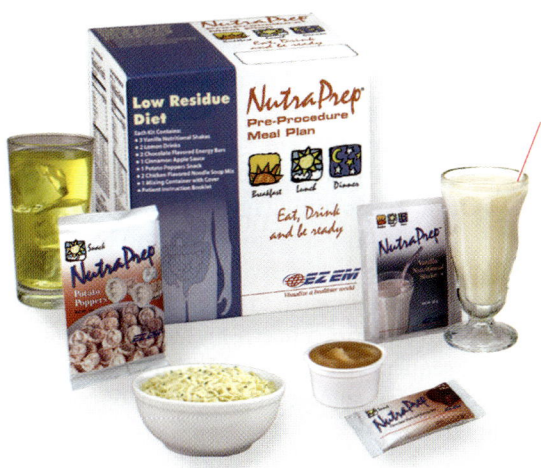

Fig. 4.2. The diet is presented in a box and provides meals and beverages on the day preceding CT colonography

frequently occur. In a recent study IANNACCONE et al. (2004) described side effects in 10% of patients using 200 ml of iodine over two days.

4.4.1.3
Mild Cathartic Cleansing

Cathartic cleansing of the colon is based on the combination of magnesium citrate and bisacodyl tablets (Loso Prep®, E-Z-EM). At 6 p.m. the patients have to ingest the magnesium citrate: 16.5 g (=single dose) dissolved in one glass of cold water. At 7 p.m. they have to take four 5-mg tablets of bisacodyl. When used at this reduced dose, magnesium citrate is a milder cathartic when compared to sodium phosphate and polyethylene glycol (VANNER et al. 1990; KOLTS et al. 1993; MACLEOD et al. 1998; TAYLOR et al. 2003b). Furthermore the magnesium citrate is dissolved in only one glass of water. Reducing the volume to drink also improves patient compliance. Magnesium citrate can be used in case of renal insufficiency, heart failure and electrolyte abnormalities which are contraindications for the use of oral sodium phosphate (MACARI et al. 2001b; TOLEDO and DIPALMA 2001).

4.4.1.4
Instruction Folder

It is accepted that availability of written information improves patient compliance (MURPHY and

COSTER 1997). In order to proceed fluently with the preparation and to avoid misinterpretation of the instructions and/or misuse of the provided items, the patients receive an information folder. This folder provides them with all the practical information necessary to bring this preparation to a good end by: 1) showing all different ingredients on a picture; 2) explaining how to proceed with the meals; 3) explaining how to ingest the barium; 4) explaining how to proceed with the cathartic cleansing; 5) giving advice when to drink additional water. A short explanation concerning the adenoma-carcinoma sequence underscoring the importance of screening for colorectal cancer encourages the patients to follow the preparation meticulously.

4.4.2
The Examination

On the day of CT colonography the patients remain sober until the examination is performed. Whenever necessary we advise the patients to take their regular medication shortly before CT colonography. CT colonography is preferably performed in the morning. Prior to the exam the patient is instructed to visit the restroom to empty the rectum. Smooth muscle relaxation is achieved using scopolamine butylbromide (Buscopan®; Boehringer Ingelheim) (TAYLOR et al. 2003a). After distending the colon with CO_2 using an automated inflator, the patients are scanned in supine and prone position using an ultra-low dose. Using a 64-slice scanner enables an ultra-low dose of 140 kV and 10 mAs without distortion of the image quality (Fig. 4.3).

If necessary, same day optical colonoscopy can be performed by preparing the patients with some additional laxatives after CT colonography (for instance 1 or 2 L of polyethylene glycol. Optical colonoscopy can be performed some 2 h after starting this additional prep (LEFERE et al. 2002).

4.4.3
Indications

This preparation is routinely used at our institution in all patients referred for: screening for colorectal cancer, change in bowel habit, iron deficiency anaemia, constipation, heme positive stool, etc. (see Chap. 2). Intravenous contrast is never used as the polyps may enhance and simulate tagged stool causing a false negative finding.

In case of an obstructing tumour, faecal tagging is not hampered. In these cases patients present with efficient tagging and the colon is relatively clean (Fig. 4.3). In our experience none of these patients suffered from post-procedural colonic impaction with baroliths.

Faecal tagging is also appropriate in case of incomplete optical colonoscopy. GRYSPEERDT et al. (2005) compared CT colonography performed immediately after incomplete optical colonoscopy (thus after a standard colonoscopy cleansing with polyethylene glycol) with CT colonography performed after faecal tagging. In the latter case CT colonography was not performed the day of incomplete colonoscopy. In the group of patients prepared with faecal tagging, there was significantly less residual fluid. This resulted in a statistically significant improvement of the colonic distension. Furthermore faecal tagging was efficient in all patients. Following these results we developed the following strategy. As the advantages of using intravenous contrast outweigh the advantages of faecal tagging in case of known tumoral pathology (staging), CT colonography is performed with IV contrast immediately after the incomplete optical colonoscopy without any addi-

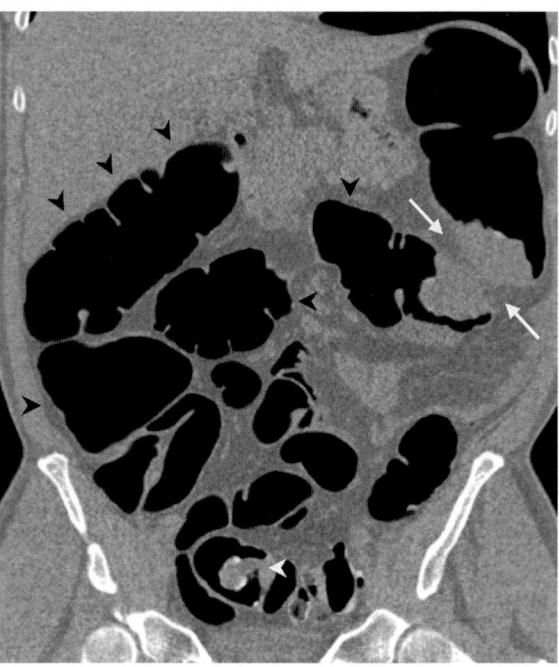

Fig. 4.3. Despite the large obstructing tumour in the transverse colon near the splenic flexure (*white arrows*), the proximal colon is clean (*black arrowheads*). There is a large stalked polyp in the sigmoid covered by a thin barium layer (*white arrowhead*). Ultra-low dose on a 64-slice scanner: 140 kV – 10 mAs

tional preparation. However, if the incomplete optical colonoscopy is related to a dolichocolon, redundancy, etc. we use faecal tagging because in these patients optical colonoscopy will probably never be complete and we want to perform CT colonography under the best conditions as possible in order to give correct advice on eventual surveillance or surgery whenever necessary.

4.5 Imaging Findings

4.5.1 Reading the Data Sets

After scanning the patient the images are sent to a dedicated workstation with regular endoluminal software. Although possible (PICKHARDT and CHOI 2003) it is important to stress that no dedicated software (stool subtraction) is needed to read and interpret the tagged data sets adequately. Reading is performed using a primary 2D read with 3D problem solving method (DACHMAN et al. 1998) (Fig. 4.4). In case of a clean colon, primary 3D read is possible. However if the colon is not clean, the residual stool causes a pseudopolypoid image on 3D and 2D problem solving is necessary (Fig. 4.5). In 2D rendering we read the data sets using lung window (W/L: 1500/–200 H.U.) and soft tissue (W/L: 400/100 H.U.)

settings. In case the tagged residue has a high density it is advisable using additional bone window settings (W/L: 3500/400). This will improve visualisation of a negative filling defect in the tagged residue. The negative filling defect can be an anatomic structure or a lesion. This is particularly helpful in the case of dense residue (Fig. 4.6).

4.5.2 Stool Tagging

4.5.2.1 Tagged Stool

With faecal tagging the residual stool appears as a bright hyperdense or white spot or mass in the colonic lumen with or without air inclusion (Fig. 4.7). This bright stool almost lights up when scrolling through the 2D images simplifying interpretation as there is no likelihood of mistaking it for a lesion. In that way the time consuming comparison between supine and prone position to detect an eventual change in location of the residual stool becomes superfluous. This shortens the reading time considerably, avoids false positives and improves polyp conspicuity because of the improved contrast difference between the non-tagged lesion and the tagged stool. When reading the tagged data sets, looking for non-tagged "material" is imperative. This non-tagged material is highly suspicious and should be

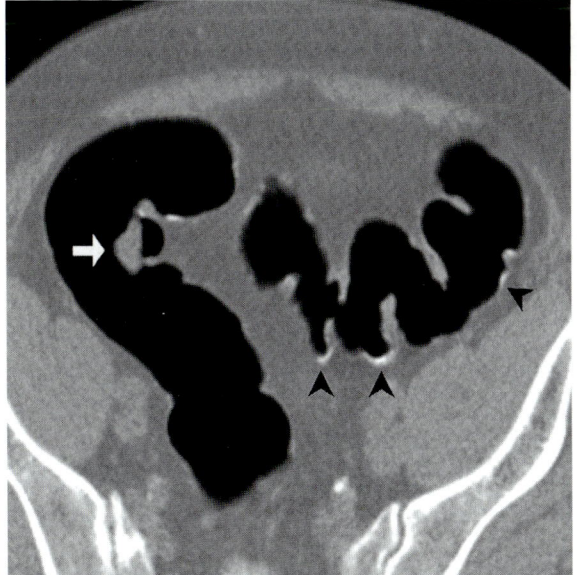 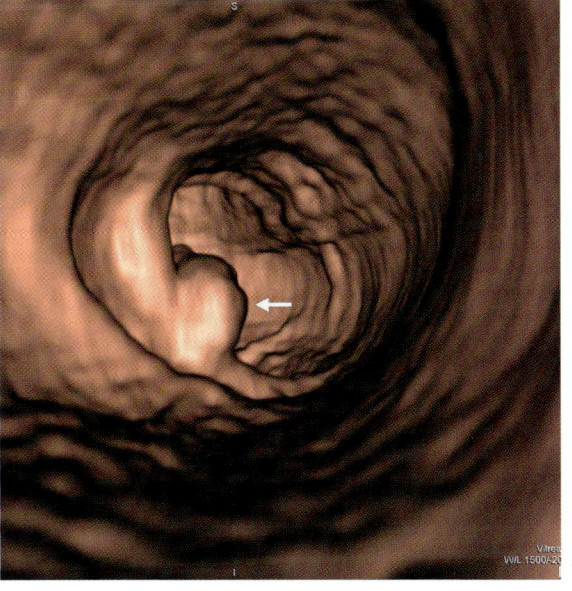

Fig. 4.4.a Stalked polyp in the sigmoid (*white arrow*) with some tagged fluid (*black arrowheads*). **b** Corresponding endoluminal view showing the head of the polyp (*white arrow*)

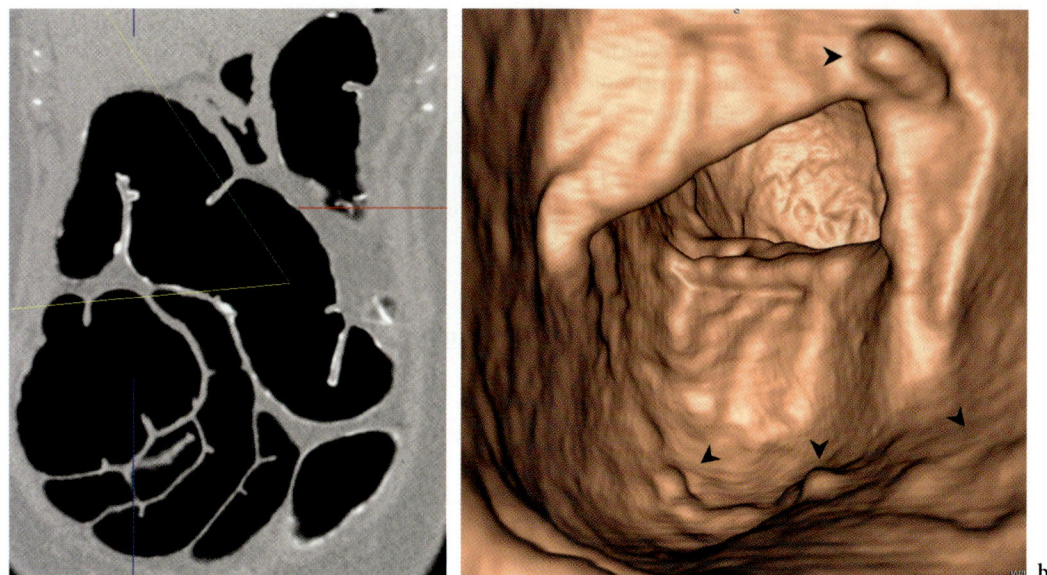

Fig. 4.5.a Coronal reformatted image of the transverse colon. *Yellow open triangle* shows the virtual camera looking in the transverse colon near the hepatic flexure. **b** Corresponding 3D view shows pseudopolypoid lesions caused by the tagged residue (*arrowheads*)

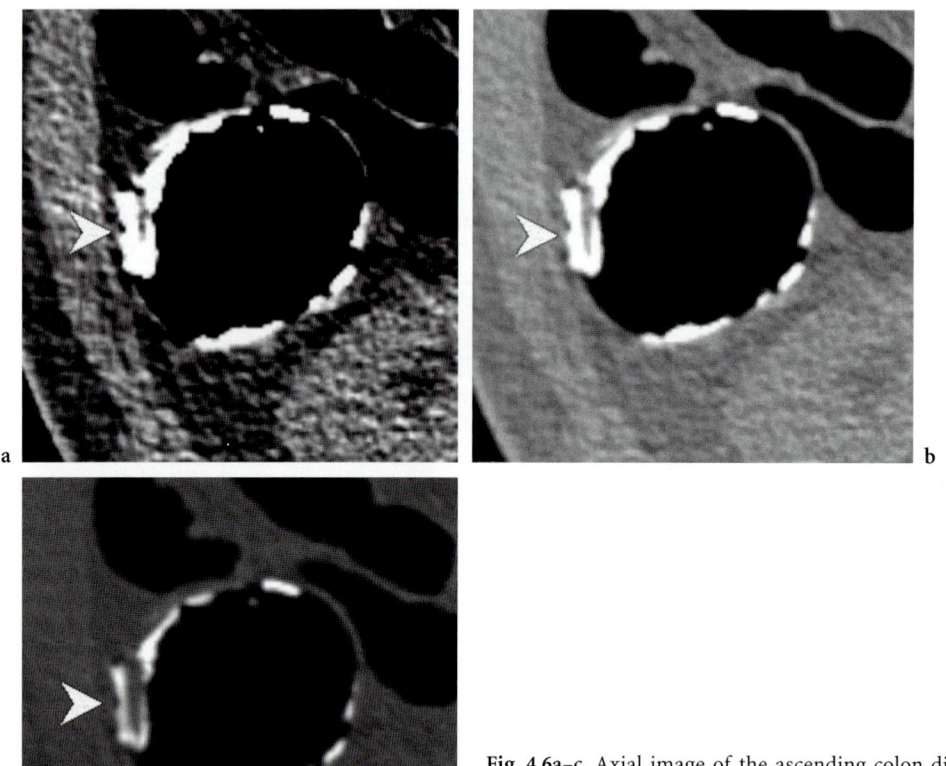

Fig. 4.6a–c. Axial image of the ascending colon displayed in different W/L settings and showing tagged residue with a very high density of 2717 H.U.: **a** soft tissue settings (W/L 400/10). The semicircular fold (*arrowhead*) is only faintly seen; **b** lung window settings (W/L 1500/–200). Slightly improved visualisation of the semicircular fold; **c** bone window settings (W/L 3500/400) with very good visualisation of the semicircular fold allowing detailed inspection

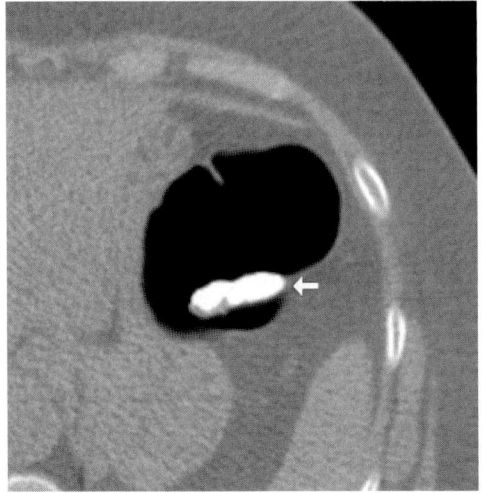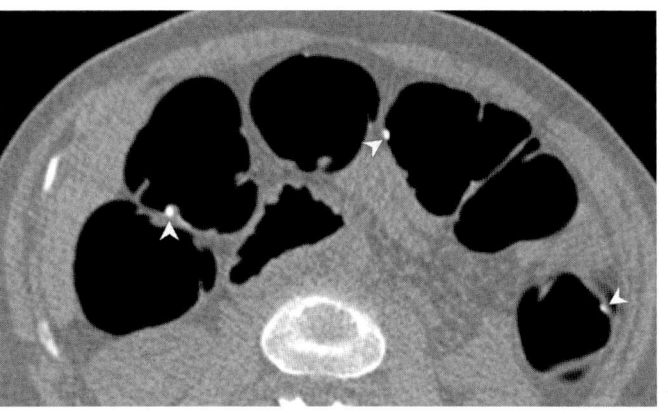

Fig. 4.7a,b. Examples of stool tagging (*arrow* and *arrowheads*). Confusion with a true lesion is excluded. No comparison between supine and prone images is necessary to exclude a lesion

considered a lesion unless it has the specific characteristics of residual stool (Fig. 4.8). Even in the case of an obvious change in position between supine and prone position, a polyp has to be excluded. In fact polyps with a long stalk may show a considerable change in location with dual positioning. A similar lesion was mistaken as stool and caused a false negative (one of the two missed lesions >1 cm) in the landmark study of FENLON et al. (1999). The density of the tagged stool varies between 100 and 3000. H.U. It is striking that there is a wide intra- and inter-patient variability. There is no apparent reason to explain this variability.

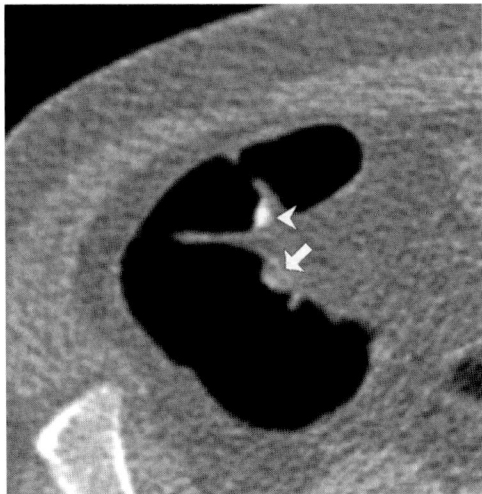

Fig. 4.8. Patient with right sided sigmoid. There is tagged stool (*arrowhead*). There is also non-tagged "material" (*arrow*). This should be considered a lesion unless the contrary is proved. A correct diagnosis of an 8-mm sessile polyp was made

As with optical colonoscopy, tagged stool frequently abuts a lesion. This makes polyps more conspicuous for detection (Figs. 4.8, 4.9, and 4.10). In these cases polyp conspicuity is improved using soft tissue settings.

4.5.2.2
Non-Tagged Stool

In a minority of cases a small amount of stool remains non-tagged.

4.5.2.2.1
Non-Tagged Stool <6 mm

Non-tagged stool <6 mm is too small too cause any concern as it is generally accepted that polyps <6 mm do not need to be removed. Hence pseudopolypoid lesions <6 mm caused by non-tagged residual stool should not be taken into consideration. This non-tagged stool appears as pinpoint filling defects abutting the colonic wall or is frequently floating in barium pools without touching the colonic wall (Fig. 4.11).

4.5.2.2.2
Non-Tagged Stool >6 mm

In our experience non-tagged stool ≥6 mm is present in 3–5% of segments. Mostly it presents as one or two non-tagged stool balls completely surrounded by some barium or floating in barium pools (Fig. 4.12). This stool may also present with the typical imaging

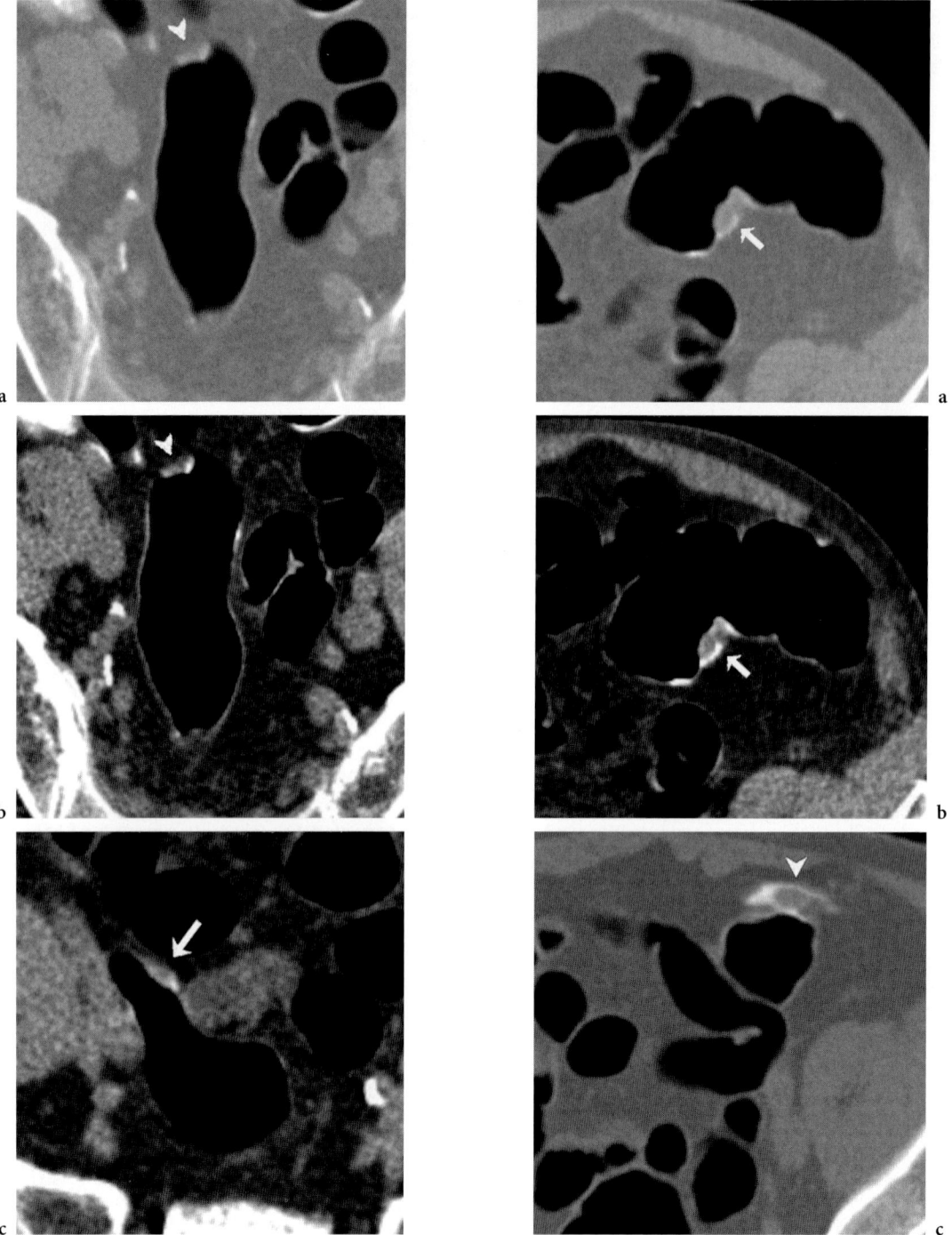

Fig. 4.9.a Small amount of barium abutting a lesion (*arrowhead*) in the sigmoid and hence improving polyp conspicuity. **b** Improved depiction of the lesion in soft tissue settings. **c** The prone view shows a partially collapsed sigmoid. The barium again delineates the lesion improving visualisation (*white arrow*)

Fig. 4.10.a Supine view of the sigmoid in lung window settings (W/L 1500/–200) showing a stalked polyp abutting the colonic wall, surrounded by a barium layer (*white arrow*). **b** Same image in soft tissue settings (W/L 400/100) showing improved conspicuity of the lesion. **c** The prone acquisition shows the corresponding segment is collapsed. The lesion is still visible as a negative filling defect as it is surrounded by tagged fluid (*white arrowhead*)

The Alternative: Faecal Tagging

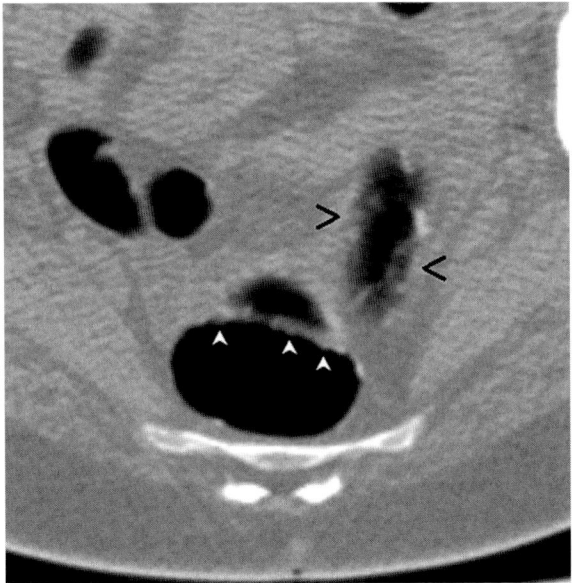
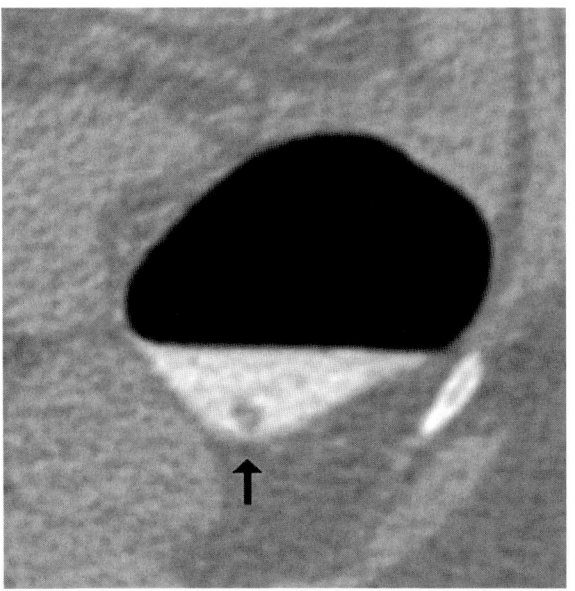

Fig. 4.11.a Supine view of the rectosigmoid showing tiny non-tagged residue in the rectum (*white arrowhead*) and sigmoid (*open black arrowhead*). This stool is too small to cause any diagnostic problem. **b** Ultra low dose scan (64-slice) showing tagged fluid level with floating non-tagged 6-mm residue (*arrow*). There is no contact with the colonic wall, so no confusion with a polyp is possible

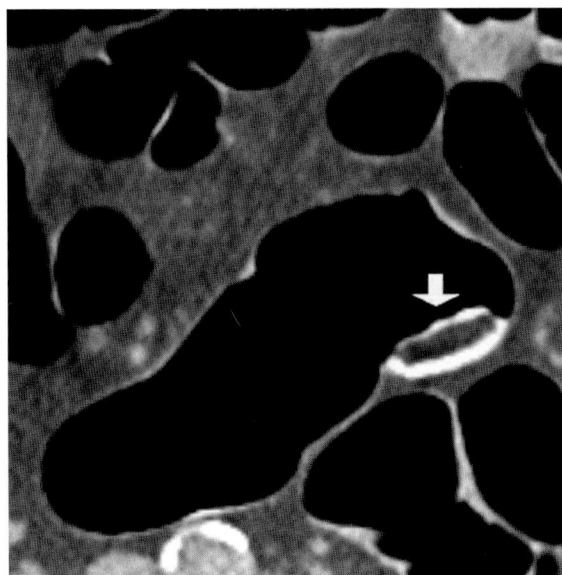

Fig. 4.12. Non-tagged stool >1 cm in the sigmoid (*arrow*). This non-tagged material shows the characteristics of non-tagged stool: completely surrounded by barium, hooked appearance, some minute air inclusions

findings of stool as seen with regular preparations without faecal tagging: 1) moving to the dependent part of the colon with dual positioning; 2) presenting with an air inclusion; 3) presenting with a hyperdense peripheral ring and central hypodensity or air inclusion; 4) having a hooked appearance; 5) having no attachment to the colonic wall.

Mostly this non-tagged stool does not cause any diagnostic problems. In a recent study of 180 patients (LEFERE et al. 2005) using this preparation no false positives were caused by non-tagged stool (see Sect. 4.6, Results).

4.5.3
Fluid Tagging

Tagged fluid typically is hyperdense or white. This enables visualisation of the colonic wall through the fluid on the 2D images and solves the issue of the drowned segment. In fact semicircular folds as well as tumoral lesions appear as negative filling defects in the fluid (Fig. 4.13). This avoids false negative findings. When tagged fluid is present in a collapsed segment, a lesion can sometimes be distinguished as a negative filling defect (Figs. 4.14 and 4.15). The semicircular folds show their typical appearance fading out in the colonic wall when scrolling through the axial slices (Fig. 4.15). Using the preparation as described above, the colon is quite dry. Fluid is detected in about 40% of segments. In most segments this fluid covers less than 25% of the colonic lumen on the axial slices. The density of the fluid is lower when compared with stool tagging and varies between 100 and 1000 H.U.

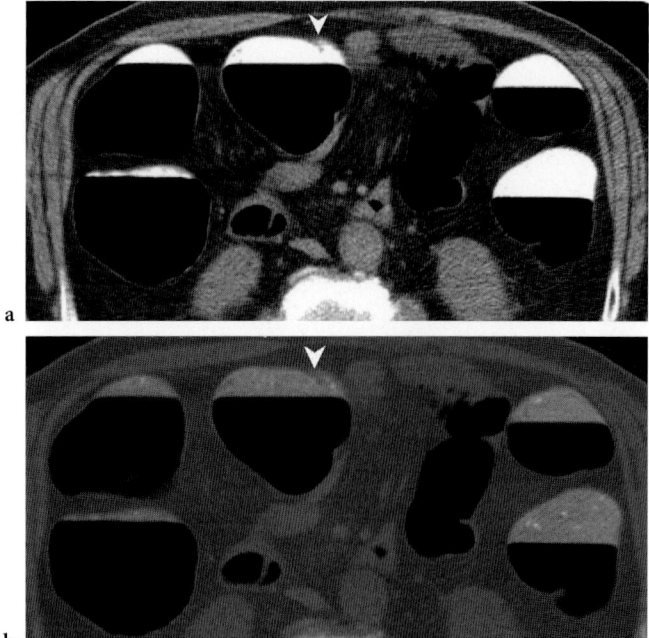

Fig. 4.13a,b. Fluid tagging in: **a** soft tissue; **b** bone window settings. The bone window setting enables visualisation of the colonic wall and semicircular folds (*arrowhead*) through the dense fluid

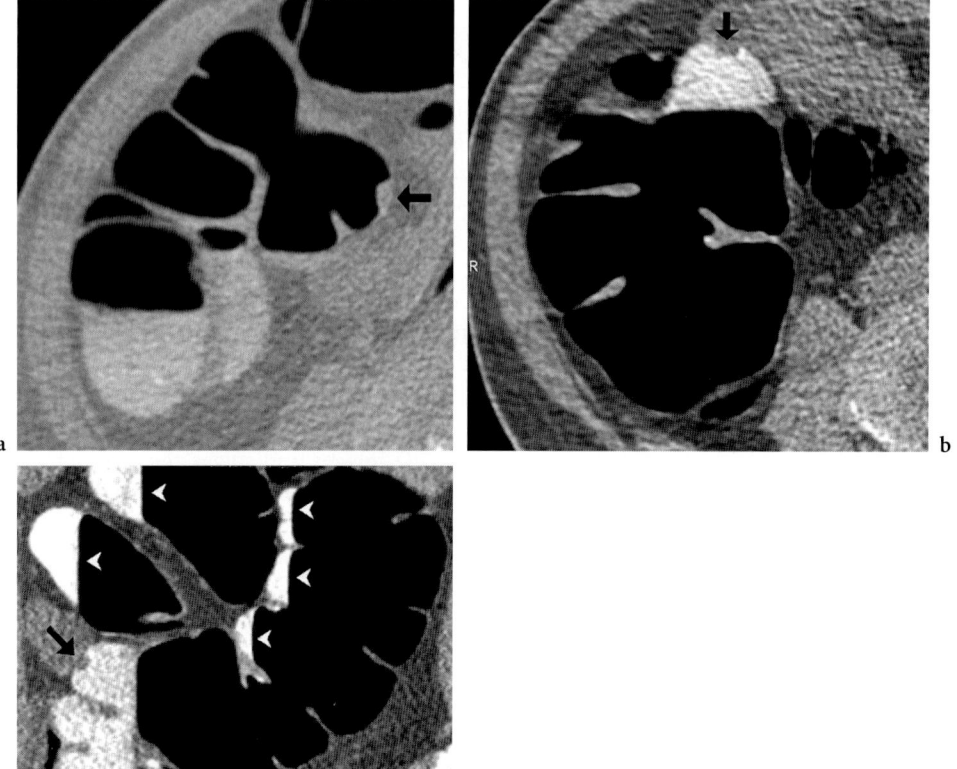

Fig. 4.14.a Supine image of the ascending colon obtained at ultra low dose (64-slice) showing sessile 8-mm polyp (*black arrow*). **b** Prone view shows the lesion covered by fluid. Because the fluid is tagged the lesion appears as a negative filling defect (*arrow*). **c** The sagittal reformatted image confirms this finding (*arrow*). This image shows different densities of tagged fluids in the same patient (*white arrowheads*)

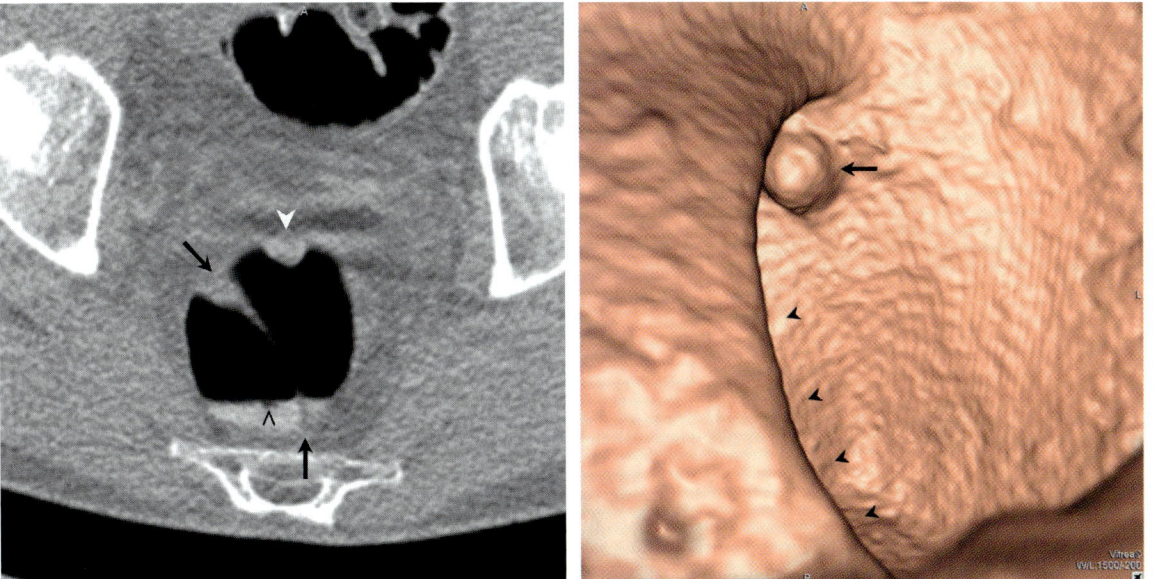

Fig. 4.15.a Ultra low dose scan (64-slice). Supine view of the rectum showing an 8-mm sessile polyp on the anterior border above a small level of tagged fluid, besides the first valve of Houston (*black arrows*). The valve of Houston is visible in the fluid as a linear filling defect. Small non-tagged residue in the fluid (*open black arrowhead*). **c** Corresponding endoluminal view. Despite the ultra low dose there are no streak artefacts. The polyp is easy to detect (*black arrow*) besides the first valve of Houston (*black arrowheads*)

The density of this fluid also shows intra- and interpatient variability (Fig. 4.14).

To assess the efficacy of fluid tagging with barium as the sole tagging agent we reviewed 200 patients. The residual fluid was evaluated on the axial slices according to its proportion to the maximal anteroposterior diameter of the segment of the colon where it was detected. In this way four different groups were generated: 0%, <25%, 25–50%, >50%. There was residual fluid in 43.9% of segments. In 14.8% of segments there was non-tagged fluid. However this fluid covered less than 25% of the colonic lumen on the axial slices in 12% of segments being 79.5% of segments with non-tagged fluid. Entire visualisation of the colonic wall was obtained in all patients as the non-tagged fluid nicely redistributed with dual positioning (i.e. supine-prone scanning) (Fig. 4.16).

4.5.4
Miscellaneous Findings

4.5.4.1
Mucous Filaments

Mucous filaments appear as thin threadlike structures crossing the colonic lumen or lying upon one or more semicircular folds. They can occur after a preparation without or with faecal tagging. In the latter case these filaments can be tagged or non-tagged. They can changed in shape with dual positioning. However they may simulate the stalk of a polyp. It is important not to misinterpret it as a polyp and vice versa. In the latter case they are not connected to the head of a polyp. However sometimes the mucous filament is attached to a semicircular fold simulating the head of a polyp on 2D images (Fig. 4.17). Care has to be taken not to misinterpret a polyp with a thin stalk as a mucous filament (Fig 4.18).

4.5.4.2
Foam

Faecal residue with a foamy appearance is mostly detected in the cecum or ascending colon. It appears as an amorphous inhomogeneous mixture mostly of air bubbles and stool. They occur in both preparations without and with faecal tagging. In the latter case the foam is tagged or non-tagged. This foam may distract the reader's attention or cover a lesion making detection difficult (Fig 4.19).

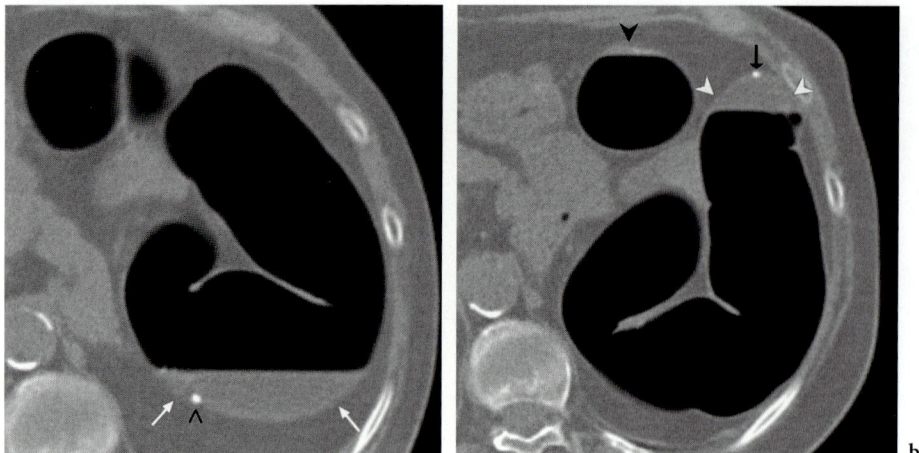

Fig. 4.16.a Non-tagged fluid covering 25–50% of the colonic lumen at the hepatic flexure in supine position (*white arrows*). Tagged residue in the fluid (*open black arrowhead*). **b** In the prone position the fluid is redistributed to the anterior part of the hepatic flexure (*white arrowheads*) and the transverse colon (*black arrowhead*) enabling complete visualisation of the colonic wall. Tagged residue is visible (*black arrow*)

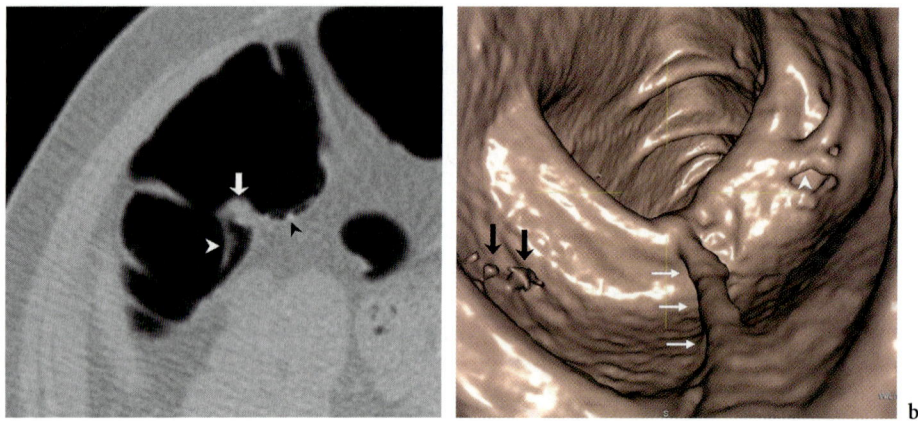

Fig. 4.17.a Supine view of the transverse colon showing a mucous filament (*white arrowhead*) attached to a prominent semicircular fold (*white arrow*), mimicking a stalked polyp. Some partially tagged foam (*black arrowhead*). **b** Corresponding endoluminal view showing the filament mimicking the stalk of a polyp (*white arrows*). The filament has an irregular shape. The foam is also visible (*black arrows*)

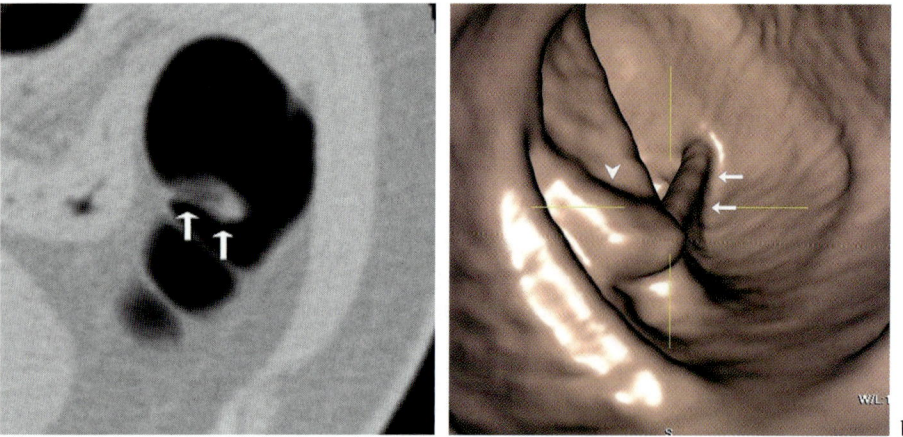

Fig. 4.18.a Polyp with a small stalk in the descending colon (*white arrows*). **b** Corresponding endoluminal view showing the stalk (*white arrows*) and the head (*white arrowhead*) of the polyp

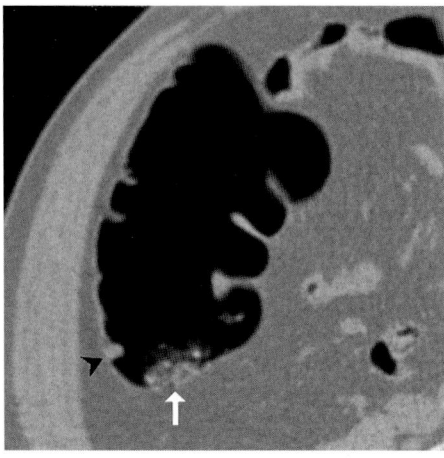 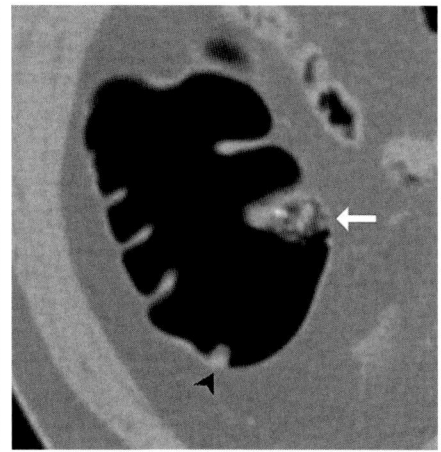

Fig. 4.19.a Non-tagged foam with some tiny tagged residue besides a possible sessile polyp (*black arrowhead*) in the ascending colon (supine view). b Corresponding prone view: the foam has moved to the anterior border of the ascending colon (*white arrow*). The sessile lesion remains unchanged (*black arrowhead*) and should be considered a sessile polyp. The lesion was confirmed on optical colonoscopy

4.6 Results

Several studies using a preparation based on faecal tagging have been performed. The results of polyp detection of these studies are listed in Table 4.1.

THOMEER et al. (2003) examined 150 patients and performed colonic cleansing using 3–5 L of an electrolyte solution on the day of CT colonography. Faecal tagging was obtained with 90–150 ml of iodinated contrast. As they were starting CT colonography in their department the results of polyp detection were clearly influenced by the learning curve. They divided the study group into 2 groups of 75 patients each. Sensitivity was clearly better in the second group of patients.

PINEAU et al. (2003) prepared patients the day before CT colonography combining a double dose of oral sodium phosphate (2×45 ml) with 30 ml of iodine and obtained good results of polyp detection.

LEFERE et al. (2002) and LEFERE and GRYSPEERDT (2005) have performed two feasibility studies with faecal tagging testing barium as the sole tagging agent. In a first study 50 patients were prepared with the low residue diet and the mild cathartic cleansing as described above. Faecal tagging was obtained with 3×250 ml of a 2.1% w/v barium suspension. In the second study 180 patients underwent faecal tagging with a 40% w/v barium suspension. In both studies good results of polyp detection were obtained.

Last but not least, PICKHARDT et al. (2003) obtained the best results of polyp detection to date with virtual colonoscopy in a large cohort of 1233 asymptomatic patients. The day before CT colonography they combined a clear liquid diet with a double dose of oral sodium phosphate and two bisacodyl tablets. Faecal tagging was performed with 2×250 ml of a 2.1% w/v barium suspension and 60 ml of Gastrografin. Excellent results of polyp detection were obtained.

The American Food and Drug Administration (FDA 2001) considers the double dose of oral sodium phosphate as an off-label use and warns not to exceed the recommended 45 ml dose. It says that people at increased risk for electrolyte disturbances (e.g. congestive heart failure, renal insufficiency, dehydration) may experience serious adverse effects using oral sodium phosphate. They advise obtaining baseline serum electrolyte values in patients ingesting more than 45 ml of oral sodium phosphate in a 24-h period in order to avoid serious electrolyte problems.

Pickhardt (HINSHAW et al. 2005) now uses two bisacodyl tablets and a single dose of oral sodium phosphate as cathartic cleansing combined with

Table 4.1. Table showing the results of polyp detection on a per patient basis

	n patients	≥6 mm	≥1 cm
THOMEER et al. (2003)	1–75	56%	50%
	75–150	80%	100%
	All (150)	64%	91.7%
PINEAU et al. (2003)	205	84%	90%
LEFERE et al. (2002)	50	92%	100%
LEFERE et al. (2005)	180	88%	100%
PICKHARDT et al. (2003)	1233	89%	94%

250 ml of the 2.1% barium suspension and 60 ml of Gastrografin to prepare the patients for CT colonography.

4.7
The Future: Laxative-Free CT Colonography

4.7.1
Principles

As with faecal tagging more residue can be left over in the colon without decreasing the accuracy of polyp detection, performing CT colonography after a preparation without cathartic cleansing is the obvious next step. Indeed, eliminating the need for cathartic cleansing prior to CT colonography would dramatically increase the adherence of an asymptomatic patient population to a colon cancer screening program (Rex 2000). This method has been called laxative-free CT colonography (Lefere et al. 2004). Several methods have been developed. These methods are based upon faecal tagging and are still at the research stage. A truly prepless method (i.e. no diet, no faecal tagging and no cathartic cleansing) has not yet been developed.

4.7.2
Results

Callström et al. (2001) performed laxative-free CT colonography without dietary restrictions in 58 patients. Faecal tagging was obtained with a combination of iodine and barium administered over one or two days. The best results of tagging were obtained by combining 6×225 ml of a 2.1% w/v barium suspension and 1×225 ml dilute diatrizoate meglumine and diatrizoate sodium. All residue with a density ≥ 150 H.U. was electronically labelled. In that way a 100% sensitivity for lesions ≥ 1 cm was obtained (5/5 lesions).

Lefere et al. (2004) performed laxative-free CT colonography in 15 patients combining the dedicated low residue diet as described above and a hydration regimen prescribed over one day and barium as tagging agent administered over one or two days. The hydration regime allowed the patients to drink a maximum of 2 L the day before CT colonography. The purpose was to obtain a dry colon with a reduced volume of residue by obtaining a balance between the fluid ingested by the patient and the fluid absorbed in the human body. Good results of tagging were obtained with 50–86 ml of a 40% w/v barium suspension. Unfortunately there was only one 8-mm polyp in this group of patients. This polyp was detected on CT colonography.

Iannaccone et al. (2004) examined successfully 203 patients with laxative-free CT colonography. They performed faecal tagging over two days with a total of 200 ml of diatrizoate meglumine and diatrizoate sodium. The patients were also on a low residue diet for two days. They obtained very good results of polyp detection: 86% for lesions ≥ 6 mm (79 lesions), 95.5% for lesions ≥ 8 mm (45 lesions), 100% for lesions ≥ 1 cm (24 lesions).

In these three studies primary 2D read was performed. Adequately reading and interpreting the data sets is an arduous task and needs a lot of experience as with laxative-free CT colonography more residue is present in the colon. For the same reason primary 3D read is impossible. To do so the faecal residue has to be removed or subtracted using dedicated software.

4.8
Conclusion

Faecal tagging is a feasible alternative to regular preparations. Up to now the best results of polyp detection were obtained using faecal tagging. Therefore faecal tagging is now advocated by an increasing number of investigators as the method of choice to prepare the colon for CT colonography. There are no problems with residual stool mimicking polyps and fluid hampering inspection of the colonic wall. Because of the contrast created between the tagged residue and the non-tagged lesion there is improved polyp conspicuity. It is also possible to improve patient compliance by reducing the cathartic part of the preparation. Barium can be used as the sole tagging agent simplifying the procedure and decreasing the side effects.

References

Barish MA, Soto JA, Ferrucci JT (2005) Consensus on current clinical practice of virtual colonoscopy. Am J Roentgenol 184:786–792

Bromer MQ, Weinberg DS (2005) Screening for colorectal cancer – now and the near future. Semin Oncol 32:3–10

Callstrom MR, Johnson CD, Fletcher JG et al. (2001) CT

colonography without cathartic preparation feasibility study. Radiology 219:693–698

Cotton PB, Durkalski VL, Pineau BC et al. (2004) Computed tomographic colonography (virtual colonoscopy): a multicenter comparison with standard colonoscopy for detection of colorectal neoplasia. JAMA 291:1713–1719

Dachman AH, Kuniyoshi JK, Boyle CM (1998) CT colonography with three-dimensional problem solving for detection of colonic polyps. Am J Roentgenol 1711:989–995

FDA (2001) Science backgrounder: safety of sodium oral phosphates oral solution. www.fda.gov/cder/drug/safety/sodiumphosphate.htm

Fenlon HM (2002) CT colonography: pitfalls and interpretation. Abdom Imaging 27:284–291

Fenlon HM, Nunes DP et al. (1999) A comparison of virtual and conventional colonoscopy for the detection of colorectal polyps. NEJM 341:1496–1502

Ferrucci J (2005a) CT colonography for detection of colon polyps and cancer. Working group on CT colongraphy. Lancet. 365:1464–1465; author reply 1465–1466

Ferrucci JT (2005b) Colonoscopy: virtual and optical – another look, another view. Radiology 235:13–16

Gryspeerdt S, Lefere P, Herman M et al. (2005) CT colonography with fecal tagging after incomplete colonoscopy. Eur Radiol 15:1192–1202

Hinshaw JL, Taylor AJ, Jones DA (2005) Prospective blind trial comparing 45-ml and 90-ml doses of oral sodium phosphate for bowel preparation prior to CT colonography. Am J Roentgenol 184(s):20

Iannaccone R, Laghi A, Catalano C et al. (2004) Computed tomographic colonography without cathartic preparation for the detection of colorectal polyps. Gastroenterology 127:1300–1311

Johnson CD, Dachman AH (2000) CT colonography: the next colon screening examination? Radiology 216:331–341

Kolts BE, Lyles WE, Achem SR et al. (1993) A comparison of the effectiveness and patient tolerance of oral sodium phosphate, castor oil, and standard electrolyte lavage for colonoscopy or sigmoidoscopy preparation. Am J Gastroenterol 88:1218–1223

Lefere P, Gryspeerdt S (2005) Fast reading of CT colonography. Am J Roentgenol 184(s):21

Lefere P, Gryspeerdt SS, Dewyspelaere J et al. (2002) Dietary fecal tagging as a cleansing method before CT colonography: initial results – polyp detection and patient compliance. Radiology 224:393–403

Lefere P, Gryspeerdt S, Baekelandt M et al. (2004) A method to perform laxative-free CT colonography. Am J Roentgenol 183:945–948

Lefere P, Gryspeerdt S, Marrannes J et al. (2005) CT colonography after fecal tagging with a reduced cathartic cleansing and a reduced volume of barium. Am J Roentgenol 184:1836–1842

Macari M, Megibow AJ (2001) Pitfalls of using three-dimensional CT colonography with two-dimensional imaging correlation. Am J Roentgenol 176:137–143

Macari M, Lavelle M, Pedrosa I (2001) Effect of different bowel preparations on residual fluid at CT colonography. Radiology 218:274–277

Macleod AJ, Duncan KA, Pearson RH et al. (1998) A comparison of Fleet Phospho-soda with Picolax in the preparation of the colon for double contrast barium enema. Clin Radiol 53:612–614

Morrin MM, Farrell RJ, Kruskal JB et al. (1999) Virtual colonoscopy: a kinder, gentler colorectal cancer screening test? Lancet 354:1048–1049

Murphy J, Coster G (1997) Issues in patient compliance. Drugs 54:797–800

Pickhardt PJ, Choi JH (2003) Electronic cleansing and stool tagging in CT colonography: advantages and pitfalls with primary three-dimensional evaluation. Am J Roentgenol 181:799–805

Pickhardt PJ, Choi JR, Hwang I et al. (2003) Computed tomographic virtual colonoscopy to screen for colorectal neoplasia in asymptomatic adults. N Engl J Med 349:2191–2200

Pineau BC, Paskett ED, Chen GJ et al. (2003) Virtual colonoscopy using oral contrast compared with colonoscopy for the detection of patients with colorectal polyps. Gastroenterology 125:304–310

Rex DK (2000) Virtual colonoscopy: time for some tough questions for radiologists and gastroenterologists. Endoscopy 32:260–263

Rockey DC, Paulson E, Niedzwiecki D et al. (2005) Analysis of air contrast barium enema, computed tomographic colonography, and colonoscopy: prospective comparison. Lancet 365:305–311

Taylor SA, Halligan S, Goh V et al. (2003a) Optimizing colonic distention for multi-row CT colonography: effect of hyoscine butylbromide rectal balloon catheter. Radiology 229:99–108

Taylor SA, Halligan S, Goh V et al. (2003b) Optimizing bowel preparation for multidetector row CT colonography: effect of Citramag and Picolax. Clin Radiol 58:723–732

Thomeer M, Carbone I, Bosmans H et al. (2003) Stool tagging applied in thin-slice multidetector computed tomography colonography. JCAT 27:132–141

Toledo TK, DiPalma JA (2001) Review article: colon cleansing preparation for gastrointestinal procedures. Aliment Pharmacol Ther 15:605–611

van Dam J, Cotton P, Johnson CD et al. (2004) AGA future trends report: CT colonography. Gastroenterology 127:970–984

Vanner SJ, McDonald PH, Paterson WG et al. (1990) A randomized prospective trial comparing oral sodium phosphate with standard polyethylene glycol-based lavage solution (Golytely) in the preparation of patients for colonscopy. Am J Gastroenterol 85:422–427

Zalis ME, Hahn PF (2001) Digital subtraction bowel cleansing in CT colonography. Am J Roentgenol 176(3):646–648

Zalis ME, Perumpillichira J, Del Frate C et al. (2003) CT colonography: digital subtraction bowel cleansing with mucosal reconstruction – initial observations. Radiology 226:911–917

5 How to Get the Colon Distended?

David Burling, Stuart Taylor, and Steve Halligan

CONTENTS

5.1 Introduction 51
5.2 Patient Preparation 52
5.3 Colonic Insufflation Methods 53
5.3.1 Manual Insufflation 53
5.3.2 Automated Insufflation 54
5.4 Carbon Dioxide or Air? 55
5.5 Choice of Rectal Catheter 56
5.6 Single vs Multidetector-row Scanners 56
5.7 Patient Positioning 57
5.8 Intravenous Spasmolytics 57
5.9 Perforation Risk 58
5.10 Recommended Technique 58
5.11 Conclusion 59
References 59

5.1 Introduction

The importance of achieving optimal colonic distension prior to CT colonography cannot be overstated, and the editors have justifiably devoted an entire chapter to the subject. Optimal luminal distension enables the reader to rapidly and confidently assess the colon, and undoubtedly improves diagnostic accuracy (Chen et al. 1999; Fletcher et al. 2000; Yee et al. 2003). Conversely inadequate distension may obliterate the colonic lumen and results in wall/haustral fold thickening (Fig. 5.1) thereby variously hiding or mimicking colorectal neoplasia (Fig. 5.2a,b) (Fletcher et al. 1999; Macari et al. 2001; Fenlon 2002). Interpretation times are increased when the colon is poorly distended but of greater importance is the potential to miss significant colonic pathology (Fig. 5.3a–c), occasionally rendering the examination non-diagnostic (i.e. necessitating requiring repeat examination or endoscopic referral) and sometimes frankly misleading. For example a review of missed significant lesions from a recent large prospective multicentre trial of CT colonography (Rockey et al. 2005; Paulson et al. 2004) found suboptimal distension, along with poor preparation, was implicated as a contributing factor in 16 of 28 (57%) false negative examinations.

Several strategies have been shown to improve distension, the most notable being dual patient positioning (i.e. prone and supine scanning). Use of faster multi-detector row scanners and administration of intravenous spasmolytics (see section below) may also help. However, despite these strategies, suboptimal distension is unfortunately frequently encountered in day-to-day clinical practice.

Unlike bowel purgation, which is largely determined by intrinsic patient-related factors such as compliance and bowel transit time, colonic distension is greatly influenced by the colonographic practitioner present at the time of examination. Distending the colon may at first appear a relatively simple and trivial procedure and, intuitively, skills acquired for barium enema should be easily transferable to CT colonography. However, the colonographer is disadvantaged. Unlike barium enema, where real time fluoroscopic screening is utilized to ensure satisfactory segmental distension, colonic insufflation prior to CT colonography is not performed under direct visualisation: A scout view must suffice. As a result, inadequate distension may only be fully appreciated once full data acquisition is complete. Furthermore, the aim for CT colonography is not simply adequate inflation but optimal distension, preferably with 'pencil-thin' wall and haustral folds. Colonic neoplasia is generally better seen when the colon is well distended, a statement that holds true for both primary 2D and 3D analysis (Pickhardt 2004). Indeed, sessile and flat lesions with minimal protrusion into the lumen or causing subtle focal wall thickening may be invisible without optimal distension.

The purpose of this chapter is to provide an evidence-based review of strategies and techniques intended to safely optimise colonic distension, and to draw readers' attention to current areas of controversy.

D. Burling, MD; S. Taylor, MD; S. Halligan, MD
Intestinal Imaging Unit, Level 4V, St. Mark's Hospital, Watford Road, Harrow, HA1 3UJ, Middlesex, UK

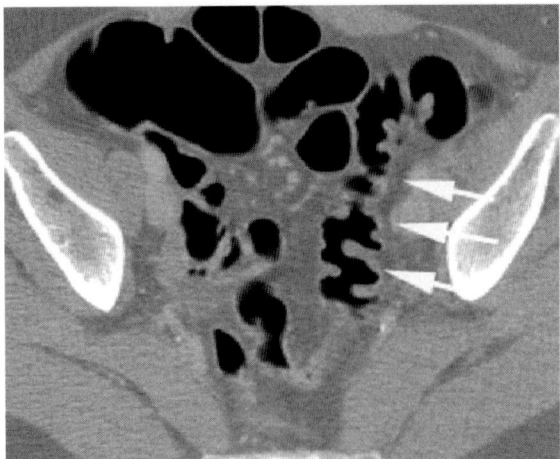

Fig. 5.1. A poorly distended sigmoid colon (*arrows*) resulting in bulbous haustral folds on this supine scan demonstrates how inadequate distension can thwart confident and time efficient interpretation. Subsequent optical colonoscopy was unremarkable

5.2
Patient Preparation

Although less invasive than endoscopic procedures, like any medical investigation, CT colonography undoubtedly generates a degree of apprehension. As for barium enema, patients should be fully appraised of what is going to happen and what is required of them (RUBESIN et al. 2000). A simple, easily understood description of the examination should ideally be made available in advance, followed by a brief reminder just before the examination itself. An appropriate discussion will prepare patients for rectal catheter insertion, the feeling of abdominal bloating, and potential mild discomfort due to retained gas. Prior to entering the CT scanner room, patients should be encouraged to empty their bowel for a final time.

Once the patient is ready and lying on the CT scanner table, a suitably qualified practitioner may choose to perform a rectal examination. This may be helpful for several reasons; detecting an occlusive tumour will avoid a potentially difficult and unsafe rectal catheter insertion and anal sphincter tone can be assessed quickly, which may influence the choice of catheter or method of insufflation. Digital rectal examination may also aid subsequent interpretation which can be particularly challenging in the rectum due to the frequent presence of haemorrhoids and redundant rectal mucosa. Despite these advantages, rectal examination may not always be appropriate, particularly for an asymptomatic screening population. One compromise is to only perform a rectal examination in patients with symptoms of rectal cancer, such as rectal bleeding or in those suspected of having poor anal tone (see section below).

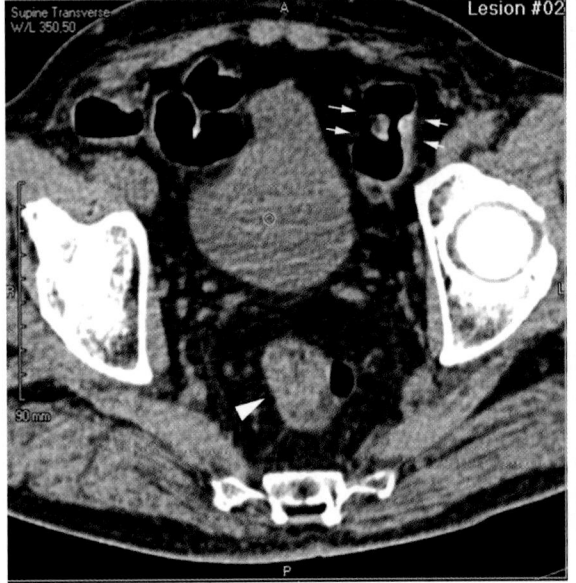
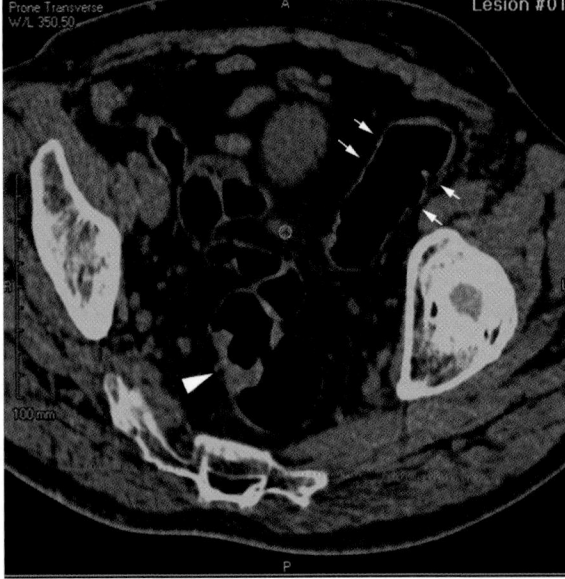

Fig. 5.2a,b. Supine and prone axial images of a 64-year-old man, obtained using a four multi-detector row scanner, demonstrating the diagnostic dilemma posed by inadequate distension and the benefit of dual scan positioning: **a** the supine scan demonstrates a possible cancer in the sigmoid colon (*arrows*) with a collapsed recto-sigmoid colon (*arrowhead*); **b** in contrast, the prone scan, in which optimal distension is achieved, reveals the area of concern in the sigmoid is normal (*arrows*) but a rectosigmoid cancer is revealed (*arrowhead*) (courtesy Drs A Laghi and R. Iannaccone)

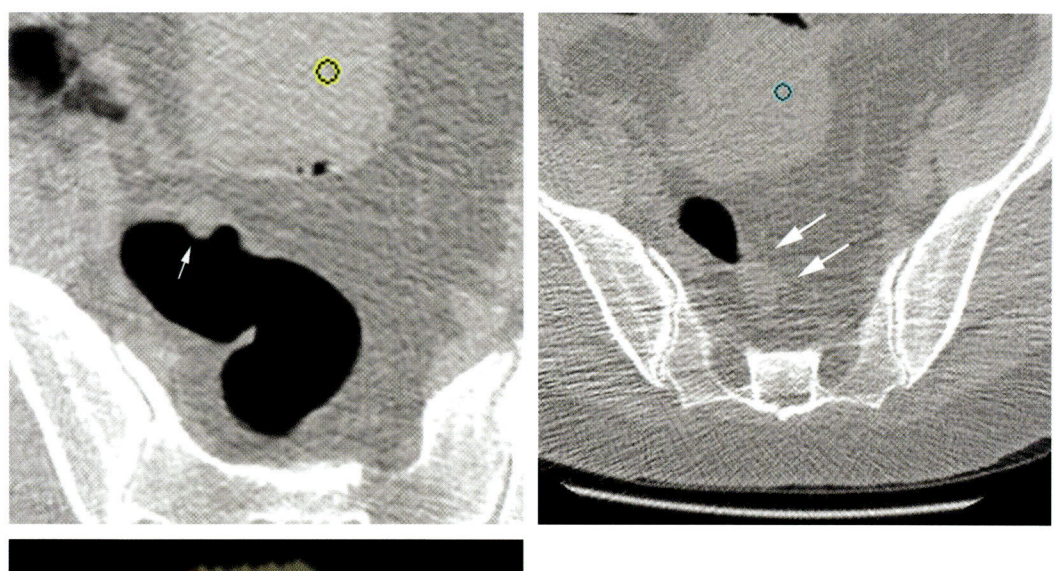

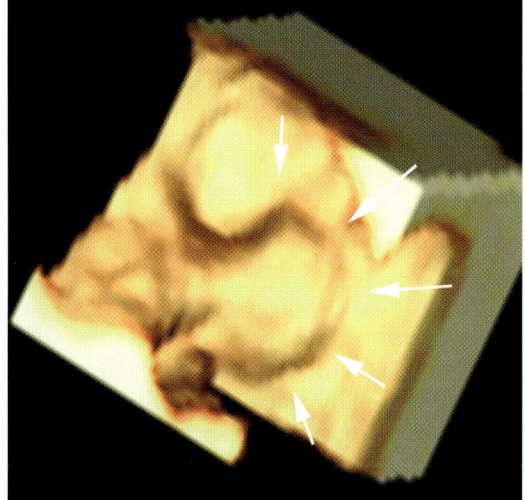

Fig. 5.3.a A 12-mm rectosigmoid polyp in a 69-year-old woman is difficult to detect as it lies partially submerged in fluid (*arrow*). **b** Unfortunately it is concealed on the supine acquisition due to segmental collapse (*arrows*). **c** However, the volume rendered endoluminal display confirms its presence (*arrows*)

5.3
Colonic Insufflation Methods

Colonic distension prior to CT colonography entails gently administering gas (air or carbon dioxide) via a rectal catheter using either manual or automated insufflation techniques. Both gases and insufflation methods are widely used and all have their advocates; some favour the least expensive and simplest method, i.e. room air insufflation by manual compression of a plastic insufflator bulb, while others prefer carbon dioxide delivered by automated insufflation devices. Until recently, there has been a lack of objective evidence to recommend one method over another but there is now data emerging that will help to guide future practice (BURLING et al. 2005; ROGALLA et al. 2004a,b; YEE et al. 2002).

5.3.1
Manual Insufflation

The easiest and cheapest method for distending the colon is to use room air, insufflated via a hand held plastic bulb. Typically patients lie on the CT scanner table in a left lateral position facing away from the operator. A lubricated rectal catheter attached to an insufflator bulb via a connecting tube is then inserted into the rectum and taped to the patient's buttocks. The patient is encouraged to retain any gas and avoid passing flatus by clenching the anal sphincter. Colonic insufflation is then performed by gently and intermittently squeezing the plastic bulb typically over a period of 1–2 min. In contrast, rapid successive squeezes can cause discomfort and may precipitate rectosigmoid spasm (RUBESIN et al. 2000)

Insufflation is continued until the operator believes the colon is optimally distended; most experts judge this by noting patient tolerance (BARISH et al. 2005), stopping when the patient feels uncomfortable or bloated. In the presence of a competent ileocecal valve, this generally occurs following the introduction of approximately 2 l of gas, usually after 30–40 compressions (MORRIN et al. 2002; MACARI 2004). Limiting insufflation to a fixed volume or number of bulb compressions is not recommended because individual patients' colonic volume and tolerance are variable. Some experts advise repositioning the patient part way through insufflation into either the prone or the supine position (CHEN et al. 1999; TAYLOR et al. 2003), depending on which scan acquisition is performed first (see below), for example first filling the non-dependant right colon in the lateral decubitus position and then the remaining distal colon after repositioning. Assessment of right sided filling by abdominal palpation is also anecdotally recommended.

Once initial colonic insufflation is deemed sufficient, a standard prone or supine CT scout image is acquired in order to assess the degree of distension and patient positioning. The sigmoid colon is typically the most difficult segment to distend optimally, and distension adequacy is often difficult to assess on the scout image due to overlapping loops in the anteroposterior plane. If suboptimal distension is encountered or doubt persists, the authors recommend additional insufflation prior to CT acquisition, repeating the scout image if necessary. Once the first scan acquisition is performed (and assuming a second is planned: see section below), the rectal catheter is left in situ and the patient repositioned. Once repositioned, and providing the patient is comfortable, the authors suggest further insufflation with approximately ten bulb compressions. We do not recommend insufflation while the patient is turning as this tends to precipitate anal leakage. Some workers advocate removing the rectal tube at this point because it may theoretically obscure rectal pathology. A repeat scout image is then performed routinely prior to the second CT acquisition (prone or supine) but patients rarely require additional insufflation following this (unless anal incontinence is present).

The ease and simplicity of this method is such that some patients can effectively insufflate their own colon using the hand held bulb (PICKHARDT et al. 2003). However, success will depend greatly on the patient population concerned, and this approach requires well motivated individuals, perhaps more applicable to a younger screening population (PICKHARDT et al. 2003).

A standard enema bag filled with approximately 3 l of gas is an alternative to the plastic bulb insufflator (Fig. 5.4), and has the additional advantage of permitting manual insufflation of carbon dioxide. The bag (filled with air or carbon dioxide via a gas cylinder) is sealed with a plastic clip and attached to a rectal catheter via a connecting tube. Once the rectal catheter is in-situ, the clip is released and the bag is gently compressed over 2–3 min, insufflating the colon. Gentle insufflation improves patient tolerance and ultimately allows greater volumes of gas to be administered. If the bag is empty and more gas required, then the plastic seal can be opened and room air introduced.

Carbon dioxide may also be insufflated directly from a gas cylinder via a tube with side hole for digitally controlling volume and pressure (ROGALLA et al. 2004a). Clearly the pressure of insufflated gas must be carefully controlled using this method.

5.3.2
Automated Insufflation

Automated insufflation devices are now widely utilised across Europe and the US, despite the additional equipment costs. Advocates suggest that insufflating carbon dioxide at controlled flow rates and pressures is convenient for the operator, and improves distension and patient compliance.

Early experience comparing a crudely modified laparoscopic insufflator to manual bulb insufflation of room air showed equivocal effects on luminal distension (RISTVEDT et al. 2003). More recently, two

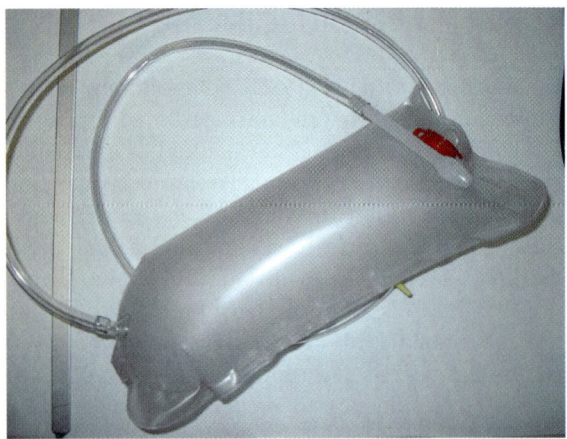

Fig. 5.4. Standard enema bag containing approximately 3 L of carbon dioxide for manual insufflation

studies (YEE et al. 2002; IAFRATE et al. 2004) compared specifically designed automated CO_2 insufflation devices with manual insufflation of room air. The first showed a modest improvement in distension using automated insufflation, particularly in the left colon (YEE et al. 2002). The second showed the insufflation methods were equivocal for luminal distension but that examination times were significantly longer (although less ileal reflux was encountered) using the automated device (IAFRATE et al. 2004). These data might suggest that only a modest benefit, if any, is derived from using an automated device. However, one significant advantage of automated insufflation is that administration has been specifically designed for use with carbon dioxide. As discussed below, there is good evidence from the colonoscopic and barium enema literature that demonstrates greater patient comfort when using carbon dioxide compared to air, because of its relatively rapid absorption by the colonic mucosa (GRANT et al. 1986; CHURCH and DELANEY 2003). Recent evidence also suggests that automated insufflation produces significantly better distension when compared to manual insufflation of carbon dioxide, again particularly in the left colon (BURLING et al. 2005; ROGALLA et al. 2004a).

At the time of writing, the authors are aware of only one commercially available device specifically designed for colonic insufflation (Fig. 5.5, Protocol colon insufflation system, E-Z-EM Inc, Westbury, NY, USA). This system electronically controls the flow rate of carbon dioxide increasing over time in a step wise fashion from 1 to 3 L/min to prevent spasm (1 L/min for the first 0.5 L, 2 L/min from 0.5 to 1.0 L, and then 3.0 L/min thereafter). The total volume of gas administered is displayed continuously and, if intracolonic pressure (measured at the rectal catheter tip) increases beyond the limit set by the user (up to a maximum of 25 mm Hg), the system automatically shuts down to prevent further insufflation and so reduces the risk of colonic perforation. In the latest version, insufflation automatically ceases when a total of 4 L of gas have been administered and then for every 2 L administered beyond this. To recommence insufflation, the operator needs to manually override this additional safety feature by pressing the start button.

The company's recommended technique is to insufflate the patient in the supine position. The pressure limit is set at 15 mm Hg initially, increasing to 25 mm Hg depending upon patient tolerance. Three litres of carbon dioxide are instilled (again dependent on patient tolerance), at which point the

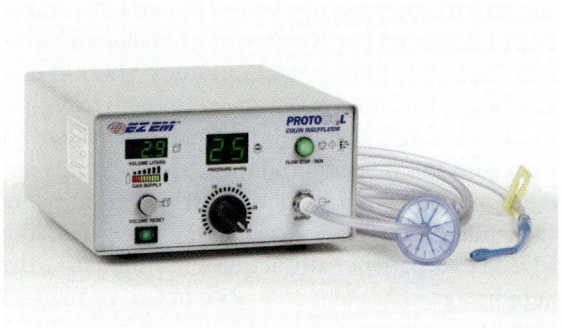

Fig. 5.5. Automated colonic insufflator, connected to a thin rectal catheter, displaying the intraluminal rectal pressure and total volume of carbon dioxide administered

patient is asked if they feel gas on the right side of their abdomen – if not, insufflation is continued until they do, or until they feel uncomfortable. A CT scout is then performed to confirm adequate distension prior to data acquisition. For the prone acquisition, propping up the patient's chest with a pillow or foam wedge helps to optimise distension of the transverse colon. The authors use a slightly modified technique (described below), setting the pressure limit at 25 mm Hg initially and pausing insufflation if the patient becomes uncomfortable. In our experience, the volume of gas administered during automated insufflation varies widely between patients (for example between 2.6 and 8.0 L with a median of approximately 4 L). Larger volumes are occasionally necessary, mostly due to anal incontinence, small bowel reflux and colonic redundancy, but are paradoxically associated with significantly poorer distension. Clearly these individuals are a challenging group to distend optimally and although the total volume of insufflated gas is a useful guide to the eventual adequacy of distension, practitioners should not limit their insufflation merely according to the volume insufflated. Interestingly, we have found no demonstrable learning curve using the automated device, suggesting that once familiar with the device's controls, practitioners can independently achieve satisfactory results despite little prior experience.

5.4
Carbon Dioxide or Air?

As mentioned above, many practitioners promulgate carbon dioxide as superior to air, largely based on barium enema and colonoscopy literature, which suggests it causes less discomfort because of its rapid mucosal absorption (GRANT et al. 1986; CHURCH and DELANEY 2003). A recent study (IAFRATE et al. 2004) also showed improved patient tolerance using automated carbon dioxide administration vs manually administered room air, although it is not clear whether the benefit was derived from using the automated device or carbon dioxide gas. Using a validated patient satisfaction questionnaire, the authors recently compared automated vs manual carbon dioxide insufflation and found virtually no difference between the two methods (BURLING et al. 2005), suggesting that in the study by IAFRATE et al. (2004), the use of carbon dioxide gas was the most important factor. An additional advantage of rapid mucosal absorption is that it significantly reduces the technical difficulties associated with a distended colon when performing colonoscopy immediately after CT colonography.

The choice of insufflated gas is ultimately dependent on the preference of the individual practitioner. Patients probably prefer carbon dioxide but the administration is relatively complicated and more expensive than bulb insufflation of room air. In a recent survey of international experts asked which gas they would advocate, 50% expressed no preference at all (BARISH et al. 2005). Of the remainder, two-thirds preferred carbon dioxide over air.

5.5
Choice of Rectal Catheter

There is wider scope for using more flexible and thinner catheters during CT colonography compared to barium enema because of the requirement to transmit only gas and because the consequences of anal incontinence are less dramatic. The choice of rectal catheter will mainly depend on local availability, method of insufflation, and individual patient but there is some evidence suggesting that thin tubes are adequate for most circumstances.

Perhaps the simplest catheter is a thin plastic or rubber tube, for example a standard 14F rectal tube (Jacques Nelaton rectal catheter; Rusch, Bucks, UK) or a Foley catheter. The former was shown to be as effective as a standard inflatable rectal balloon catheter (Trimline DC; E-Z-EM, Westbury, NY) for achieving adequate distension (TAYLOR et al. 2003). Alternatively, the Foley catheter is almost ubiquitous and can be used effectively when attached to a bulb insufflator. The soft tip allows safe insertion and it has a relatively small inflatable balloon, which can be used to assist continence if necessary.

Routine use of an inflated rectal balloon catheter is discouraged for barium enema following evidence that the risk of rectal perforation is increased (BLAKEBOROUGH et al. 1997), usually due to tearing the rectal wall either during insertion of the stiff catheter or due to the radial force applied by inflating the balloon. This also likely holds true for CT colonography, not least because insufflation of the balloon cannot be performed under fluoroscopic control. Most experts recommend choosing the most appropriate catheter according to an individual's requirements; for example, most patients can be optimally scanned using a thin, flexible rectal tube whereas those with anal incontinence may require judicious use of an inflated rectal balloon catheter. In the latter situation, most complications can be avoided by performing a rectal examination (see section above), careful catheter insertion and gentle balloon inflation.

Automated insufflation systems demand specific tubes which are designed to simply plug into the front of the device. Even here there is a choice of both standard larger bore balloon catheter and the slimmer so-called paediatric tip. In our experience, insertion of the larger catheters is, for many patients, the most uncomfortable part of the study. In response to this, the manufacturers have recently developed thin balloon catheters.

Some groups advocate removing the tube for the second acquisition to enhance patient comfort and to facilitate subsequent rectal assessment. However, this issue is much less relevant with thin catheters. Even if using larger catheters, the advantage of being able to insufflate additional gas likely outweighs any potential benefit of early removal.

5.6
Single vs Multidetector-row Scanners

Multidetector row scanners allow considerably reduced scan times, facilitating single breath hold studies for the majority of patients. As a consequence, image misregistration is practically eliminated and respiratory artefact significantly reduced (HARA et al. 2001). Moreover, distension also seems to be improved with a study by HARA et al. (2001) showing that suboptimal distension in at least one colonic segment was significantly more common with single detector row CT (40 of 77 patients, 52%) compared to multi-detector row CT (26 of 160 patients, 19%). This finding was presumably because patients do not have to retain the gas for as long and mucosal absorption is less critical.

5.7 Patient Positioning

Despite unanimous consensus in favour of dual position scanning amongst 27 international experts in 2003 (Barish et al. 2005), a minority still promulgate single position scanning.

However, the evidence in support of dual position scanning is strong (Yee et al. 2003; Fletcher et al. 2000; Chen et al. 1999; Morrin et al. 2002). These studies have found that colonic segments obscured by either faecal residue/fluid or poor distension will be revealed by redistribution in the complementary position; for example, the rectum is usually optimally distended with the patient lying prone while the transverse colon is usually best distended on the supine acquisition since it is least dependent in this position. Unsurprisingly, improved segmental visualisation significantly increases polyp detection. An early study (Chen et al. 1999) using manual insufflation to distend the colon with room air, showed the majority of colonic segments (59%) were inadequately distended if only one acquisition (prone or supine) was assessed. However when data from both acquisitions were combined, a large majority of segments (87%) were adequately distended and polyp detection rates were increased. Later studies (Yee et al. 2003; Fletcher et al. 2000) confirmed these findings and demonstrated significantly improved polyp detection with dual position scanning owing to improved distension and therefore segmental visualisation.

Advocates of single position scanning stress the additional radiation burden of scanning patients twice routinely, and choose to perform an additional scan only if visualization is deemed inadequate on the initial study. By necessity, this approach requires constant supervision. Moreover, studies of luminal visualisation (Yee et al. 2003; Chen et al. 1999; Morrin et al. 2002) suggest that a second scan will be required frequently. It is possible that in the future scanning may be performed routinely in a single position but this will require improved automated insufflation methods and possibly electronic subtraction of tagged faeces and fluid. However, at the time of writing most authorities would strongly recommend routine dual position data acquisition.

Almost all published descriptions of CT colonography techniques recommend acquiring the supine dataset first, followed by the prone scan (Ristvedt et al. 2003; Yee et al. 2003; Gluecker et al. 2003; Svensson et al. 2002). This anecdotal recommendation is likely a result of insufflation being performed in the supine position, which subsequently dictates the initial scan acquisition. Also, if intravenous contrast is utilised, this is frequently administered with the first scan and usually the supine position is chosen for convenience despite some evidence suggesting distension may be better overall on the prone scan (Morrin et al. 2002). However, in the authors experience, the grade of distension is independent of the initial scan position (Burling et al. 2005). Left lateral decubitus positioning is an effective alternative to the prone position for the second CT acquisition (following the supine scan), particularly for immobile and elderly patients, or patients with respiratory disease (Gryspeerdt et al. 2004).

5.8 Intravenous Spasmolytics

There are two intravenous spasmolytics available for CT colonography; hyoscine butylbromide and glucagon hydrochloride. Both produce hypotonia in smooth muscle within the colonic wall and are used widely to improve distension during double contrast barium enema. However, while both agents have been shown to improve patient perception during barium enema, only hyoscine butylbromide reliably improves distension (Goei et al. 1995; Bova et al. 1993). As a result, it is widely utilized for barium enema across Europe (hyoscine butylbromide is not licensed for use in the USA).

The use of spasmolytics prior to CT colonography has been widely investigated. In one randomised study (Taylor et al. 2003), intravenous administration of 20 mg hyoscine butylbromide immediately prior to gas insufflation was associated with significantly improved distension in all colonic segments proximal to the sigmoid. Moreover, for all segments combined, the colon was over six times more likely to be adequately distended compared to using no spasmolytic. Interestingly, there was no additional benefit gained by increasing the dose to 40 mg. A smaller study (Bruzzi et al. 2003) also showed significantly improved transverse and descending colonic distension in patients given hyoscine butylbromide, but only in patients with diverticular disease. The authors postulated that hyoscine butylbromide might relieve diverticulosis related spasm. More recently, data has been presented comparing hyoscine butylbromide and glucagon hydrochloride to no spasmolytic (Rogalla et al. 2004b). These authors found that both spasmolytics conveyed benefit, an effect most marked when using hyoscine butylbromide. In contrast, two previous studies failed to demonstrate any benefit when glucagon hydrochloride was administered prior to CT colonography (Yee et al. 1999; Morrin et al. 2002).

While the authors would recommend routine use of hyoscine butylbromide prior to CT colonography, some caution needs to be exercised prior to administration. Glaucoma, cardiac ischaemia and urinary retention may all be precipitated and minor self limiting effects of dry mouth and blurred vision are also associated. Consequently, patients should be questioned about any relevant past medical history and advised not to drive for a short time following administration.

5.9
Perforation Risk

The morbidity and mortality of colonoscopy are well recognised and described (Vallera and Bailie 1996; Bowles et al. 2004; Waye et al. 1992; Muhldorfer et al. 1992), and larger series report perforation rates in the region of approximately 0.2% (i.e. 1/500). Since its introduction, proponents of CT colonography have proclaimed an excellent safety profile in comparison to endoscopy, assumptions based on its relatively non-invasive nature and the ability to perform the investigation without a need for intravenous sedation. However two recent case reports of colonic perforation during CT colonography have questioned its safety. The first case of perforation followed CT colonography in a patient two weeks after a deep rectal biopsy in the presence of a near obstructing rectosigmoid tumour (Kamar et al. 2004). A rectal balloon catheter and manual insufflation of room air were also utilised. It is generally accepted that clinically non-obstructing tumours can prevent the retrograde passage of both liquid and gas due to a change in morphology when under distal pressure. Given this, an inflated rectal balloon could generate critically high intraluminal pressure during inflation. The second case was performed in a patient with fulminant ulcerative colitis, generally considered a contraindication to CT colonography (Coady-Fariborzian et al. 2004). Indeed, the referring gastroenterologist had requested CT colonography because of concerns that colonoscopy would involve a higher risk of perforation. Again, an inflated rectal balloon catheter was used with manual insufflation of room air. These case reports further underline the principle that rectal balloon catheters should be used judiciously and with great care. They are contraindicated in patients with inflammatory bowel disease and in patients with potentially obstructing tumours. It is possible that the use of automated insufflator devices may have prevented perforation in these two cases by automatically terminating insufflation at a safe intracolonic pressure.

CTC is a relatively new technique and no large scale studies of complication rates have appeared in the peer-reviewed literature. Because of this, it is difficult to determine accurately the overall perforation rate in clinical practice. Given the well-defined, albeit small, risk during barium enema, it seems inevitable that CT related perforations will occur. Recently, abstracted data has been presented that investigated the perforation rate in 3 USA centres, finding 3 perforations out of 7180 patients studied (0.04%), and again the use of rectal balloon catheters were implicated in these (Sosna et al. 2004). There are now international efforts to establish the true perforation rate for CT colonography but preliminary data suggests the rate will lie between barium enema (0.01%; Gharemani 2000) and colonoscopy (0.2%; Vallera and Bailie 1996; Bowles et al. 2004; Waye et al. 1992; Muhldorfer et al. 1992).

5.10
Recommended Technique

It is clear form the above discussion that the practitioner has many options available when attempting to optimise colonic distension prior to scan acquisition. While some techniques have an established evidence-base, others are largely a matter of personal preference. Whatever regime is chosen, it is clear that good distension is absolutely pivotal to the success of any CTC examination. The follow section will provide the reader with details of the authors' preferred methods.

Written patient information is provided and posted to the patient along with the bowel preparation approximately two weeks prior to examination. On the day of the examination, the radiologist or radiology resident greets the patient, checks they have understood what the procedure involves, they have no contraindications to hyoscine butylbromide or intravenous contrast and are happy to proceed. They are asked to evacuate the rectum just prior to entering the scanner room. In an attempt to improve compliance, patients are routinely warned that they will experience abdominal bloating and mild discomfort and the importance of good colonic distension for the accurate interpretation of their scan is stressed.

The authors favour carbon dioxide as the distension agent and in the past have slowly administered this via gentle compression of a filled enema bag as described in the section above. However, we now utilize an automated insufflator delivering carbon dioxide via a narrow calibre catheter, reserving a balloon catheter for the very occasional patient with anal incontinence. The patient is asked to lie supine initially so that an intravenous catheter can be sited if intravenous contrast is to be used, and for administration of Buscopan if not contraindicated. The patient is then asked to lie in the left lateral decubitus position and a lubricated rectal catheter, already attached to the insufflation device, is inserted. For all patients the maximum pressure shutdown dial is set initially at 25 mm Hg. Insufflation is commenced and after approximately 1.5 L have been introduced, the patient is turned into the supine position. Distension is then continued, titrated to patient tolerance, and sustained if rectal pressure remains low (i.e. below 15 mm Hg), providing the patient does not complain of undue abdominal discomfort. Once either the patient is mildly uncomfortable or intraluminal pressure consistently remains above 25 mm Hg (such that further insufflation is automatically prevented, which usually occurs following administration of 2–4 L of gas), a first CT scout image is acquired. If distension is deemed optimal by the supervising radiologist, then the full supine scan is acquired in a single breathhold. As long as the patient is comfortable the authors prefer to leave the insufflator device switched on during scanning, but turn down the pressure limit to 15 mm Hg so that this minimal rectal pressure is maintained. If the patient is uncomfortable, the device is paused to ensure that no further gas is insufflated until such time as the patient is happy for it to be recommenced. If distension is suboptimal despite the device recording rectal pressures exceeding 25 mm Hg, the catheter is checked and repositioned because it may be that its tip is occluded against the rectal wall. If unsuccessful, we will either then reposition the patient (e.g. prone) or gently manually palpate the abdomen to encourage redistribution of gas.

Once the supine study has been acquired, the rectal catheter is left in situ and the patient asked to turn prone. A second scout is performed and if distension is deemed suboptimal, the pressure limit will be increased to 25 mm Hg to encourage further gas insufflation. A further scout is performed and when this demonstrates optimal insufflation, the second study is acquired. The examination is then complete and the rectal catheter removed. The patient is reassured that much of the insufflated gas will be absorbed (rather than expelled), and that any abdominal cramping should ease within a few minutes.

5.11
Conclusion

There are several strategies available to the practitioner for optimising colonic distension and, if used appropriately, the time and effort invested will be rewarded by easier and more accurate interpretation. The authors recommend ongoing quality assurance measures are adopted by all departments performing CT colonography in order to minimise failure rates due to inadequate distension. Finally, safety concerns about CT colonography will likely diminish with more judicious use of rectal balloon catheters.

References

Barish MA, Soto JA, Ferrucci JT (2005) Consensus on current clinical practice of virtual colonoscopy. AJR 184:786–792

Blakeborough A, Sheridan MB, Chapman AH (1997) Retention balloon catheters and barium enemas: attitudes, current practice and relative safety in the UK. Clin Radiol 52:62–64

Bova JG, Jurdi RA, Bennett WF (1993) Antispasmodic drugs to reduce discomfort and colonic spasmduring barium enemas: comparison of oral hyoscyamine, i.v. glucagon and no drug. AJR 161:965–968

Bowles CJ, Leicester R, Romaya C et al. (2004) A prospective study of colonoscopy practice in the UK today: are we adequately prepared for national colorectal cancer screening tomorrow? Gut 53:277–283

Bruzzi JF, Moss AC, Brennan DD et al. (2003) Efficacy of IV Buscopan as a muscle relaxant in CT colonography. Eur Radiol 13:2264–2270

Burling D, Taylor SA, Halligan S et al. (2005) Automated colonic insufflation for Multi-Detector Row CT colonography: distension and patient experience in comparison to manual carbon dioxide insufflation. AJR (in press)

Chen SC, Lu D, Hecht JR et al. (1999) CT colonography: value of scanning in both the supine and prone positions. AJR 172:595–599

Church J, Delaney C (2003) Randomized controlled trial of carbon dioxide insufflation during colonoscopy. Dis Colon Rectum 46:322–326

Coady-Fariborzian L, Angel LP, Procaccino JA (2004) Perforated colon secondary to virtual colonoscopy: report of a case. Dis Colon Rectum 47:1247–1249

Fenlon HM (2002) CT colonography:pitfalls and interpretation. Abdom Imaging. 27:284–291

Fletcher JG, Johnson CD, Maccarty RL, Welch TJ, Reed J, Hara AK (1999) CT colonography: potential pitfalls and problem solving techniques. AJR 172:1271–1278

Fletcher JG, Johnson CD, Welch TJ et al. (2000) Optimization of CT colonography technique: prospective trial in 180 patients. Radiology 216:704–711

Ghahremani G (2000) Iatrogenic gastrointestinal disorders. In: Gore RM, Levine MS (eds) Textbook of gastrointestinal radiology, 2nd edn. W.B Saunders Co., Philadelphia, pp 2228–2242

Gluecker T, Johnson D, Harmsen W et al. (2003) Colorectal cancer screening with CT colonography, colonoscopy, and double contrast barium enema examination: prospective assessment of patient perceptions and preferences. Radiology 227:378–384

Goei R, Nix M, Kessels AH et al. (1995) Use of antispasmodic drugs in double contrast barium enema examination: glucagon or buscopan? Clin Radiol 50:553–557

Grant DS, Bartram CI, Heron CW (1986) A preliminary study of the possible benefits of using carbon dioxide insufflation during double contrast barium enema. Br J Radiol 59(698):190–191

Gryspeerdt SS, Herman MJ, Baekelandt MA (2004) Supine/left decubitus scanning: a valuable alternative to supine/prone scanning in CT colonography. Eur Radiol 14:768–777

Hara AK, Johnson CD, MacCarty RL et al. (2001) CT colonography: single versus multi-detector row imaging. Radiology 219:461–465

Iafrate F, Laghi A, Paolantonio P et al. 2004 Colonic distension using mechanical CO2 insufflator versus manual air distension. In Radiological Society of North America scientific assembly and annual meeting program. Oak Brook, Ill: Radiological Society of North America, p 432

Kamar M, Portnoy O, Bar-Dayan A, Amitai M, Munz Y, Ayalon A, Zmora O (2004) Actual colonic perforation in virtual colonoscopy: report of a case. Dis Colon Rectum 47:1242–1244

Macari M (2004) Techniques for CT colonography. In: 5th International Symposium Virtual Colonoscopy course handbook, Boston, pp 45–48

Macari M, Megibow AJ (2001) Pitfalls of using 3D CT colonography with 2D imaging correlation. AJR 176:137–143

Morrin M, Farrell R, Keogan M et al. (2002) CT colonography: colonic distension improved by dual positioning but not intravenous glucagons. Eur Radiol 12:525–530

Muhldorfer SM, Kekos G, Hahn et al. (1992) Complications of therapeutic gastrointestinal endoscopy. Endoscopy 24:276–283

Paulson EK, Foster WL, Thonpson WM et al. (2004) Causes of errors in CT Colonography (CTC) and Air Contrast Barium Enema (ACBE) in detection of colonic lesions 1 cm or larger (abstr). In: Radiological Society of North America scientific assembly and annual meeting program. Oak Brook, Ill: Radiological Society of North America, p 618

Pickhardt PJ (2004) Differential diagnosis of polypoid lesions seen at CT colonography (virtual colonoscopy). Radiographics 24:1535–1556

Pickhardt PJ, Choi JR, Hwang I et al. (2003) Computed tomographic virtual colonoscopy to screen for colorectal neoplasia in asymptomatic adults. NEJM 349:2191–2200

Ristvedt S, McFarland E, Weinstock L et al. (2003) Patient preferences for CT colonography, conventional colonoscopy, and bowel preparation. Am J Gastroenterol 98:578–585

Rockey DC, Paulson EK, Niedzwiecki D et al. (2005) Analysis of air contrast barium enema, computed tomographic colonography, and colonoscopy: prospective comparison. Lancet 365:305–311

Rogalla P, Bauknecht HC, Hein PA et al. (2004a) Pressure-controlled colonic insufflation for CT colonography. In: Radiological Society of North America scientific assembly and annual meeting program (abstr). Oak Brook, Ill: Radiological Society of North America, p 432

Rogalla P, Lembcke A, Hein PA et al. (2004b) Spasmolysis with butyl scopolamine versus glucagon in CT colonography. In: Radiological Society of North America scientific assembly and annual meeting program (abstr). Oak Brook, Ill: Radiological Society of North America, p 433

Rubesin S, Levine MS, Laufer I et al. (2000) Double-contrast barium enema examination technique. Radiology 215:642–650

Sosna J, Bar-Meir E, Amitai M, Blachar A, Peled N (2004) Assessment of the risk of perforation at CT colongraphy (abstr). In: Radiological Society of North America scientific assembly and annual meeting program (abstr), Oak Brook, Ill. Radiological Society of North America, p 280

Svensson MH, Svensson E, Lasson A et al. (2002) Patient acceptance of CT colonography and conventional colonoscopy: prospective comparative study in patients with or suspected of having colorectal disease. Radiology 222:337–345

Taylor SA, Halligan S, Goh V et al. (2003) Optimizing colonic distension for multi-detector row CT colonography: effect of hyoscine hydrobromide and rectal balloon catheter. Radiology 229:99–108

Vallera R, Bailie J (1996) Complications of endoscopy. Endoscopy 28:187–204

Vos F, Van Gelder R, Serlie I et al. (2003) Three dimensional display modes for CT colonography: conventional 3D virtual colonoscopy versus unfolded cube projection. Radiology 228:878–885

Waye JD, Lewis BS, Yessayan S (1992) Colonoscopy: a prospective report of complications. J Clin Gastroenterol 15:347–351

Yee J, Hung RK, Akerkar GA et al. (1999) The usefulness of glucagon hydrochloride for colonic distension in CT colonography. AJR 173:169–172

Yee J, Galdino G, Kumar N et al. (2002) Comparison of colonic distention using electronic CO2 insufflation and manual atmospheric insufflation on CT colonography (abstr). In: RSNA Scientific Assembly and Annual Meeting program

Yee J, Kumar N, Hung R et al. (2003) Comparison of supine and prone scanning separately and in combination at CT colonography. Radiology 226:653–661

6 The Right Scanner Parameters to Use

Andrea Laghi and Pasquale Paolantonio

CONTENTS

6.1 Introduction 61
6.2 Collimation 62
6.3 Image Reconstruction 64
6.4 Pitch 64
6.5 Tube Current Setting and Low Dose Protocols 65
6.6 Practical Guidelines 68
    Appendix. Glossary of Terms 69
    References 70

6.1 Introduction

The advent of CT colonography (CTC) (or, virtual colonoscopy) in 1994 was made possible by the development of spiral CT technology, which provides a volumetric coverage of a cleansed and air-distended colon within a single breath-hold (Vining et al. 1994).

The introduction of multidetector row computed tomographic (MDCT) scanners in late 1998 opened a new era for CT in general and CTC in particular (Berland and Smith 1998). The use of multiple detector arrays along the z-axis offers substantial benefits related to anatomic coverage, scanning time and longitudinal spatial resolution compared with single-slice spiral CT (SSCT) (Beaulieu et al. 1998; Fenlon et al. 1999; Hara et al. 2001).

In principle, using similar parameters on both SSCT and MDCT results in wider anatomic coverage and faster scanning time with MDCT. On the other hand, MDCT provides sub-millimeter collimation, improves z-axis resolution and generates isotropic voxels, thus resulting in better image quality of reformatted planes as well as three-dimensional reconstructions. The drawback is represented by data explosion, with generation of over 1000 images per scan per patient, making data viewing and analysis ("data workflow") a key issue to be solved within the next period of time (Sherbondy et al. 2005).

Another major issue is represented by dose delivery, usually higher with CTC compared with a standard abdominal CT study due to routine use of prone and supine scans (Chen et al. 1999). Radiation exposure has also substantially increased over the past few years due to the widespread use of thinner collimations and the consequent increase of tube current setting in order to reduce image noise. Low or ultra-low dose MDCT protocols together with new automatic dose modulation software may help in solving this problem representing a crucial issue for proposing VC as a screening method for colonic polyp in healthy subjects (Iannaccone et al. 2003a).

A further variable in CTC scanning parameters is due to technological differences among CT vendors and MDCT generations. It does exist quite a large experience on investigations using 4-slice MDCT scanners, but, on the other hand, there are only few manuscripts on 16-slice MDCT and almost no experience, at the time of this paper, on new 64-slice scanners. As technology continues to advance, there will be a continuing need to reassess the relative tradeoffs between scan width, image noise, patient dose, image artefacts, breath-hold times, and the number of reconstructed images to be viewed and archived.

As a consequence of what is discussed above, the "panorama" of technical approaches is expanding, offering a wide spectrum of different possibilities. For these reasons, the answer to the question "which are the right parameters to be used for CTC?" may be puzzling.

A. Laghi, MD; P. Paolantonio, MD
Department of Radiological Sciences, University of Rome "La Sapienza", Polo Didattico Pontino, I.C.O.T., Via Franco Faggiana 34, 04100 Latina, Italy

6.2 Collimation

Collimation is the parameter that – more than the others – has dramatically changed since the development of CTC in parallel with continuous evolution of scanner technology.

"Thin" collimation is a mandatory pre-requisite for a CTC study. The question is how thin is a thin collimation? The answer may be either political or technical. In fact, collimation is strictly related to the size of the target lesion. Since on CT you are not able to detect a lesion smaller than the effective slice thickness due to partial volume effect, the size of the ideal target lesion should be defined. This should avoid the risk of searching for the thinnest possible collimation as soon as a new equipment becomes clinically available.

On a technical point of view, a consensus was achieved (Barish et al. 2005). If considering SSCT, the maximum accepted collimation is 5 mm with overlapped image reconstruction (usually set at 3 mm) (Hara et al. 1997a). In the first CTC studies, due to limited tube capacity, two or three consecutive breath-holds were needed to cover the entire colon. With the progress in tube technology a single breath-hold of 40–50 s was made possible on SSCT scanners (Taylor et al. 2003).

One of the major benefits of MDCT was represented by the possibility of further reducing the collimation compared with SSCT. Although some authors, at the beginning of the era of MDCT, still proposed 5 mm as an optimal collimation due to acquisition time, breathing artefacts as well as image workload (Hara et al. 2001), it is now widely accepted that a collimation no thicker than 3 mm is mandatory (Barish et al. 2005).

A major drawback of the use of thin collimation is the increased current tube setting, necessary in order to reduce image noise and to maintain an acceptable image quality. This is the reason why several researchers have performed investigations on the potential benefits of thin collimation protocols (Whiting et al. 2000; Fletcher et al. 2000; Rogalla and Meiri 2001; Gillams and Lees 2002; Macari et al. 2002; Taylor et al. 2003; Wessling et al. 2003) looking for the clinical impact of thin collimation protocols in terms of polyp detection and characterization.

Several in-vitro evaluations were reported. Although phantom models have inherent limitations represented by the ideal conditions of the study design (a true colon is a "moving" organ, with peristaltic motion as well as motion related to the anatomic location, partly intra-peritoneal and partly retroperitoneal) they may provide useful data to be tested on patients.

In a personal experience (Laghi et al. 2003), we built a phantom model with 12 lesions ranging in size between 3.2 mm and 12 mm; lesion morphology simulated sessile polyps and flat and depressed lesions. Different scanning protocols were compared based on 1.0-mm, 2.5-mm and 5-mm collimations with effective slice thicknesses of respectively 1.25 mm, 3 mm and 5 mm. Results showed the best performance when using 1.0-mm collimation protocol (no lesions missed), although a statistically significant difference was observed only among 1.0/2.5-mm protocols in comparison with 5.0-mm protocol. If only lesions larger than 10 mm were considered no differences were observed among the three different protocols (Fig. 6.1).

In another study (Wessling et al. 2003), a phantom with simulated polypoid lesions ranging in size between 2 mm and 12 mm was built. Different protocols were compared with collimation ranging between 1.25 mm and 5 mm. Results showed no significant differences for detection of lesions larger than 10 mm, but for lesions smaller than 6 mm a clear benefit was observed when a thin collimation protocol (1.25 mm) had been used.

Finally, in another in-vitro experience (Taylor et al. 2003), where a human colonic specimen of a patient with familiar adenomatous polyp syndrome after total colectomy was used as a phantom, collimation had a significant effect on the polyp detection rate which, when unadjusted for size, was 50% higher at 1.25 mm collimation than at 2.5 mm. This effect was most marked for polyps less than 5 mm, for which a small but significant improvement in detection also occurred with increased tube current. For polyps 5 mm or larger the benefit of decreased collimation was significant resulting in 7% improved detection rate. The use of thin collimation is also associated with a possible increase of specificity, especially of small lesions, since the detection of tiny air bubbles might be easier.

Although thin collimation protocols may provide benefits in terms of detection of small polypoid lesions, the application to patients is limited by technical restrictions of four-slice MDCT. In fact, with four-slice MDCT a compromise between scanning time and collimation is necessary since the use of 1 mm is associated with scanning time over 30 s (Fig. 6.2). On the other hand, the increased radiation exposure as compared with thicker collimation

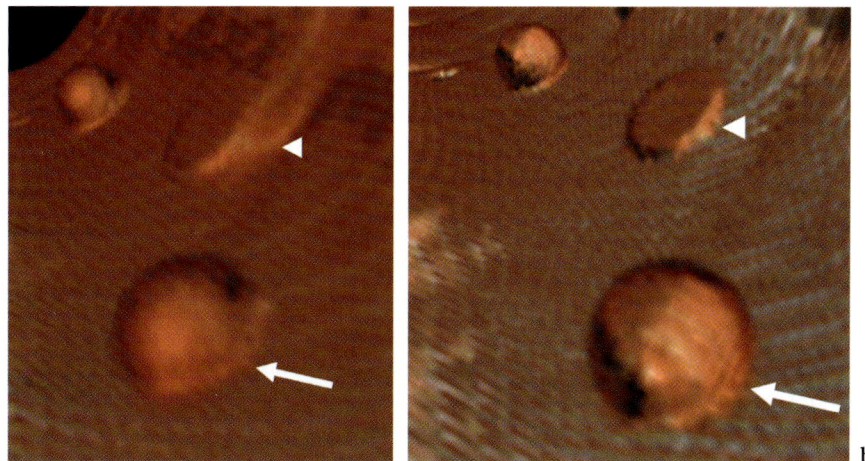

Fig. 6.1a,b. Colonic phantom containing three different simulated lesions: 9.6-mm and 5.5-mm sessile polyps and 8-mm "flat" lesion. Using: **a** a thick collimation protocol lesions' sharpness is definitely reduced compared with; **b** a thin collimation protocol. Note edge blurring (*arrow*) directly related to the increase of effective slice thickness as well as geometric distortion. This artefact particularly affects simulated "flat" lesion (*arrowhead*)

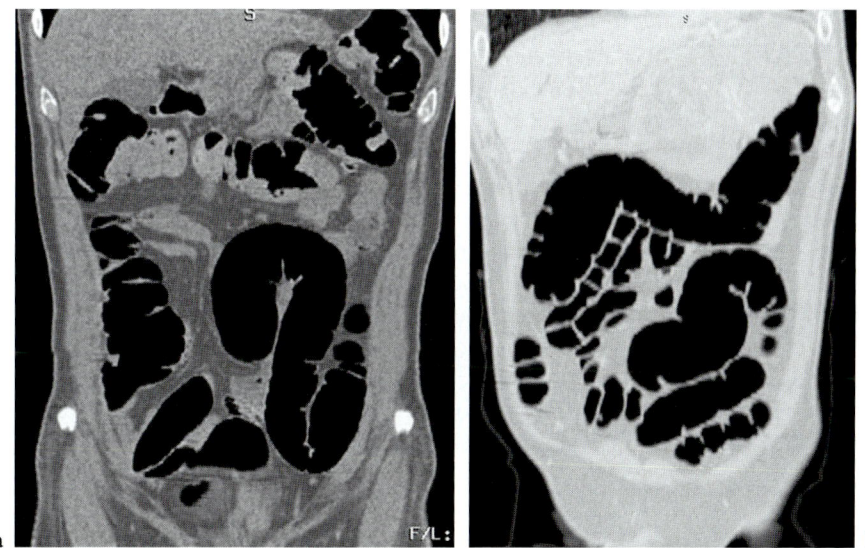

Fig. 6.2a,b. Four-slice MDCT scan of the abdomen and pelvis: "high-resolution" protocol with 1-mm collimation and 1.25 mm effective slice thickness vs "fast scanning" protocol with 2.5-mm collimation and 3 mm effective slice thickness (**b**). The quality of coronal reformatted image is much improved on high-resolution scanning protocol although the acquisition time is much longer

protocols as well as the unclear benefits of detecting small polypoid lesions (smaller than 5 mm) generated controversies among different research groups. As an example, some authors reported the benefits of 1-mm collimation (MACARI et al. 2002) whereas others recommended 2.5 mm (effective slice thickness, 3 mm) (POWER and PRYOR 2002) or even 5 mm (HARA et al. 2001; MCCOLLOUGH 2002). The theoretical effect of changing collimation on polyp detection was also investigated by reconstructing 1-mm data sets at various section thicknesses; sensitivity for polyps measuring 3–5 mm decreased from 96% at a 1 mm section thickness to 74% at a 5 mm section thickness (ROGALLA and MEIRI 2001).

To summarize, data from both phantoms and patient populations suggest that, for four-slice MDCT, a collimation no larger than 3 mm should be implemented. Thinner collimations may provide benefits in terms of detection of small polypoid lesions (smaller than 5 mm) although the effects on false positive rates as well as on radiation exposure have not been fully evaluated.

First results on 16-slice MDCT scanners confirm these data, suggesting a scanning protocol with 1-mm collimation for the detection of lesions smaller than 3 mm and with 3-mm collimation for lesions larger than 3 mm (ROTTGEN et al. 2003).

The advent of new 64-slice MDCT has completely solved the scanning problems, since no compromise between collimation and scan time is necessary any more (Fig. 6.3). Collimation is routinely ranging between 1.2 mm and 0.6 mm and scanning time is below 10 s (FLOHR et al. 2005). Results are expected in the next few months, with a possible consistent improvement in the detection of tiny polyps. Problems to be face with are image noise of sub-millimetre collimation protocols, dose delivery and the huge datasets needing powerful workstations to be managed. At the time of this chapter, there is not enough experience to answer these raising issues.

6.3
Image Reconstruction

Resolution in the z-direction is particularly important for three-dimensional reconstructions. With SSCT a compromise between slice thickness, anatomical coverage and scanning time is necessary. The result is a relative thick collimation (3–5 mm) and consequently slice thickness negatively affecting the quality of reconstructed images. A possible solution, in order to improve z-axis resolution using SSCT, is to reconstruct raw data in order to obtain overlapped slices. Usually, 60% overlap is recommended (PAUL et al. 1999).

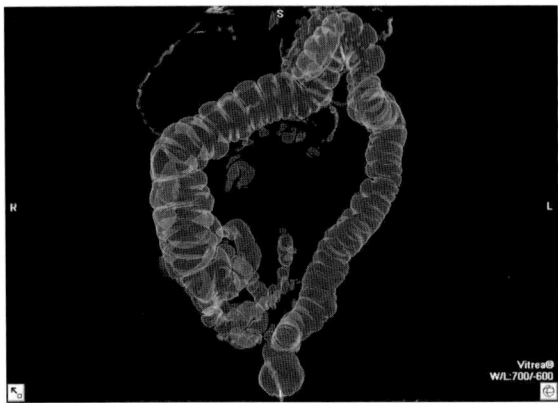

Fig. 6.3. Tissue Transition Projection (TTP) (or "virtual double contrast enema") showing the entire colon scanned with sub-millimetre collimation during an acquisition time of less than 10 s

The technical approach with MDCT is completely different. The reconstruction process for MDCT makes use of multiple-row data collection to minimize image degradation induced by rapid patient translation using reconstruction algorithms (TAGUCHI and ARADATE 1998; FLOHR et al. 2005). MDCT makes use of data interpolation and different reconstruction algorithms in order to obtain from an original data set of images acquired with a fixed collimation different data sets with different slice thickness (HU 1999; HU et al. 2000). Of course, the reconstructed images cannot be thinner than detector collimation. With this approach the reconstruction of overlapped slices is no longer recommended as for SSCT.

6.4
Pitch

Pitch is a technical parameter intrinsic to spiral CT correlating table travel, collimation and gantry rotation time. In other terms, pitch=TS RT/C, where TS is table speed, expressed in mm/s, RT is gantry rotation time, expressed in seconds and C is collimation expressed in mm. Pitch directly affects image quality, since the higher the pitch value the broader the Slice Sensitivity Profile (SSP) (see Appendix). It means that the effective scan width increases with increasing pitch. High pitch values introduce artefacts especially along the z-axis, resulting in blurred images. For this reason, a maximum pitch value of 2 is advisable.

In colon imaging, spiral artefacts induced by high pitch values may affect, in particular, those structures changing dramatically the anatomic position along the *z* axis (i.e., hepatic and splenic flexures, sigmoid colon) as well as polyp visualization. This is the case of rippling artefacts which are introduced in the images when increasing angle relative to the z axis as well as when pitch is increased; rippling artefacts result in a negative effect on the depiction of sessile polyps (WHITING et al. 2000) (Fig. 6.4).

Moreover, the degree to which partial volume effects distort polyp morphology is determined by polyp size relative to the effective section thickness and section sensitivity profile, which are primarily a function of collimation, pitch and interpolation algorithm. For SSCT protocols with 3 mm and 5 mm collimation and pitch ranging between one and two, excellent depiction of 6-mm and 13-mm pedunculated polyps and 10 3 mm sessile polyps can be

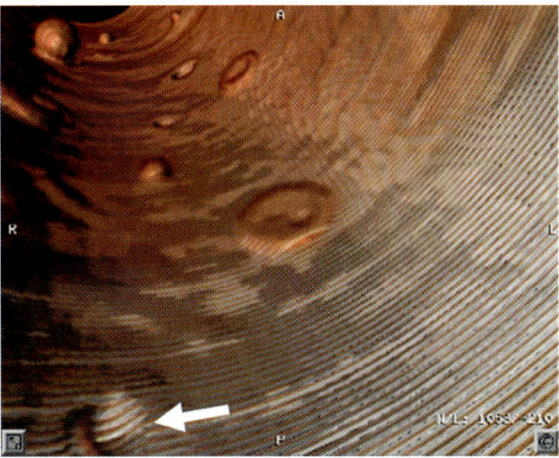

Fig. 6.4. Example of rippling artefacts induced by high pitch value. The small sessile polyp in a simulated colonic phantom (*arrow*) is barely seen

achieved. With a protocol including 5-mm collimation and pitch two, flat lesions of 11 mm 1 mm and 6 mm 2 mm can be degraded by rippling artefact (Whiting et al. 2000).

It has been observed that polyp conspicuity decreases when pitch increases, in particular on three-dimensional reconstructions (Dachman et al 1997).

In a different study using a pig colon phantom the prevalence of adverse CT artefacts over a range of scanning parameters was assessed, demonstrating that smoothing becomes more evident when collimation increases, whereas stair-step artefacts and longitudinal distortion are more dependent on increasing pitch (Springer et al. 2000).

Pitch is also correlated to dose delivery to patients, expressed in mGy, as CT Dose Index (CTDI) (see Appendix).

CTDI is inversely proportional to pitch (e.g. doubling pitch halves the CTDI). This is true only if mA value remains constant. This is not the case for all manufacturers, since in some scanners mA is automatically adjusted for pitch so CTDI remains constant.

The introduction of MDCT has also modified the concept of pitch, which can be defined either relative to total X-ray collimation ($pitch_x$) or to individual detector width ($pitch_d$). Consequently $pitch_d = pitch_x$ number of slices. As an example, on 4-slice MDCT, with 12.5 mm/s table speed of 2.5 mm collimation, $pitch_d$ is 2.5 (12.5 mm/s/2.5 mm 0.5 sec) whereas $pitch_x$ is 0.625 (12.5 mm/s/10 mm 0.5 s) where

10 mm is total X-ray beam (2.5 mm 4). For the sake of clarity and uniformity, the detector pitch should no longer be used. For both single-section CT and multi-detector row CT, the pitch (p) is given by p=TF/w, where TF is table feed per rotation, and w is total width of the collimated beam, according to International Electrotechnical Commission specifications. For p<1, data acquisition occurs with overlap in the z-axis direction; for p>1, data acquisition occurs with gaps.

Some remarkable differences about the influence of pitch on image quality between SSCT and MDCT do exist. In fact, on MDCT the influence of pitch on image quality depends on the scanner. Some manufacturers recommend particular pitch values, whilst others allow any pitch to be used. The difference depends on data interpolation properties. However, in general, MDCT allows the use of faster table speed compared with SSCT.

On a human colonic specimen phantom, for polyps of 5 mm or larger the effect of pitch on detection is insignificant on MDCT using pitch value ranging from 0.75 to 1.5 (Taylor et al. 2003). However this is not true for small lesions, smaller than 5 mm for whom the detection rate is higher with lower pitch value.

Finally, although pitch in MDCT is a less essential parameter in terms of section sensitivity profile, image noise in MDCT depends on pitch (for fixed tube current-time product in mAs). This is opposite to SSCT scanning where image noise is virtually pitch-independent. To account for that difference, MDCT systems automatically increase mA/s as the pitch is increased to maintain comparable image noise.

6.5
Tube Current Setting and Low Dose Protocols

One of the major limitations preventing CTC from being used in screening programs for patients at risk for colorectal carcinoma is its relatively high radiation exposure. There are three main reasons that account for the high radiation dose of CTC. First, the technique is usually performed in the prone and supine positions, because both positions have been found to detect the highest number of lesions; this, of course, doubles the radiation dose to the patient (Chen et al. 1999). Second, CTC examinations are currently performed with MDCT scanners, which tend to have a higher effective dose level for the same dose compared with SSCT, due to geometric inefficiency (Giacomuzzi et al. 2001). This is especially true if considering 4-row scanners, although geometric efficiency has much improved on 16- and 64-MDCTs. Third, there is a trend to use narrower collimations (1.0 mm or even less instead of 2.5 mm or 5.0 mm); this has the great advantage of near isotropic spatial resolution (i.e., the voxels have almost identical sides along the three axes) but, at the same time, leads to an increase in effective dose (Van Gelder et al. 2002).

In a single experience, a higher number of small polyps (<5 mm) was detected using thin collimation (1.25 mm), low pitch, and high tube current (150 mA) (Taylor et al. 2003). Unfortunately, the associated dose penalty was prohibitive, with an effective dose of 20.0 mSv for combined supine and prone scanning. Strategies to reduce patient radiation exposure although working at thin collimation include high pitch value as well as low tube current. Thus doubling the pitch and reducing the tube current setting to 50 mA would deliver an effective dose for combined supine and prone scans of 3.4 mSv, lower than the dose of either a standard abdominopelvic CT scan (6–24 mSv) or a barium enema study (6.4 mSv).

Indeed, in a recent study, Van Gelder et al. showed that the median effective dose for complete (i.e., prone and supine acquisitions combined) CTC in 12 different institutions is about 8.8 mSv. CTC at 8.8 mSv may result in a risk of up to 0.02% for inducing cancer in the population over 50 years (who are currently considered the target population for colorectal cancer screening) (Van Gelder et al. 2002). Considering these factors, increasing attention has been focused on the optimization of low-dose protocols for CTC.

In theory, in view of the inherently high contrast between the air-filled lumen of the colon and the soft-tissue attenuation of the colonic wall, a relevant dose reduction should be achievable without loss of diagnostic accuracy. The low-dose technique is associated with an increase in image noise because of the reduced number of X-rays reaching the detectors. The increase in image noise may deteriorate lesion conspicuity in terms of detectability on low-contrast imaging. The noise level on CT images depends on the accuracy of the transmission measurements used in the reconstruction of the images, which in turn depends primarily on the number of transmitted photons. This number is proportional to the dose used for the CT scan and also depends strongly on the size of the patient.

The imaging of high-contrast structures allows a higher noise level with a satisfactory image quality and diagnostic reliability. Thus, it seems feasible to decrease the dose in CTC because endoluminal lesions show an inherently high contrast to the surrounding colonic air or gas (Figs. 6.5 and 6.6). Because subjectively perceived noise is inversely related to window width, image analysis is usually performed with a wide window centre and setting.

The first attempt was performed in 1997, when it was proposed to reduce data size and radiation dose delivery for SSCT colonography (Hara et al. 1997b), using 70 mA.

Subsequently, the same authors took advantage of the faster data acquisition provided by MDCT and demonstrated better bowel distension and fewer respiratory artefacts with a beam collimation (5.0 mm) and an effective radiation dose (4.7 mSv for men; 6.7 mSv for women) comparable to those of SSCT (Hara et al. 2001). A different proposed approach was to use a thin (i.e., 1.0 mm) beam collimation protocol to obtain images with near isotropic voxels, but simultaneously decrease the effective mAs to 50 in order to keep the effective radiation dose to a level comparable to that of SSCT (5.0 mSv for men and 7.8 mSv for women) (Macari et al. 2002). Such a protocol provided excellent sensitivity for detection

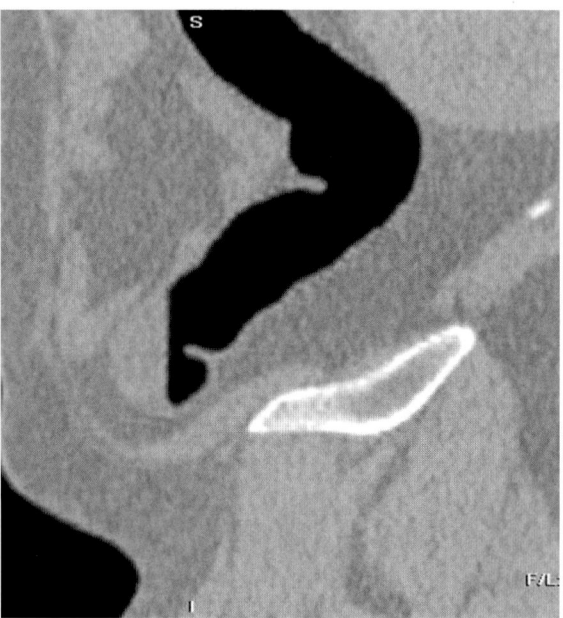

Fig. 6.5. Low dose scan of normal sigmoid colon. Due to inherently high contrast between colonic surface and endoluminal air, image quality of colonic lumen is still optimal, in particular if image analysis is performed with a wide window centre and setting

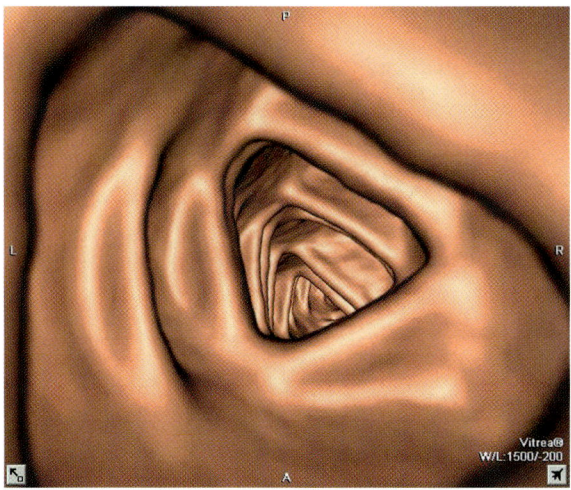 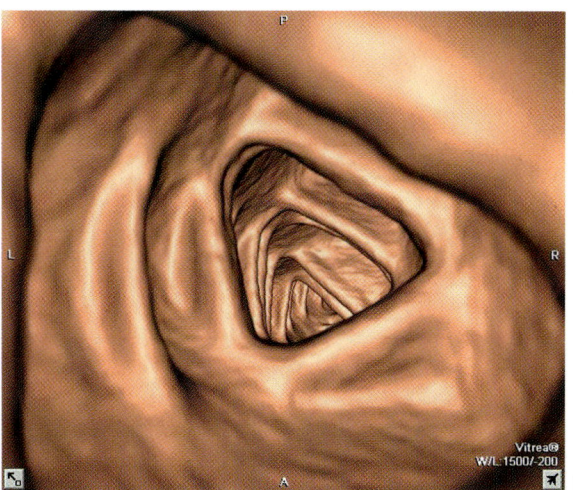

Fig. 6.6a,b. The increase in image noise is perceived more on three-dimensional endoluminal views: **a**, standard dose scan; **b**, low dose scan. Note sharpness of endoluminal surface negatively affected by dose reduction in **b**

of polyps 10 mm in diameter or larger and improved differentiation of colorectal polyps from residual stool and hypertrophied folds (with a consequent reduction of false positive diagnoses).

Other authors used a 2.5-beam collimation protocol and demonstrated that, despite a perceptible worsening of image quality, the sensitivity for detection of polyps was equal at 100, 50, and 30 effective mAs (Van Gelder et al. 2002). These results indicated that CTC with MDCT can be reliably performed with an effective dose of 3.6 mSv.

In our experience we used an effective mAs value of 10, demonstrating that MDCT technology can achieve a further, substantial radiation dose reduction for CTC with a total (i.e., prone and supine acquisitions combined) effective dose of 1.8 mSv for men and 2.4 mSv for women. These values are substantially lower than previously published data, both as reported for SSCT and MDCT, and also lower than those of barium enema (5–7 mSv) (Kemerink et al. 2001). This technical approach (defined as "ultra low-dose" technique) was subsequently validated in a large population of patients with results comparable with full dose imaging protocols (Iannaccone et al. 2003b) (Fig. 6.7). Potential criticisms to the use of an ultra low-mAs protocol are as follows: (1) imaging of obese patients, which might be unfeasible although this issue has not been well evaluated yet; (2) poor assessment of low contrast structures, such as liver, pancreas, kidneys, and lymph nodes (Fig. 6.8). This can be expected because the quality of low contrast structures is affected more by noise than that of high contrast structures (i.e., colonic mucosa-air interface). Thus, this imaging protocol will prevent the detection of extra-colonic findings unless deionising filters are implemented.

Another feasible way to reduce patient dose delivery might be a combined approach of ultra low-dose protocol for prone scan and normal tube current setting for supine scan in order to achieve reduction of patient exposure, having at the same time a consistent evaluation of extra-colonic findings. This might be an optimal solution for symptomatic patients, especially if contrast medium injection is required. In a non-symptomatic screening population, both the acquisitions might be achieved using low dose protocols (Nicholson et al. 2005).

A recent technological advancement is represented by the development of automatic dose delivery system, able to modulate the tube current on the basis of the depth of tissues to be scanned. In other words, this technique allows one to reduce patient radiation dose modifying the tube output according to the patient geometry during each rotation and in the longitudinal direction.

Another technical parameter influencing dose delivery is tube potential. Tube potential is expressed as kilovolt peak (kVp). Modification of kVp leads to changes of the photon beam energy expressed as kiloelectron volt (keV). Increasing tube potential, photon beam are more penetrating resulting in an enhancement of detector energy fluency. Modification of tube potential leads to changes in image noise, contrast resolution and patient dose exposure. The most important effect of kVp changes is represented by increase of patient radiation exposure. CTDI increase linearly with mAs and exponentially with kVp ($\oplus kVp^2$). Increase in tube potential

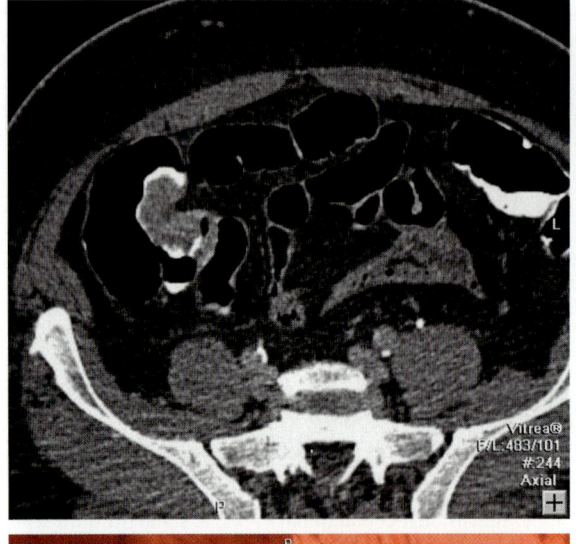
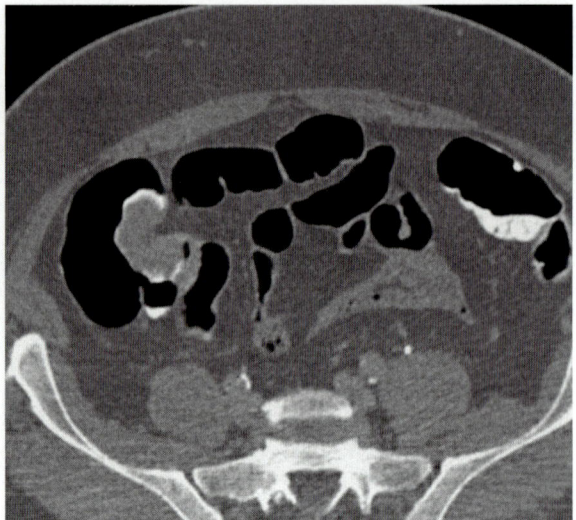
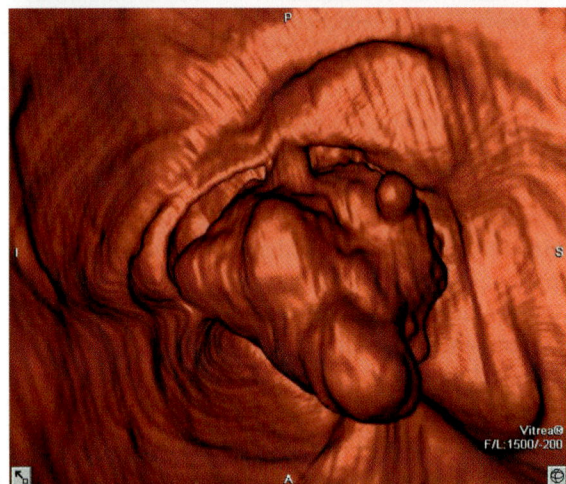

Fig. 6.7a–c. Low dose scan of carcinomatous polyp of the right colon. Although: a noise clearly degrades image quality, the evaluation using: b wide window centre and setting as well as: c three-dimensional endoluminal view are not significantly affected

produces decrease of image noise but also decrease of HU values of different structures due to a stronger detector energy fluency. Decrease of HU values using high values of tube potential is more pronounced for structures with intrinsic high Z, like bone or iodine rather than fat or muscles. Thus increase of tube potential leads to reduction of contrast-resolution for high density materials (HUDA et al. 2000). Due to huge impact on patient radiation exposure, increase of kVp in order to reduce image noise should not be used.

6.6
Practical Guidelines

A single scanning protocol with identical parameters for all scanners and patients cannot be recom-

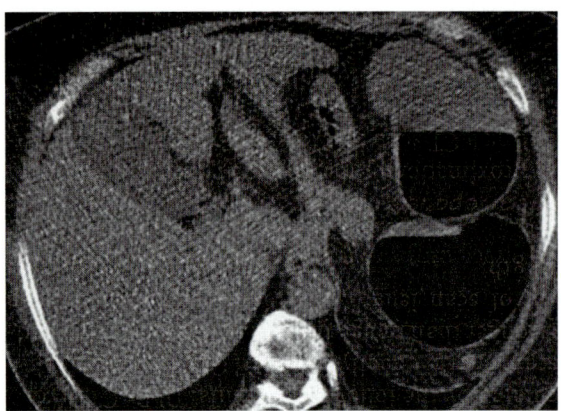

Fig. 6.8. Low dose scan of liver parenchyma. Image noise prevents the assessment of focal liver lesions and makes difficult even the visualization of the gallbladder

mended due to technological differences as well as different clinical indications to CTC.

General guidelines are provided by the recently published Consensus Statement (BARISH et al. 2005). If considering basic parameters (i.e., collimation and mAs values) recommendations propose a collimation no larger than 5 mm for SSCT and no larger than 3 mm for MDCT. With the advent of 64-slice MDCT, sub-millimeter collimation will be mandatory, although clinical benefits are still unclear.

Image reconstruction should be overlapped with SSCT: it is usually set at 3 mm for 5-mm collimation protocols and at 1 mm for 3-mm collimation protocols (SANJAY 2004). On MDCT, when using 3 mm effective slice thickness, images are usually reconstructed at 1 mm; when 1 mm or sub-millimeter effective slice thicknesses are used, 1 mm might be the best compromise considering also the number of images to be managed on the workstation.

Considering dose exposure, if CTC is performed as a screening method in asymptomatic population, tube current must be set at the minimum level possible that allows adequate visualization of the colonic wall even if visualization of parenchymatous organs is reduced. There is no consensus at the moment regarding the value of detecting the extra-colonic findings.

If patient is symptomatic or he/she requires i.v. injection of contrast medium for any other clinical reason, mAs should be set at the standard value for an abdomen and pelvis CT scan. In order to reduce dose delivery, patient might be scanned in prone position using a low or an ultra-low dose protocol, and at full dose only in supine scan when contrast medium is injected.

Appendix. Glossary of Terms

Adapted from FLOHR et al. (2005)

Automatic exposure control
This is a recently developed technique that allows one to reduce patient radiation dose, modifying tube output according to the patient geometry during each rotation and in the longitudinal direction.

Collimated section thickness
Active width of one detector row in the longitudinal direction, measured at the isocenter. The collimated section thickness can be different from the effective section thickness established in the spiral reconstruction process.

Cone angle
With multi-detector row CT system, the measurement rays are no longer perpendicular to the longitudinal axis but are tilted by the cone angle with respect to the center plane. The cone angle is largest for the sections at the outer edges of the detector.

Weighted CT dose index (CTDI$_w$)
Dose measure that uses the absorbed dose in an acrylic plastic phantom. Weighted CTDI (CTDIw) is approximation to average dose in the x-y plane for phantom and so is an approximation of the dose delivered to a cross section of the patient's anatomy. CTDI$_w$ is measured in milligrays. CTDIw does not consider exposure variation along the z-axis.

CTDIvol
CTDIvol takes account of exposure variation in the z axis and is calculated by the following formula: CTDIvol=CTDIw Pitch

Deionising filters
Filters implemented from some vendors in the processing of raw data with the aim of reduce image noise.

DLP
Dose length product: is measure of total radiation exposure for the whole series of image and is calculated by the following formula: DLP=CTDIvol scan length. Usually in helical CT irradiated length is longer than imaged length. CTDIvol is independent of scan length. DLP is proportional to scan length.

Effective patient dose
Approximation of the dose delivered to the patient during a CT scan that takes into account the different organ sensitivities to radiation. Effective patient dose is measured in millisieverts.

Effective section thickness
Section thickness that is established in the spiral reconstruction process, measured at the isocenter. It is equal to or larger than the collimated section width.

Hyperplane
Intermediate image plane used in a reconstruction method for multi–detector row spiral CT.

Using MDCT, X-ray beam is no longer perpendicular to detector. To overcome this problem vendors have developed different reconstruction algorithms; some of them use an intermediate image plane to reconstruct the final axial image. This algorithm is represented by the so-called hyperplane weighted reconstruction.

Isocenter
Centre of the measurement field of view of a CT scanner. Physical parameters such as section thickness and resolution are usually determined at the isocenter.

Longitudinal resolution
Spatial resolution in the patient (z-axis) direction, determined by the effective section thickness and the image increment.

Pitch
Parameter that characterizes a spiral scan, defined as table feed per rotation divided by the total width of the collimated beam. In the early days of four-section CT, the term detector pitch had been additionally introduced, which accounts for the width of a single section in the denominator. In this way two different pitch can be defined relative to total X-ray collimation ($pitch_x$) or to individual detector width ($pitch_d$). Consequently $pitch_d = pitch_x$ number of slices. For the sake of clarity and uniformity, the detector pitch should no longer be used. For both single-section CT and multi-detector row CT the pitch (p) is given by $p = TF/w$, where TF is table feed per rotation, and w is total width of the collimated beam, according to International Electrotechnical Commission specifications. For $p<1$, data acquisition occurs with overlap in the z-axis direction; for $p>1$, data acquisition occurs with gaps.

Prepatient collimation
Collimation system between X-ray tube and patient that limits the width of the collimated beam in the longitudinal direction.

Section sensitivity profile (SSP)
Function indicating the signal contribution of an infinitesimal object to each position along the z axis. SSP is determined by section collimation, size of the focal spot, and the spiral reconstruction algorithm.

Tube current
Acquisition parameter expressed in terms of milliAmpere (mA) strictly related to image noise and patient dose exposure.

Tube potential
Acquisition parameter expressed in terms of kilovolts peak strictly related to image noise and patient dose exposure (kVp).

Voxel
Basic 3D element of a volume image. A value, the CT number, is assigned to each voxel.

Volume-rendering technique (VRT)
Three-dimensional postprocessing method based on a weighted display of all voxels along each ray in the view direction. Transfer functions assign opacity and color to each CT number.

Weighted hyperplane reconstruction (WHR)
Reconstruction method for multi-detector row spiral CT that accounts for the cone angle of the measurement rays by introducing intermediate hyperplanes for image reconstruction.

Z-filter reconstruction
Method for multi-detector row spiral interpolation that uses all direct and complementary rays within a selectable distance from the image plane. Z-filter reconstruction allows establishment of different SSPs to trade off longitudinal resolution and image noise.

References

Barish MA, Soto AJ, Ferrucci JT (2005) Consensus on current clinical practice of virtual colonoscopy Am J Roentgenol 184:786–792

Beaulieu CF, Napel S, Daniel BL et al. (1998) Detection of colonic polyps in a phantom model: implications for virtual colonoscopy data acquisition. J Comput Assist Tomogr 22:656–663

Berland LL, Smith JK (1998) Multidetector-array CT: once again, technology creates new opportunities. Radiology 209:327

Calhoun PS, Kuszyk BS et al. (1999) Three-dimensional volume rendering of spiral CT data: theory and method. RadioGraphics 19:745

Chen SC, Lu DSK, Hecht JR et al. (1999) CT colonography: value of scanning in both the supine and prone positions. Am J Roentgenol 172: 595–599

Dachman AH, Lieberman J, Osnis RB et al. (1997) Small simulated polyps in pig colon: sensitivity of CT virtual colography. Radiology 203:427–430

Fenlon HM, Nunes DP, Schroy PC III, Barish MA et al. (1999) A comparison of virtual and conventional colonoscopy for the detection of colorectal polyps. N Engl J Med 341:1496–1503

Fletcher JG, Johnson CD, Welch TJ et al. (2000) Optimization of CT colonography technique: prospective trial in 180 patients. Radiology 216:704–711

Flohr TG, Schaller S, Stierstorfer K et al. (2005) Multi-detector row CT systems and image-reconstruction techniques. Radiology 235:756–773

Giacomuzzi SM, Torbica P, Rieger M et al. (2001) Radiation exposure in single slice and multi-slice spiral CT (a phantom study). Fortschr Rontgenstr (ROFO) 173(7):643–649

Gillams AR, Lees WR (2002) What collimation is necessary for polyp detection at VC? Proceedings of the 3rd International Workshop on Multislice CT, 3D Imaging, Virtual Endoscopy, June 5–8, 2002, Rome, Italy

Hara AK, Johnson CD, Reed JE et al. (1997a) Reducing data size and radiation dose for CT colonography. Am J Roentgenol 168:1181–1184

Hara AK, Johnson CD, Reed JE et al. (1997b) Detection of colorectal polyps with CT colography: initial assessment of sensitivity and specificity. Radiology 205:59–65

Hara AK, Johnson CD, MacCarty RL et al. (2001) CT colonography: single-versus multi-detector row imaging. Radiology 219:461–465

Hu H (1999) Multi-slice helical CT: scan and reconstruction. Med Phys 26:5–18

Hu H, He HD, Foley WD et al. (2000) Four multidetector-row helical CT: image quality and volume coverage speed. Radiology 215:55–62

Huda W, Scalzetti EM, Galina L et al. (2000) Technique factors and image quality as functions of patient weight at abdominal CT. Radiology 217:430–435

Iannaccone R, Laghi A, Catalano C et al. (2003a) Feasibility of ultra-low-dose multislice CT colonography for the detection of colorectal lesions: preliminary experience. Eur Radiol 13(6):1297–1302

Iannaccone R, Laghi A, Catalano C et al. (2003b) Performance of lower dose multi-detector row helical CT colonography compared with conventional colonoscopy in the detection of colorectal lesions. Radiology 229(3):775–781

Kemerink GJ, Bortslap AC, Frantzen MJ et al. (2001) Patients and occupational dosimetry in double contrast barium enema examinations Br J Radiol 74(881):420–428

Laghi A, Iannaccone R, Mangiapane F et al. (2003) Experimental colonic phantom for the evaluation of the optimal scanning technique for CT colonography using a multidetector spiral CT equipment. Eur Radiol 13:459–466

Macari Ml, Bini EJ, Xue X et al. (2002) Colorectal neoplasms: prospective comparison of thin-section low-dose multi-detector row CT colonography and conventional colonoscopy for detection. Radiology 224:383–392

McCollough CH (2002) Optimization of multidetector array CT acquisition parameters for CT colonography. Abdom Imaging 27:253–259

Nicholson FB, Taylor S, Halligan S et al. (2005) Recent developments in CT colonography. Clin Radiol 60: 1–7

Power NP, Pryor AM (2002) Optimization of scanning parameters for CT colonography. Br J Radiol 75:401–408

Rogalla P, Meiri N (2001) CT colonography: data acquisition and patient preparation techniques. Semin Ultrasound CT MR 22:405–412

Rottgen R, Schroder RJ, Lorenz M et al. (2003) CT-colonography with the 16-slice CT for the diagnostic evaluation of colorectal neoplasms and inflammatory colon diseases. Fortschr Rontgenstr (ROFO) 175:1384–1391

Sanjay S (2004) Multi-detector row CT: principles and practice for abdominal applications. Radiology 233:323–327

Sherbondy AJ, Holmlund D, Rubin GD et al. (2005) Alternative input devices for efficient navigation of large CT angiography data sets. Radiology 234(2):391–398

Springer P, Stohr B, Giacomuzzi SM et al. (2000) Virtual computed tomography colonoscopy: artefacts, image quality and radiation dose load in a cadaver study. Eur Radiol 10:183–187

Taguchi K, Aradate H (1998) Algorithm for image reconstruction in multi-slice helical CT. Med Phys 25:550–561

Taylor SA, Halligan S, Bartram I et al. (2003) Multi-detector row CT colonography: effect of collimation, pitch, and orientation on polyp detection in a human colectomy specimen. Radiology 229:109–118

Van Gelder RE, Venema HW, Serlie IW et al. (2002) CT colonography at different radiation dose levels: feasibility of dose reduction. Radiology 224:25–33

Vining DJ, Gelfand DW, Bechtold RE et al. (1994) Technical feasibility of colon imaging with helical CT and virtual reality. Am J Roentgenol 62 Suppl:104

Wessling J, Fischbach R, Meier N et al. (2003) CT colonography: protocol optimization with multi detector row CT – study in an anthropomorphic colon phantom. Radiology 228:753–759

Whiting BR, Mc Farland EG, Brink JA et al. (2000) Influence of image acquisition parameters on CT artefacts and polyp depiction in spiral CT colonography: in vitro evaluation. Radiology 217:165–172

7 How to Interpret the Data Sets?

Beth G. McFarland

CONTENTS

7.1 Introduction 73
7.2 Current and Future Image Display Techniques 73
7.2.1 2D Multiplanar Reformation (2D MPR) 74
7.2.2 3D Endoscopic Fly-Through 75
7.2.3 3D Transparency View (Edge-Enhanced View) 76
7.2.4 Future Advances in Image Display Techniques 76
7.3 Different Categories of Colorectal Morphologies 76
7.3.1 Focal Polypoid Lesions (r/o stool) 76
7.3.2 Pedunculated Lesions 79
7.3.3 Sessile/Flat Lesions (r/o thick or confluent Folds) 79
7.3.4 Advanced Mural Lesions (r/o collapse) 81
7.4 Standardization of Reporting of Clinically Significant Colorectal Findings 82
References 85

7.1 Introduction

CT colonography (CTC) image acquisition and image display capabilities continue to evolve. Concordant with such changes is the need to re-evaluate how to interpret the data. From 2002 to 2005, validation studies have reported a range of results in different patient cohorts using different methods. Important differences in acquisition methods have varied in stool tagging and CT dose techniques, while image display techniques have ranged from primary use of 2D multiplanar reformation to 3D endoscopic fly-through techniques. Specifically the largest cohort to date of 1233 patients reported excellent results using rigorous tagging and electronic subtraction, with reader evaluation of primary 3D fly-through review (Pickhardt et al. 2003). Three other multi-institutional studies reported less good results using no tagging or subtraction and predominant use of 2D MPR as primary review (Cotton et al. 2004; Johnson et al. 2003; Rockey et al. 2005). Recently a series of 200 patients with excellent results used stool tagging without catharsis or subtraction, exploiting ultra low dose techniques and 2D MPR as a primary review (Iannaccone et al. 2004). Certainly the differences in these studies are complex; however key influences of image display techniques for data interpretation are important to understand.

This chapter will focus on 1) current and future image display techniques for data interpretation, 2) application of these techniques in the major categories of colorectal morphologies, and 3) issues of standardization of reporting clinically significant colorectal findings in CTC (C-RADS).

7.2 Current and Future Image Display Techniques

After years of diligent use of 2D multiplanar reformation (2D MPR) as a primary review with 3D to problem solve, the success of the study of Pickhardt et al. (Pickhardt et al. 2003), aided by improved computer graphics, eclipsed the field in 2003 to demonstrate that 3D as a primary review was not only feasible but may be better. Unfortunately, there has been somewhat of a binary debate of whether 2D vs 3D is better, rather than an understanding of how to apply each of these techniques cohesively in the appropriate setting.

How are we now to approach data interpretation? Currently, the answer probably is a seamless interaction between 2D MPR and 3D endoscopic fly-through techniques, which may vary across patients or within specific colonic segments of a patient. The 3D fly-through as a primary review uses 3D to detect, with 2D MPR to help characterize. Conversely, use of 2D MPR as a primary review uses 2D to detect,

B. G. McFarland, MD
Diagnostic Imaging Associates, Center for Diagnostic Imaging, St. Luke's Hospital, 232 S. Woods Mill Rd, Chesterfield, MO 63017, USA and Adjunct Professor, Washington University School of Medicine, Mallinckrodt Institute of Radiology, 510 S. Kingshighway Blvd, St. Louis, MO 63110, USA

with 3D MPR to help characterize. In addition to these techniques, the 3D transparency view allows an overall view of the colonic anatomy, simulating a barium enema visualization. In order to apply optimally techniques best, it is important to understand the uses, advantages and disadvantages.

7.2.1
2D Multiplanar Reformation (2D MPR)

Primary 2D MPR review for lesion detection can provide a time efficient evaluation of the colon, exploiting an extra-colonic field of view for improved orientation. This visualization is based on a real time sectoring through the colonic sub-segments in cine mode, in a continuous direction typically from the rectum to the cecum. Two window levels settings are typically utilized. The polyp window (width 1500, level −200) imparts the high contrast interface to detect intraluminal colorectal polypoid lesions. The soft tissue window setting (width 400, level 10) is critical to evaluate more advanced wall lesions, discern the high density of false positives or the fat density of lipomas, and to evaluate the extra-colonic findings. In some areas of retained dense fluid, a narrower window setting may be needed to better see within the fluid level.

When a lesion is detected in the polyp window of 2D MPR, the following steps can be taken to most efficiently characterize a lesion. First, the *density* of the lesion in the soft tissue window is directly available. If the lesion is dense (i.e., false positive of stool) or fatty (lipoma), typically no further evaluation is needed. If however the lesion is soft tissue in density, both the 2D MPR additional views (e.g., sagittal and coronal) and the 3D endoscopic view can then be used to assess *morphology* of a focal finding better. The use of 3D to further characterize can be very helpful to evaluate the common dilemma of discernment of a thickened fold (or confluence of folds) from a polyp on a fold. Lastly, confirmation of a lesion's *anatomic location* on the corresponding prone (or supine) data set is needed. Although automated registration of supine and prone data sets is becoming technically feasible, the in vivo range of change in position of a focal finding between prone and supine positions might make 2D MPR with its extra-colonic field of view most efficient to localize a given area. Confirmation of the same location on both prone and supine data sets (when image quality permits) greatly increases confidence of a true positive lesion.

To use 2D MPR as a primary review, it can be helpful to perform initially a one minute coronal cine of both the prone and supine data sets to get the "lay of the land". This allows the reader to determine the degree of tortuosity and the colonic course, as well as the image quality of colonic distention and fluid/stool retention. The data set with the best image quality can be chosen to evaluate first. Typically, as each lesion is detected, characterization of the lesion on the other 2D MPR views and 3D views can be made between prone and supine data sets. Images of true positive lesions are taken and an internet report of findings for future dictation can be started. This type of organization of effort, involving lesion detection and characterization, followed by image capture of important findings, along the continuous retrograde path of the colon from rectum to cecum, allows an efficient and thorough evaluation of the colonic surface area. If interrupted by another task, the colon segment reached can be recorded and then evaluation can be reinitiated at this segment, once the interpretation can be resumed. After finishing the first data set (typically supine) with characterization of each lesion detected, the other data set (typically prone) can be briefly viewed with an axial cine to see potentially any additional findings. Using embedded arrows for lesions already detected prevents one wasting time re-evaluating the same lesions between data sets.

What are the advantages and disadvantages of 2D MPR? The use of 2D MPR offers several important advantages. First there is the direct display of the source attenuation data of a focal lesion to determine density. Specifically, the density of a focal lesion, such as fat in a lipoma or high density or focal pockets of air in stool, provides the most important characteristics to confirm false positive lesions. Another advantage of 2D MPR is the ability to visualize the location of a lesion from an extraluminal viewpoint, rather than the immersed endoscopic view of 3D fly-through. This can be helpful to confirm whether a lesion is in the same segment between prone and supine data sets (especially helpful in tortuous colons), as well as whether the lesion is dependent or non-dependent within a given segment. If a lesion shifts in position to different segments or changes to a dependent position on both prone and supine views without a visualized stalk, the concern for a false positive (e.g., retained stool) increases. Another advantage is that 2D MPR can be a time efficient evaluation of the colonic findings, since a thorough cine of both data sets is done once, compared to the need of forward and retrograde 3D fly-through views in both prone and supine data sets. Subtle mural lesions can often best be seen in the MPR soft tissue window settings. The disadvantages of 2D MPR as a primary review may be decreased sensitivity compared to the increased surface area visualization of 3D fly-through. Although this has not been directly confirmed in validation studies, the improved results of 3D as a primary review in the PICKHARDT et al. study are compelling. Reader fatigue can also be greater with 2D MPR, given the potentially more subtle and briefer visualization of lesions during the cine method of sectoring through the data.

7.2.2
3D Endoscopic Fly-Through

The use of 3D fly-through as a primary review provides a continuous fly-through of the colon, using the endoscopic field of view. The exciting advances of this technique have become more generalizable across 3D workstations; however differences still exist. In some 3D workstations, preprocessing of the data with segmentation (i.e., selective extraction) of the colon is first done, followed by calculation of the central path through the entire colon. Other workstations do not segment the colon or calculate the central path. For the reader, the review typically begins within the rectum, with continuous retrograde fly-through to the cecum.

When a focal lesion is found in 3D, further characterization can be done in several ways. First the 3D *morphology* is initially directly viewed, which can efficiently display overall anatomy and relationship of a lesion to surrounding folds. Second, assessment of *density* can then be performed with simultaneous registration of the finding in 2D MPR to display directly the density of the lesion. Some vendors provide an opacity map of the lesion within the 3D endoscopic view, which helps display the profile of density differences across the lesion. Finally, confirmation of the position and *anatomic location* of the lesion in both supine and prone data sets is again needed to increase confidence of a true positive lesion. This may best be performed with comparison of the lesion between MPR views for extraluminal orientation.

To use 3D as a primary review, endoscopic fly-through in antegrade and retrograde paths for both supine and prone data sets are necessary. Some advocates of 3D however state that if excellent visualization with no lesions found is present after forward and backward fly-through paths of the supine data set, only a retrograde fly-through is needed in the prone data set (e.g., eliminates antegrade fly-through in the second data set). Similar to 2D MPR, use of embedded arrows in lesions already evaluated keeps evaluation of additional lesions efficient between prone and supine data sets. A critical point is the need to also sector through the axial MPR data in soft tissue settings (done at start or end of review) to exclude any subtle or advanced mural lesion. Circumferential narrowing or partial wall involvement of the colon in advanced cancers can be more subtle in the immersed 3D endoscopic view, whereas soft tissue wall thickening or irregularity can be better seen in the extraluminal viewpoint of 2D MPR.

What are the advantages and disadvantages of 3D endoscopic fly-through techniques? A strong advantage is the increased surface area visualization, which continues to be aided by improved navigational tools. In non-tortuous segments of colon, there is a longer period of visualization of a focal colorectal lesion over the course of the fly-through, compared to the brief visualization seen while sectoring through a sub segment of the colon using 2D MPR cine techniques. This advantage however is diminished in marked areas of tortuosity or areas of collapse. Also focal polypoid lesions can be more visibly apparent within the colon lumen, compared to 2D, and thus can be easier to see in 3D fly-through. Both the potential advantages of longer visualization and increased ease of visualization of a lesion can lead to greater detection rates with less reader fatigue. The disadvantages of 3D endoscopic fly-through can include longer length of evaluation to complete review of the antegrade and retrograde paths. In tortuous colons, surface areas visualization around the inner curve of a turn can be initially missed. Importantly, any increased sensitivity to detect more lesions needs to be scrutinized relative to specificity. Namely, improvements in lesion detection with increased surface area visualization must be achieved, without increased false positive rates.

In summary, use of 2D MPR and 3D display techniques optimally are best used with seamless integration to exploit their inherent advantages and diminish their disadvantages. Although there is increasing use of the 3D fly-through technique with improved computer graphics and navigational aids, use of 2D MPR as a primary review may still be needed in specific segments or sub-segments not amenable to 3D. Specifically, areas best evaluated with 2D MPR primarily may include areas of marked muscular hypertrophy from diverticulosis, sharp hairpin turns, colonic collapse, or marked fluid retention. In these areas, the 3D fly-through may be suspended, with transition to 2D MPR through a given region. In addition, in areas where multiple focal findings are being detected in 3D raising the concern for stool retention, evaluation in 2D MPR may allow a better overall characterization. Thus, given differences in image quality and anatomy which vary within or between patients, complementary use of 2D or 3D can be selectively utilized for improved visualization.

Appropriate training is important to acquire the new skills of these techniques. Currently both academic and commercial programs for reader training are available. A highly recommended source of these sites is available at the International Symposium of Virtual Colonoscopy held each fall in Boston. With training, primary review of the colorectal lesions (not including extra-colonic findings) using either technique to complete a normal data set with good to excellent image quality has been stated by experts to range from five to ten minutes. A recently developed clinical service may benefit initially from double reading of cases among trained colleagues.

7.2.3
3D Transparency View (Edge-Enhanced View)

In addition to the primary modes of interpretation, the 3D transparency view provides an effective visualization to display the overall colonic anatomy and to demarcate where focal findings are. Although this view is not helpful in making the diagnosis, its role to summarize the findings in a consistent and accurate way is important for current management and future surveillance of lesions. Similar to the barium enema in appearance, this view can give an effective roadmap for the gastroenterologist or surgeon. Even in cases with no lesions, standard AP and bilateral oblique views can be helpful for future reference.

7.2.4
Future Advances in Image Display Techniques

How we interpret virtual colonography in 2005 will probably change dramatically in the next five to ten years. Important influences will be the further refinement of computed aided diagnosis and molecular imaging. Computed aided diagnostic algorithms in CTC are being actively explored in academic and commercial efforts. If sensitivity can be achieved across the complexity of colorectal morphologies, without a compromise of specificity, remarkable efficiency of the data evaluation will be achieved. Whether CAD is used optimally as a primary read or a secondary read will be interesting to evaluate. As molecular imaging techniques continue to evaluate functional information at cellular and molecular levels, colorectal applications may shift to other modalities, such as MR and optical imaging. Certainly the success of molecular imaging could lead to a phenomenal break-through of detection of clinically significant lesions in the polyp-carcinoma pathological continuum, along with focused therapy.

7.3
Different Categories of Colorectal Morphologies

There are common types of colorectal morphologies evaluated in CT colonography. These include the focal polypoid lesion, pedunculated lesion, flat or sessile lesion and advanced mural lesions. This section will describe these morphologies and their corresponding false positive counterparts. The differential application of 2D and 3D image displays to assess these morphologies will also be reinforced.

7.3.1
Focal Polypoid Lesions (r/o stool)

One of the most common colorectal morphologies is the focal polypoid lesion. This is also the most common morphology of the false positive lesion of retained stool. Thus discernment between a focal polyp and stool are critical. Key features include the following:

The morphology of a focal polyp is typically smooth and round (Fig. 7.1). Although stool can also be similar in morphology, margins which are more geometrical or angular are highly suggestive of stool (Fig. 7.2). A polypoid lesion is typically soft tissue in density; however lesions which are increased in density are highly specific of stool. Stool can also be low attenuation or opaque; however this can overlap with the partial volume effects of smaller polyps, depending on the collimation used. A focal polyp can have air around the edges where it abuts the wall; however central focal pockets of air within a lesion

How to Interpret the Data Sets?

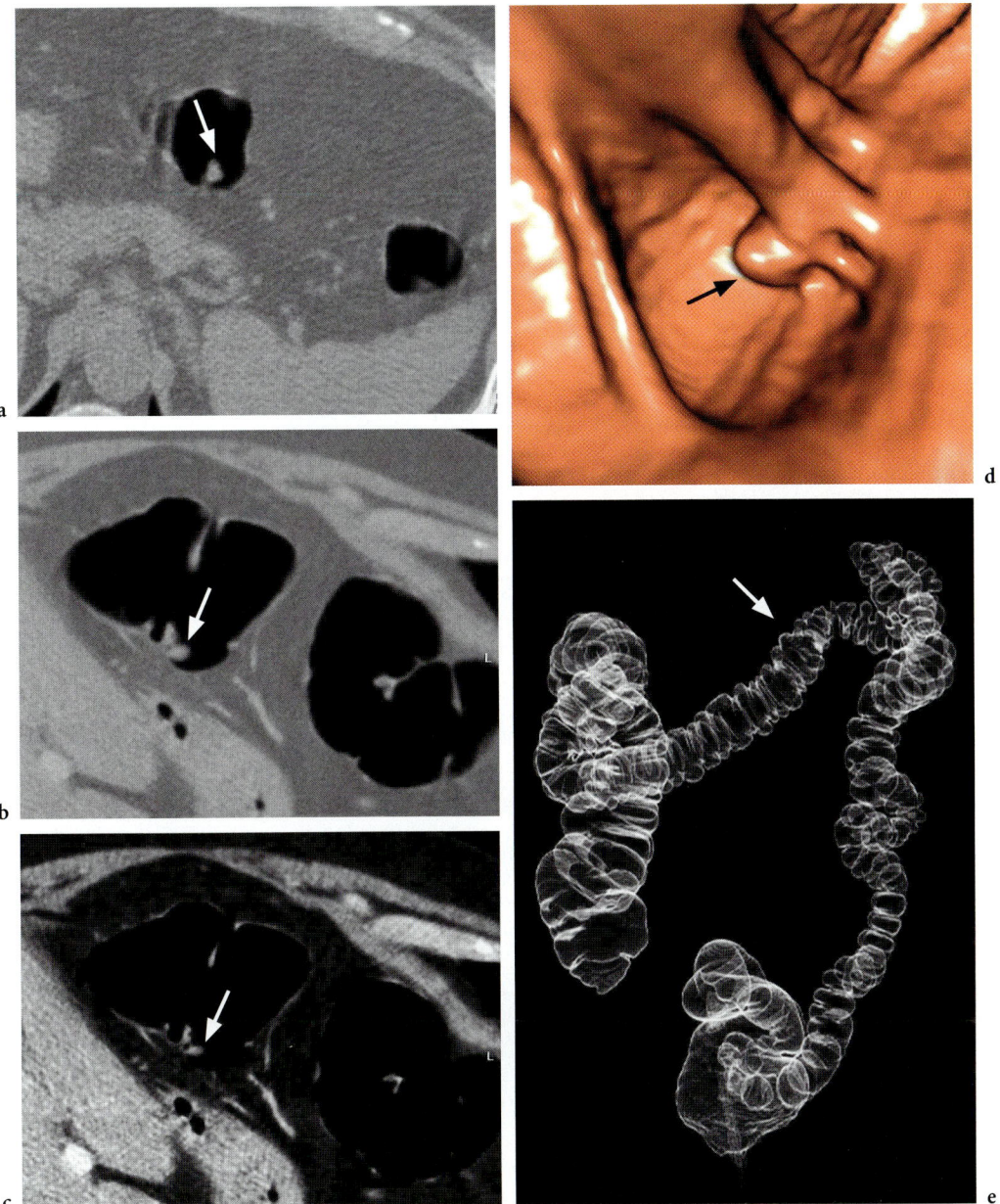

Fig. 7.1a–e. Typical features of a true positive polypoid morphology (*arrows*), demonstrating smooth margins, soft tissue density and constant location between prone and supine positions: **a** prone axial 2D MPR and **b** supine axial 2D MPR in polyp settings (W 1500, L −200); **c** axial 2D MPR with soft tissue settings (W 400, L 10) confirms polyp density; **d** 3D perspective volume rendered view demonstrates smooth polypoid morphology; **e** 3D transparency view gives roadmap of colonic anatomy, with arrow demarcating location of lesion

is diagnostic of stool (Fig. 7.3). Shift vs constancy of location of a focal finding relative to the colon wall is important. A polypoid lesion will stay fixed in the same position relative to the wall between prone and supine images. In contrast, the finding of stool which drops dependently is highly characteristic (Fig. 7.4). There are exceptions to this. A sigmoid polyp may appear to shift dependently on prone and supine images, but actually the redundancy of the sigmoid mesentery is what shifts (Laks et al. 2004). Stool can be adherent to the wall, which has been described with the phospha-soda bowel preparations. Also, a pedunculated polyp which does not demonstrate its stalk can appear to drop dependently. Finally, if intravenous contrast is used, differences in enhancement can be seen. Polyps potentially can enhance,

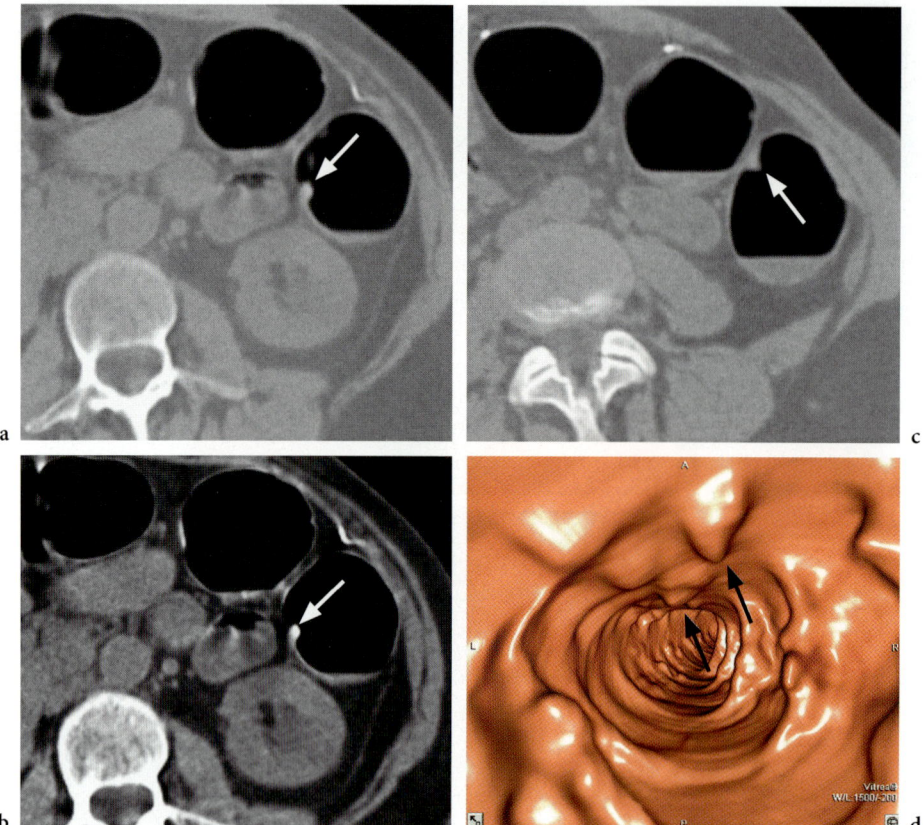

Fig. 7.2a–d. Typical features of false positive retained stool (*arrows*), demonstrating high density or angular margins: **a** axial 2D MPR (W 1500, L –200) shows focal polypoid lesion, compared to **b**; **b** axial 2D MPR (W 400, L 10) in soft tissue settings better demonstrates high density of stool; **c** axial 2D MPR view shows angular margins of another area of stool; **d** 3D perspective volume rendered view demonstrates dilemma of detection of multiple focal lesions, some demonstrating angular margins of stool

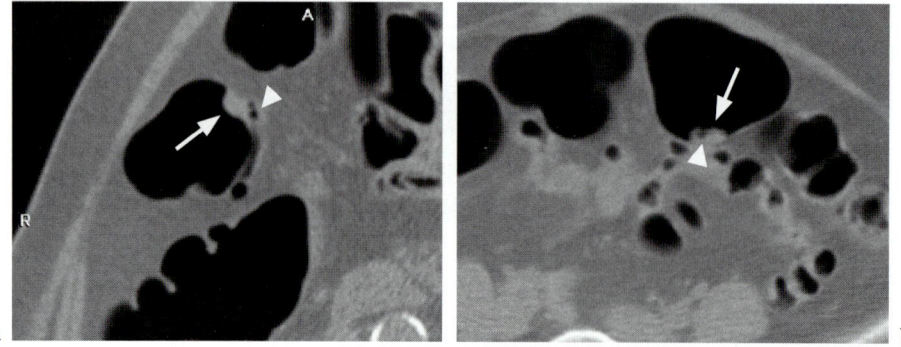

Fig. 7.3a,b. Polypoid lesions with focal pockets of air seen in true polyp vs stool, best shown in axial 2D MPR: **a** true positive sessile polyp (*arrow*) with air around edges of lesion (*arrowheads*), where lesion abuts the wall; **b** false positive of stool (*arrow*) with central pockets of air (*arrowheads*)

whereas stool will not enhance. As diagnostic CT is exploited to stage the liver along with evaluation of the colorectal lesions, the increasing use of IV contrast may lead to better understanding of the enhancement characteristics of polyps.

Both 2D and 3D techniques help to evaluate these characteristics. The morphologic features of round or smooth vs angular or geometric margins are best seen with 3D endoscopic views. Inherent density, location, focal pockets of air, and degree of enhance-

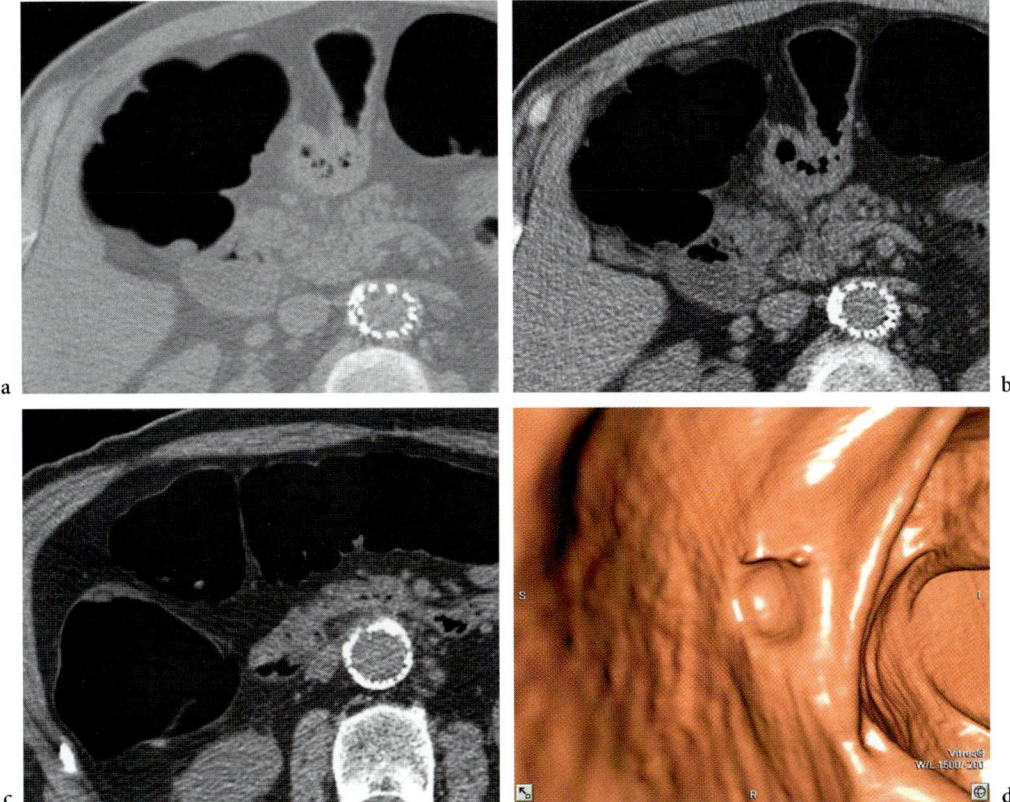

Fig. 7.4a–d. False positive lesion of retained pill (*arrow*) with characteristic shift of position: **a** axial 2D MPR supine image (W 1500, L –200) demonstrates a polypoid lesion; **b** axial 2D MPR view in soft tissue window settings (W 400, L 10) better shows low density of pill; **c** axial 2D MRP prone image in soft tissue settings better demonstrates shift to dependent position of pill, consistent with false positive; **d** 3D volume rendered view of pill mimics a polyp

ment is best evaluated with 2D MPR. As stool tagging continues to be developed, the ability to see high density within residual stool will further aid differentiation of polyp from stool.

7.3.2
Pedunculated Lesions

The pedunculated lesion, comprised of a round polyp head with a linear stalk, is a very distinguishable lesion. The challenge is how different these lesions can appear between prone and supine data sets (Fig. 7.5). On one data set, the polyp head can be suspended dependently from the stalk, whereas on the corresponding data set both polyp head and stalk can lie dependently together along the wall. If the stalk is long enough, lesions on the border between two segments can lie in different adjacent segments between prone and supine views. Also of importance is the variability in lesion measurement with such morphological differences between views.

A consistent reporting style is to measure the polyp head, with exclusion of the stalk. Thus, choosing the image where the polyp head and stalk are best discerned provides the more accurate and reproducible measurement (Fig. 7.5).

In general, 3D endoscopic views can provide improved visualization of these morphological features. One exception would be the visualization of the highly characteristic stalk of a pedunculated lesion in a segment with marked muscular hypertrophy of diverticulosis. In this setting, 2D MPR may offer an advantage, due to the impaired endoscopic visualization within the thickened folds (Fig. 7.6).

7.3.3
Sessile/Flat Lesions
(r/o thick or confluent Folds)

These lesions are currently considered the most challenging lesions to detect (Fig. 7.7). One important issue is the variability in definition of the terms.

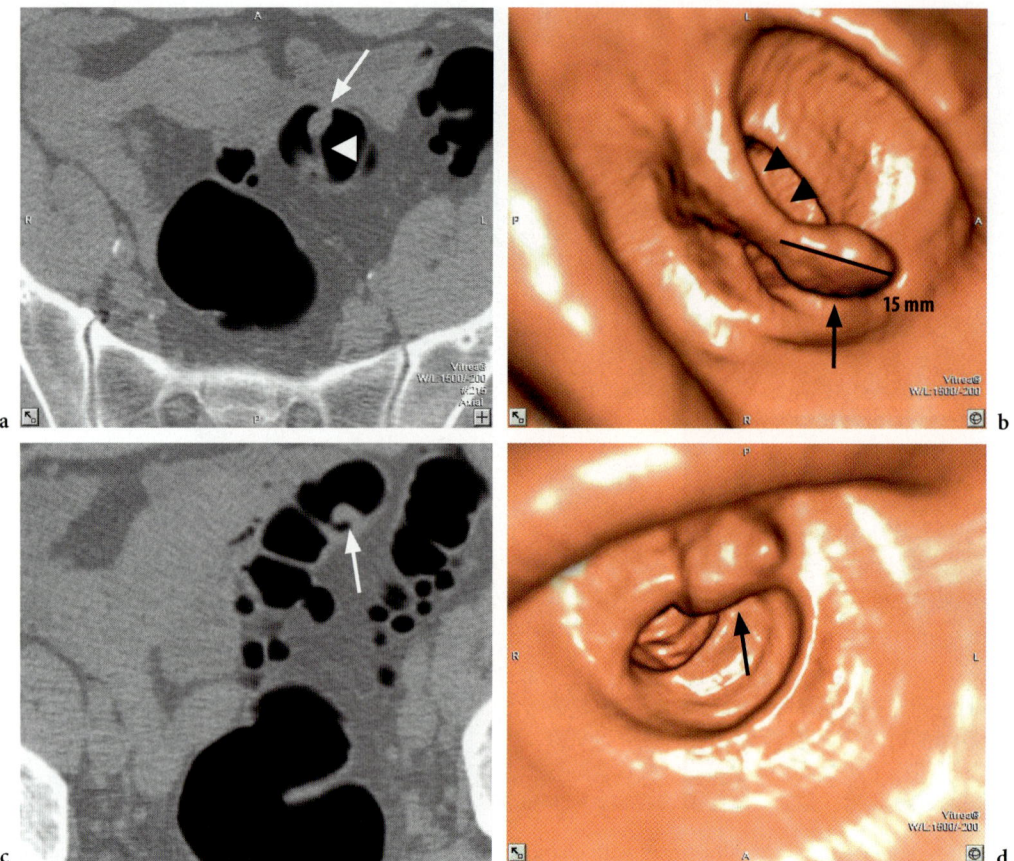

Fig. 7.5a–d. Typical features of a pedunculated polyp in sigmoid colon, demonstrating polyp head (*arrow*) and characteristic stalk (*arrowheads*), with marked changes between positions: **a** axial 2D MPR and **b** 3D volume rendered view in prone position demonstrates polyp head and stalk. Accurate measurement of long axis of polyp head, excluding the stalk, is shown; **c** axial 2D MPR and **d** 3D volume rendered view in prone position shows shift to dependent position with corresponding change in morphology

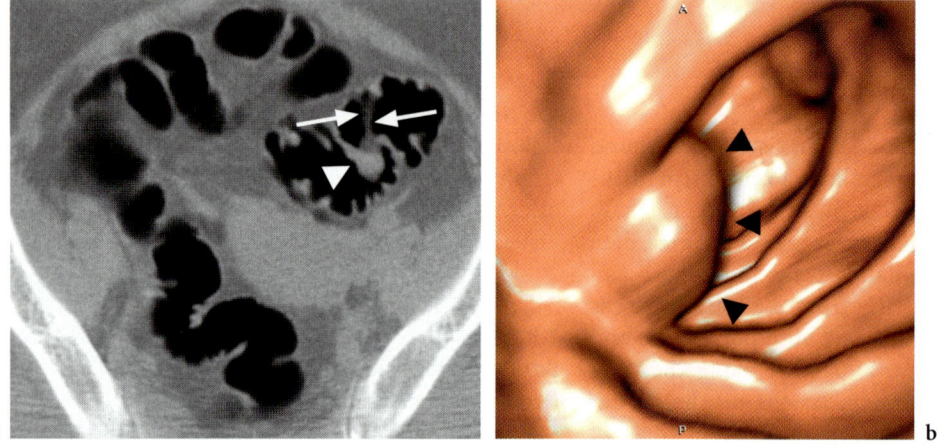

Fig. 7.6a,b. Pedunculated lesion in area of luminal narrowing and marked diverticulosis: **a** axial 2D MPR view best visualizes the characteristic stalk (*arrows*) from the polyp head (*arrowhead*), compared to **b**; **b** 3D volume rendered view, with polyp head shown (*arrowheads*), but stalk obscured by luminal narrowing and muscular hypertrophy

How to Interpret the Data Sets?

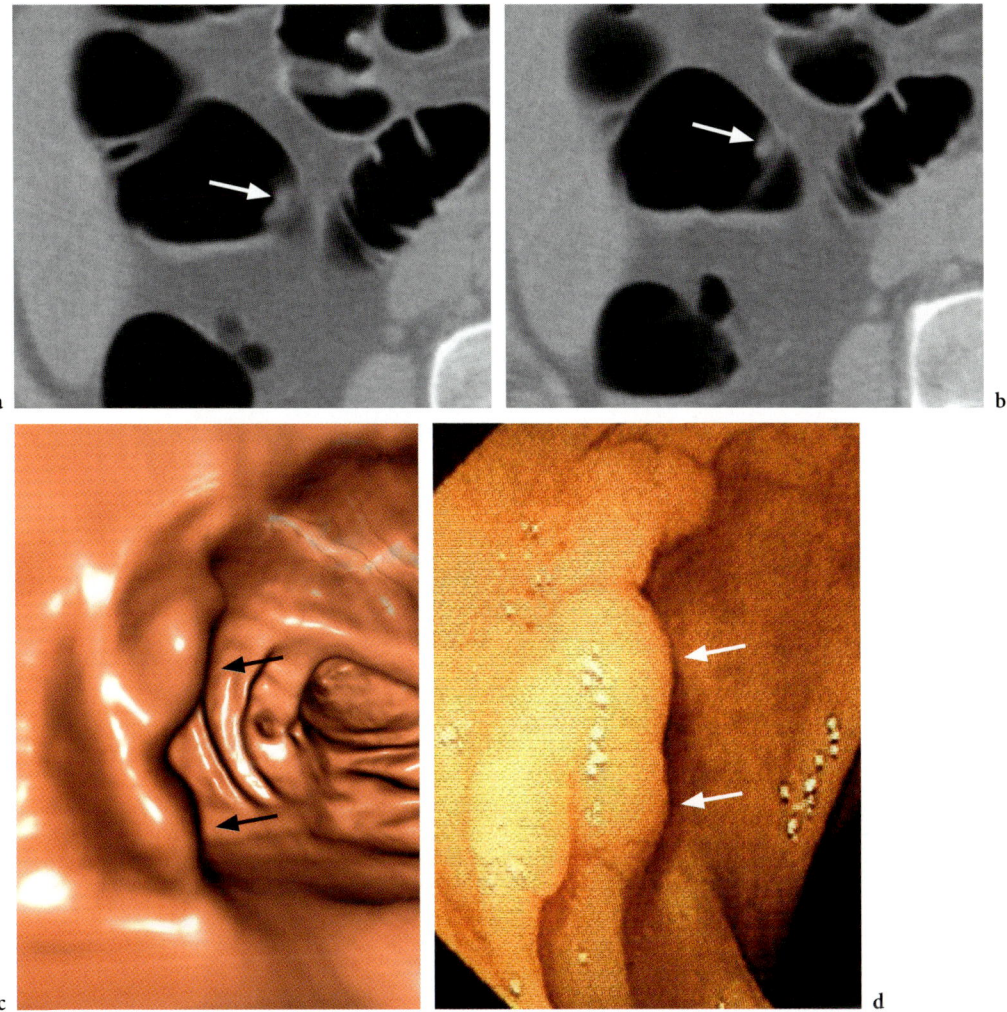

Fig. 7.7a–d. Sessile lesion (*arrows*) along a fold poses a challenge in detection: **a,b** axial 2D MPR images partially demonstrate the sessile lesion as an asymmetric bulge along the fold (best demonstrated with cine motion not shown); **c** 3D volume rendered view better demonstrates overall morphology of lesion; **d** correlative view from optical colonoscopy (copyright given by *Radiology* for MCFARLAND et al. 2002)

"Sessile" is generally defined as a lesion with a polyp base that is twice as long as the polyp height. Thus a 1 cm high lesion with a 2-cm base could be defined as sessile. This is very different from a "flat" lesion which is generally defined as a lesion measuring 1–3 mm in height. Unfortunately, the literature is inconsistent with these definitions and reported sensitivities have varied. FIDLER et al. (2002) reported a sensitivity range of 15–65% to detect 22 sessile polyps (size range of 0.4–3.5 cm) in a cohort of 547 patients. PICKHARDT et al. (2004) reported a sensitivity of 80% (47/59 polyps) to detect sessile lesions (defined as lesions with a base greater than height) in the cohort of 1233 screening patients.

The most common false positive counterpart to the flat or sessile lesion is a thickened fold or conflu-ence of folds (Fig. 7.8). For these types of challenging lesions, both 2D MPR (in soft tissue window-level settings) and 3D views have advantages and disadvantages. Both techniques should be explored to detect and characterize these lesions best.

7.3.4
Advanced Mural Lesions (r/o collapse)

CT colonography has reliably shown high sensitivity to detect advanced mural lesions (Fig. 7.9). A potential challenge in CT colonography is the discernment between an advanced mural lesion of advanced cancer from an area of focal collapse with relative wall thickening (often seen at points of flex-

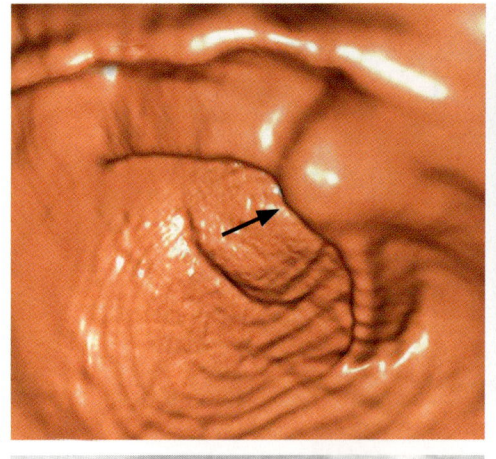
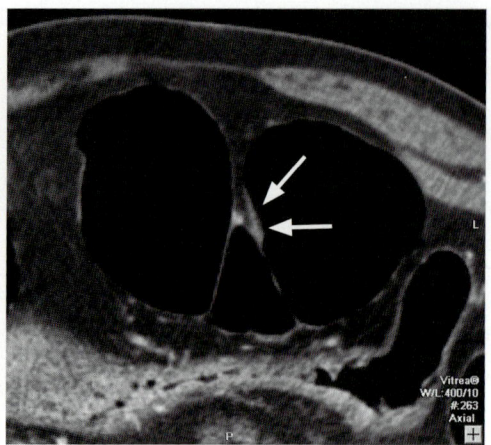
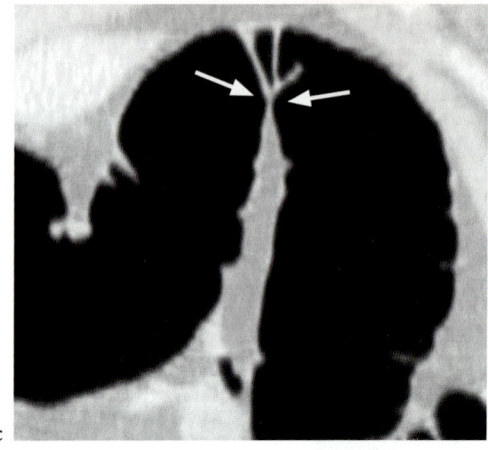

Fig. 7.8a–c. False positive of confluence of folds (*arrows*) mimicking a flat lesion: **a** 3D volume rendered view raises concern for a flat lesion; **b** axial 2D MPR in soft tissue settings also demonstrates flat morphology; **c** sagittal 2D MPR best demonstrates confluence of folds

ures, tortuosity, or muscular hypertrophy). At CT colonography, an advanced cancer will tend to stay fixed between prone and supine imaging, whereas an area of collapse can change in distention between positions. A cancer will typically have irregularity of the soft tissue rind along the wall, whereas focal collapse or muscular hypertrophy will be more smooth and symmetric (Fig. 7.10). If intravenous contrast is given, a cancer may have more irregular enhancement, whereas focal collapse of normal colon will enhance symmetrically.

The importance of 2D MPR with soft tissue settings (window 400, level 10) needs to be emphasized with these types of lesions. Whether this is subtle mural thickening or advanced, the 2D MPR views give valuable information of the mural relationships, which extend beyond the "lumenography" of the 3D fly-through (Fig. 7.11). In addition the 3D transparency view, which simulates the barium enema, can be a powerful view to display the lesion for others to appreciate the size and location of the cancer.

7.4 Standardization of Reporting of Clinically Significant Colorectal Findings

The Virtual Colonoscopy Working Group, represented by an organized group of CTC investigators at the International Virtual Colonoscopy annual meeting, recently published a consensus statement regarding the early development of a reporting structure of colorectal findings (Zalis et al. 2005). This reporting structure, named "C-RADS" helps to lay the groundwork for structured reporting of lesion morphology, size, and location, and preliminary recommendations of lesion surveillance. Although this effort now needs to be refined with multi-disciplinary consensus, it represents an important step towards more consistent and reproducible reporting at CT colonography.

C-RADS describes the use of *three morphologies* of lesions: sessile (broad based lesion whose width is greater than its vertical height), pedunculated (polyp with a separate stalk), and flat (polyp with vertical

How to Interpret the Data Sets?

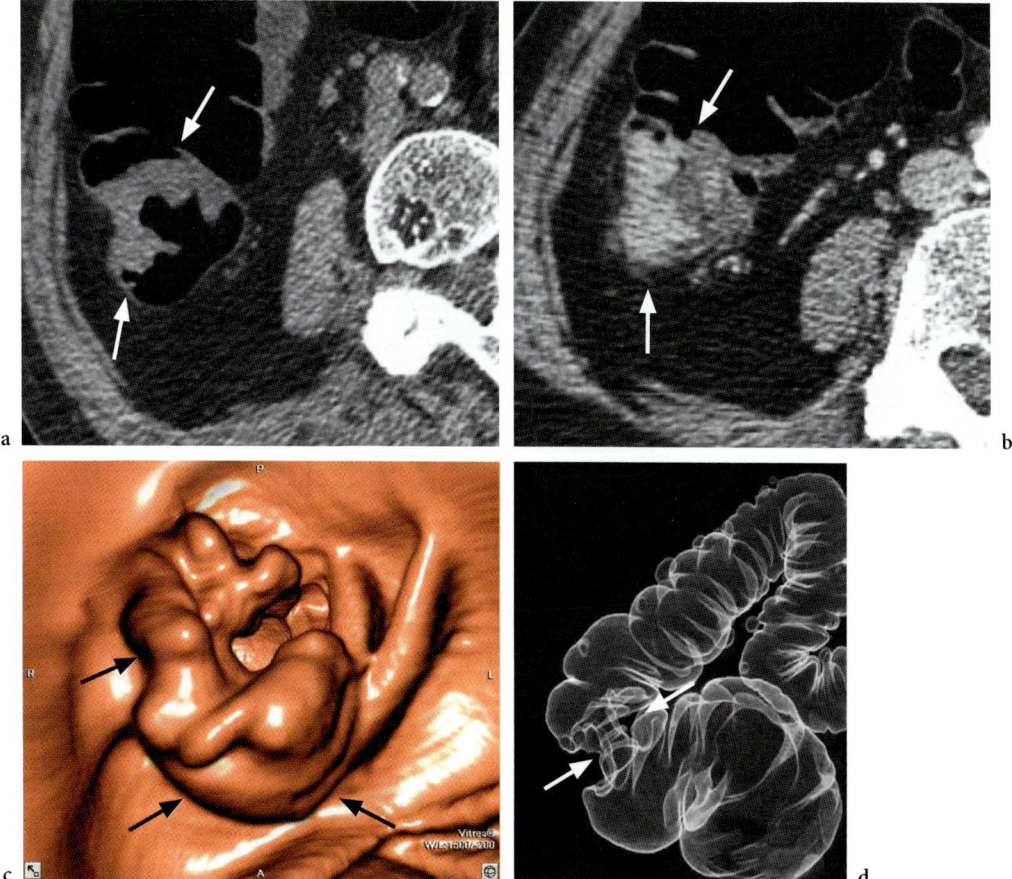

Fig. 7.9a–d. Advanced mural lesion (*arrows*): **a** prone non-contrast axial 2D MPR demonstrates advanced mural lesion; **b** supine contrast enhanced axial 2D MPR shows enhancing mass immersed in fluid; **c** 3D volume rendered intraluminal view demonstrates mural mass of cancer; **d** 3D transparency view shows classic apple-core lesion

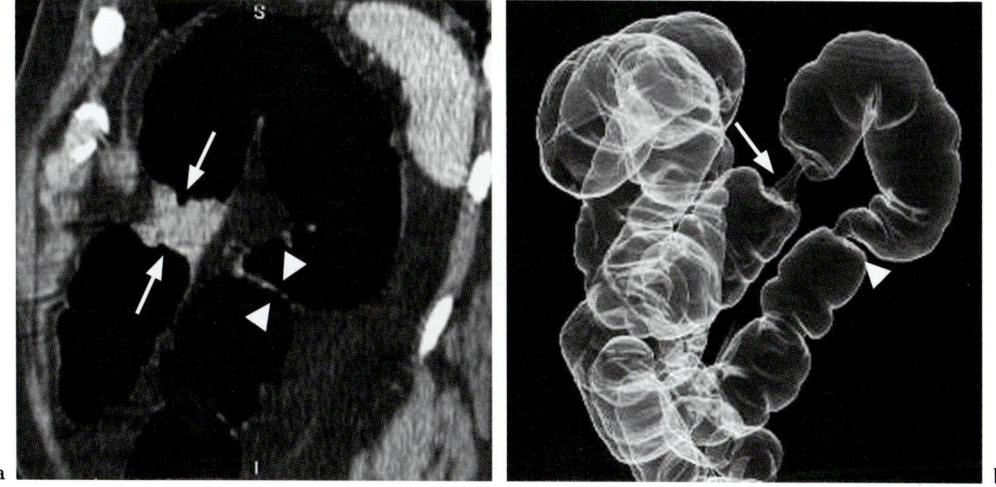

Fig. 7.10a,b. Advanced mural lesion (*arrows*) vs collapse (*arrowheads*): **a** sagittal 2D MPR view shows mural thickening of advanced cancer vs area of luminal collapse without mural thickening; **b** 3D edge enhanced view also demonstrates these two areas

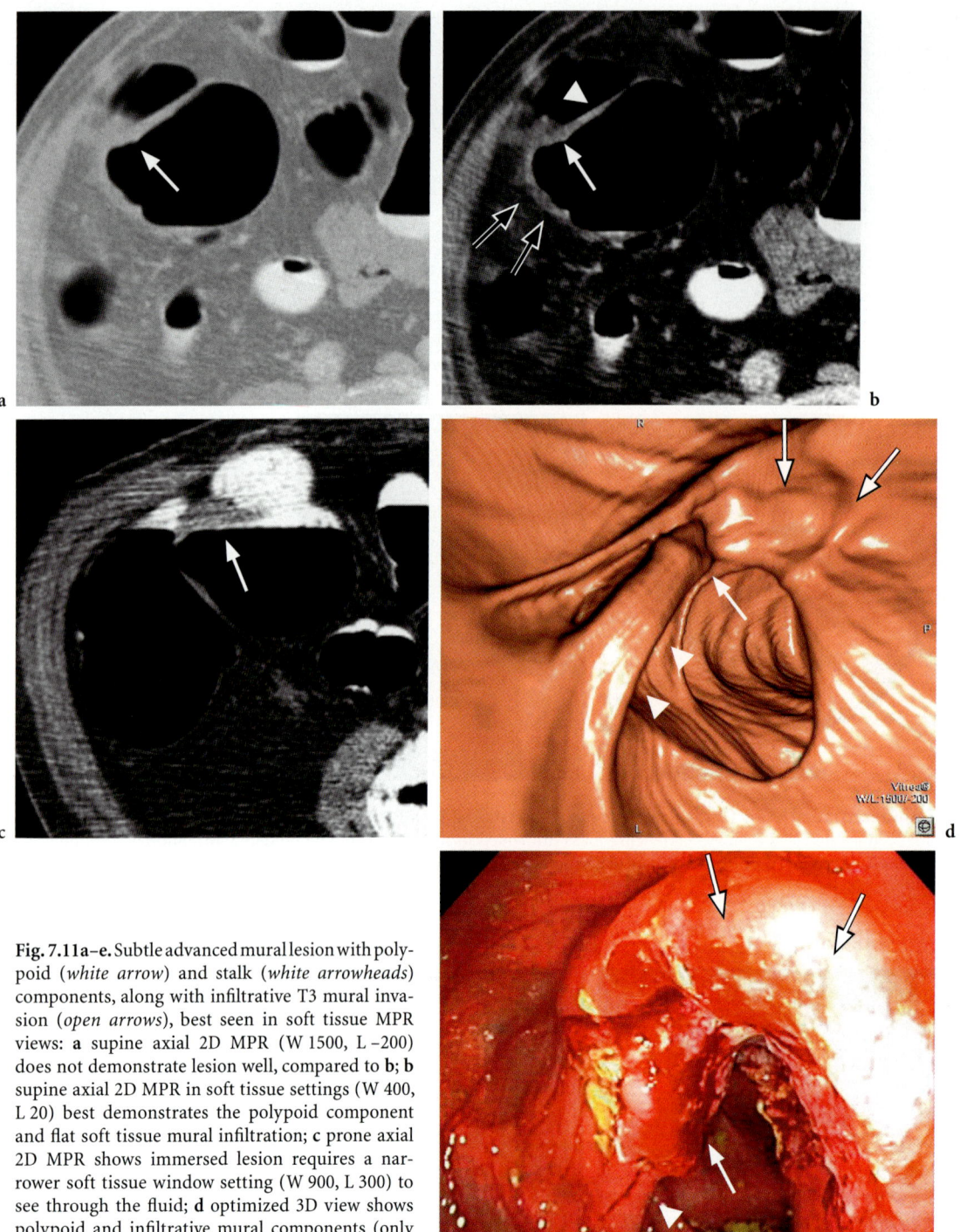

Fig. 7.11a–e. Subtle advanced mural lesion with polypoid (*white arrow*) and stalk (*white arrowheads*) components, along with infiltrative T3 mural invasion (*open arrows*), best seen in soft tissue MPR views: **a** supine axial 2D MPR (W 1500, L –200) does not demonstrate lesion well, compared to **b**; **b** supine axial 2D MPR in soft tissue settings (W 400, L 20) best demonstrates the polypoid component and flat soft tissue mural infiltration; **c** prone axial 2D MPR shows immersed lesion requires a narrower soft tissue window setting (W 900, L 300) to see through the fluid; **d** optimized 3D view shows polypoid and infiltrative mural components (only seen retrospectively); **e** corresponding view at optical colonoscopy

height less than 3 mm). Lesion *measurement* is critical for clinical management and can vary among readers. C-RADS defines the measurement of a polypoid lesion to be the maximal long axis of the polyp head, with exclusion of the stalk if present. For more sessile lesions, the maximal length along the base of the polyp should be used. Both 2D MPR and 3D techniques have been advocated for measurement, both of which certainly are felt to exceed the accuracy of axial measurements (Pickhardt 2005).

Lesion *location* refers to the standardized colonic segmental divisions of rectum, sigmoid, descending, transverse, ascending and cecum.

Recommendations of *lesion surveillance* are of active debate. At the heart of this issue is the controversy of what is the clinical index lesion of significance. In a recent future trends report initiated by the American Gastroenterology Association, the clinical significance of the intermediate 6–9 mm polyp poses the largest debate (Van Dam et al. 2004). Further multi-disciplinary consensus will now be needed to refine these recommendations.

The suggested *categories of lesions* are as follows. A **C0** category represents an inadequate study (e.g., inadequate prep or insufflation) or a study awaiting prior comparisons. A **C1** category is a normal colon (no lesions or lesions <5 mm) or a benign lesion (e.g., lipoma). A **C2** category is an intermediate polyp (e.g., less than three 6- to 9-mm polyps) or indeterminate finding (e.g., cannot exclude a polyp ≥6 mm). A **C3** category designates clinically significant polyps (e.g., polyps ≥10 mm or greater than three 6- to 9-mm polyps). A **C4** category is a colonic mass, which is likely malignant. Surveillance guidelines are still being refined; however each patient needs to be evaluated in the clinical context of age, comorbidity, colorectal symptoms and a priori concern for colorectal cancer.

Finally, C-RADS discusses the reporting of *extra-colonic findings*. To achieve cost effectiveness, the judicious reporting of extra-colonic findings to minimize unnecessary additional imaging tests will be critical. Significant extra-colonic findings, such as abdominal aortic aneurysms, solid renal or liver masses, adenopathy and lung nodules (greater than 1 cm) are emphasized. Less significant findings, such as small liver and renal cystic lesions (common findings which are often difficult to characterize without contrast), and gallstones hopefully will be under-reported. Further definition of how to categorize and follow these findings will be important.

In summary, C-RADS begins the process of standardization during the continuum of change and improvement. The RSNA initiative of RADLEX will mature the elements of informatics to this process. Multi-disciplinary consensus of radiologists, gastroenterologists, internists, surgeons, pathologists, and epidemiologists will hopefully continue to define and standardize clinical issues of importance. At the core of these issues will be definition of what constitutes a clinically significant lesion, with appropriate surveillance recommended within the clinical context of comorbidity, age and colorectal symptoms. As standardization is refined during ongoing evolution of the technique, an active process of quality assurance will be helpful for community implementation.

References

Cotton PB, Durkalski VL, Pineau BC, Palesch YY, Mauldin PD, Hoffman B et al. (2004) Computed tomographic colonoscopy (virtual colonoscopy): a multi-center comparison with standard colonoscopy for detection of colorectal neoplasia. JAMA 291:1713–1719

Fidler JL, Johnson CD, MacCarty RL, Welch TJ, Hara AK, Harmsen WS (2002) Detection of flat lesions in the colon with CT colonography. Abdom Imaging 27:292–300

Iannaccone R, Laghi A, Catalono C, Mangiapane F, Lamazza A, Schillaci A et al. (2004) Computed tomographic colonography without cathartic preparation for the detection of colorectal polyps. Gastroenterology 127:1200–1211

Johnson CD, Harmsen WS, Wilson LA, Maccarty RL, Welch TJ, Ilstrup DM et al. (2003) Prospective blinded evaluation of computed tomographic colonography for screen detection of colorectal polyps. Gastroenterology 125:311–319

Laks S, Macari M, Bini E (2004) Positional changes in colon polyps at CT colonography. Radiology 231:761–766

McFarland EG, Pilgram TK, Brink JA, et al. (2002) CT colongraphy: multi-observer diagnostic performance. Radiology 225:380–390

Pickhardt PJ, Choi JR, Hwang I, Butler JA, Puckett ML, Hildebrandt HA et al. (2003) Computed tomographic virtual colonoscopy to screen for colorectal neoplasia in asymptomatic adults. N Eng J Med 349:2191–2200

Pickhardt PJ, Nugent PA, Choi JR, Schindler WR (2004) Flat colorectal lesions in asymptomatic adults: implications for screening with CT virtual colonoscopy. AJR 183:1343–1347

Pickhardt PJ, Lee AD, McFarland EG, Taylor AJ (2005) Linear polyp measurement at CT colonography: in vitro and in vivo comparison of two-dimensional and three-dimensional displays. Radiology 236:872–878

Rockey DC, Paulson E, Niedzwiecki D, Davis W, Bosworth HB, Sanders L et al. (2005) Analysis of air contrast barium enema, computed tomographic colonography, and colonoscopy: prospective comparison. Lancet 365(9456):305–311

Van Dam J, Cotton P, Johnson CD, McFarland BG, Pineau BC, Provenzale D, Ransohoff D, Rex D, Rockey D, Wootton T (2004) AGA future trends report: CT colonography. Gastroenterology 127:970–984

Zalis ME, Barish MA, Choi JR, Dachman AH, Fenlon HM, Ferrucci JT, Glick SN, Laghi A, Macari M, McFarland EG, Morrin MM, Pickhardt PJ, Soto J, Yee J (2005) CT colonography reporting and data system: a consensus proposal. Radiology 236:3–9

8 How to Avoid Pitfalls in Imaging. Causes and Solutions to Overcome False Negatives and False Positives

STEFAAN GRYSPEERDT and PHILIPPE LEFERE

CONTENTS

8.1 Introduction 87
8.2 False Negative Diagnosis 87
8.2.1 Failure to Detect the Lesion 88
8.2.1.1 Preparation Related False Negative Diagnosis 88
8.2.1.2 Technical Artefacts 88
8.2.1.3 Normal Anatomy and Areas of Danger 89
8.2.1.4 Diverticular Disease 90
8.2.1.5 Sessile Polyps 94
8.2.1.6 Small Lesions and Small Flat Lesions 94
8.2.2 Failure to Characterise the Lesions 96
8.2.2.1 Annular Stricturing Lesions 96
8.2.2.2 Larger Flat Lesions 96
8.2.2.3 Small Sessile Polyps 96
8.2.2.4 Sessile Cancers 96
8.2.2.5 Pedunculated Lesions 99
8.3 False Positive Diagnosis 99
8.3.1 Preparation Related False Positive Findings 99
8.3.2 Technical Artefacts Causing False Positive Findings 101
8.3.2.1 Breathing Artefacts 101
8.3.2.2 Spasm 104
8.3.3 Pitfalls Related to Normal Anatomy and Non-Tumoral Lesions 104
8.3.3.1 Ileocecal Valve 104
8.3.3.2 Extrinsic Impression 106
8.3.3.3 Complex or Thickened Folds 106
8.3.3.4 Lipoma 107
8.3.3.5 Vascular Lesions 107
8.3.3.6 Appendiceal Orifice 107
8.3.3.7 Scar after Polypectomy 107
8.3.3.8 Spasm of the Internal Sphincter 110
8.3.3.9 Intermittently Prolapsing Rectal Mucosa 110
8.3.3.10 Diverticular Disease 110
References 114

8.1 Introduction

A major requisite, prior to the use of CTC as a screening tool, is to achieve an accuracy level comparative to that of conventional colonoscopy. Until now, a wide range of sensitivities has been reported (FLETCHER et al. 2005), even for the largest lesions (>9 mm): Johnson et al. (JOHNSON et al. 2003) reported a major inter-observer variability, with sensitivity ranges between 32% and 73%, whereas Pickhardt et al. (PICKHARDT et al. 2003) reported excellent sensitivities of 93.8%. This wide range of reported sensitivities is one of the major reasons for gastrointestinal endoscopists not to advocate the technique as screening tool yet (HWANG and WONG 2005; PICKHARDT 2005).

In depth analysis of the different results has shown numerous possible causes for the reported differences in accuracy, including a learning curve, influencing sensitivity (SPINZI et al. 2001), as well as specificity (GLUECKER et al. 2002). This learning curve includes the whole process of CTC: patient preparation, scanning technique (including patient positioning, colon insufflation, and scanning parameters), image manipulation and interpretation (TAYLOR et al. 2004).

Each step in the process of a CTC examination has its own potential dangers of hindering a final correct diagnosis.

In this chapter, different causes of false positive and false negative diagnosis are reviewed, and possible solutions to overcome these problems are proposed.

In the first part, false positive diagnosis will be reviewed, in the second part, false negative diagnosis are reviewed.

The figures represent a pictorial review of the different pitfalls, with lessons to overcome those pitfalls, marked italic in the figure legend.

8.2 False Negative Diagnosis

Overall, false negative diagnosis can be related to errors in characterisation, failure to detect the lesions, or a combination (FIDLER et al. 2004).

S. GRYSPEERDT, MD; P. LEFERE, MD
Stedelijk Ziekenhuis, Bruggesteenweg 90, 8800 Roeselare, Belgium

8.2.1
Failure to Detect the Lesion

8.2.1.1
Preparation Related False Negative Diagnosis

There are two main bowel preparations available: cathartics, such as magnesium citrate and phosphosoda, and gut lavage solutions, such as polyethylene glycol (PEG).

PEG is known as a "wet prep", leaving a clean colon filled with residual fluid. Residual fluid does not hinder colonoscopic evaluation because of the ability of the colonoscopist to aspirate the residual fluid. In CTC however, PEG results in fluid filled segments, impeding full mucosal visibility, resulting in false negative diagnosis.

Prone supine imaging might overcome this problem in some way (Fig. 8.1), but is still insufficient to guarantee a complete colon evaluation (GRYSPEERDT et al. 2002).

Fluid tagging has been proposed to overcome the problem of drowned segments: the fluid can be tagged either by barium, iodinated contrast material, or a combination (LEFERE et al. 2002; ZALIS et al. 2003; PICKHARDT et al. 2003; PINEAU et al. 2003). As a result, the polyp can be detected as a hypodense structure in the tagged, hyperdense fluid levels (Fig. 8.2). Additionally, there is the possibility of electronic cleansing, removing the tagged fluid level, resulting in complete mucosal visibility (ZALIS et al. 2003; PICKHARDT et al. 2003).

Preparation without cathartic cleansing, so-called "dry preparation" is currently being evaluated as the ultimate reduced preparation, further improving patient compliance, and almost eliminating residual fluid (BIELEN et al. 2003; CALLSTROM et al. 2001; LEFERE et al. 2004; McFARLAND and ZALIS 2004; PICKHARDT et al. 2003; ZALIS et al. 2003).

8.2.1.2
Technical Artefacts

A major technical artefact is caused by suboptimal distended or even undistended segments, possibly hiding polyps.

Spasmolytic agents can be used to improve colonic distention.

There are two main spasmolytic agents: glucagon (a single chain polypeptide hormone that increases blood glucose and relaxes the smooth muscle of the gastrointestinal tract), and butylhyoscine (Buscopan) used in Europe and Asia to induce bowel hypotonia.

The rationale to use spasmolytic agents is a possible improved colonic distention, and reduced procedural pain.

Goei et al. (GOEI et al. 1995) found Buscopan to be more effective in distending the colon than glucagon, which is in agreement with the findings of both Yee et al. (YEE et al. 1999) and Morrin et al. (MORRIN et al. 2002) who found that colonic distention was not improved after glucagon administra-

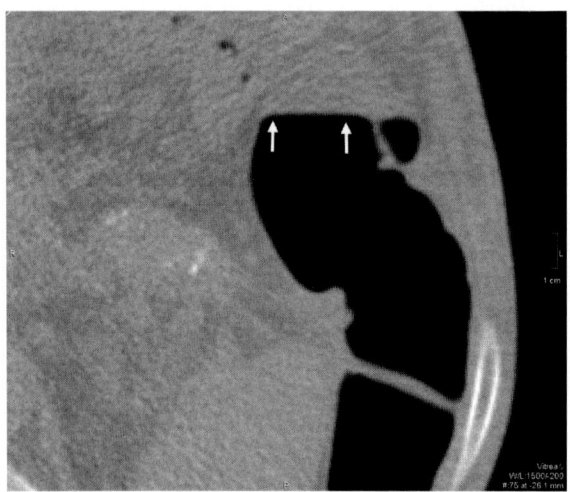 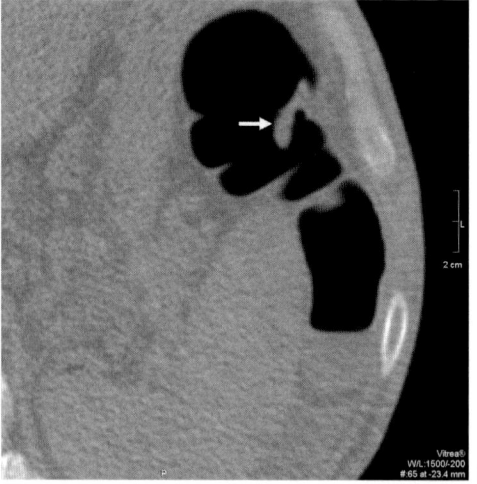

Fig. 8.1a,b. False negative diagnosis due to a non-tagged, fluid drowned segment: **a** prone image shows a fluid level (*arrows*), impeding visualisation of a stalked polyp; **b** the stalked polyp is clearly seen on the supine image (*arrow*). *Lesson:* Prone/supine imaging is useful to prevent false negative diagnosis in case of fluid filled segments

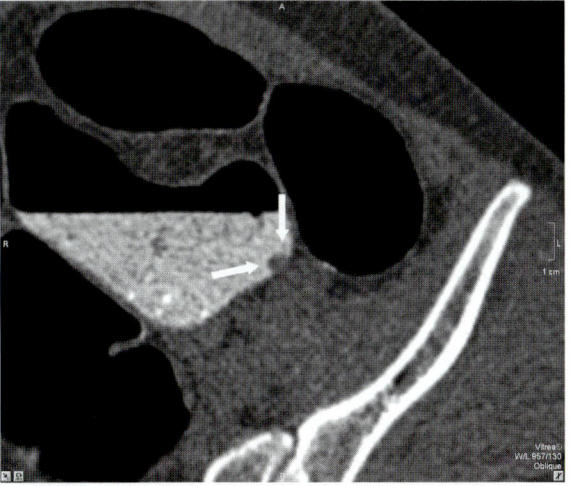
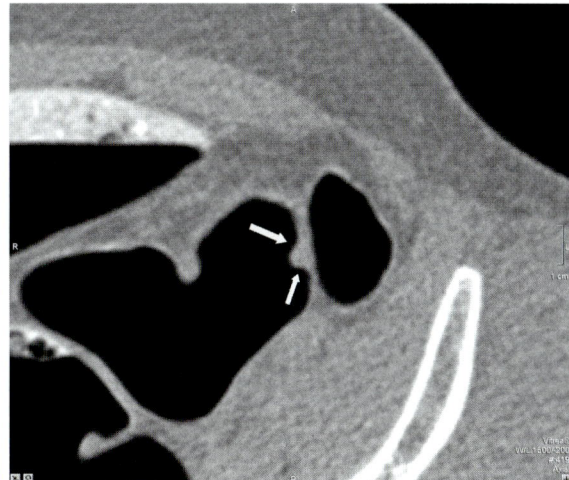
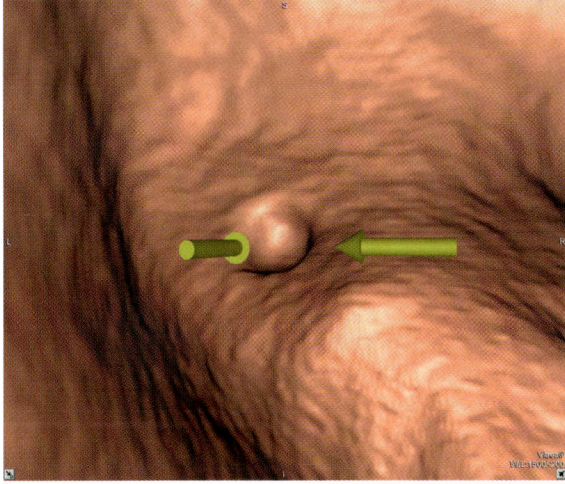

Fig. 8.2a–c. True positive diagnosis in a tagged, fluid drowned segment: a supine image shows a hypodense structure in a tagged, hyperdense fluid level (*arrows*), suspicious for a sessile polyp; b,c the presence of a 5-mm sessile polyp (*arrows*) is confirmed on prone (b) and endoluminal 3D image (c). *Lesson:* Fluid tagging can be used to overcome the problem of drowned segments: polyps can be detected as a hypodense structure in a tagged, hyperdense fluid level

tion. Therefore, the use of glucagon is abandoned at this moment.

Bruzzi et al. (Bruzzi et al. 2003) found that Buscopan should not be used routinely, but is useful in patients with diverticular disease. Taylor et al. (Taylor et al. 2003a) on the other hand found the effect of Buscopan also extends to those without diverticular disease.

Orally administered Buscopan has also proven useful during barium enema (Bova et al. 1999).

In our institution, we routinely use Buscopan: 10 mL diluted in 100 mL of 0.9% sodium chloride and administered intravenously at a rate of 10 mL/min.

The reason is the subjective impression of reduced procedural pain, and the fact that procedural spasm can mimick tumor (see below) or impedes adequate evaluation.

A persistent spasm can be differentiated from tumoral lesions by its smooth contours, and the absence of surrounding lymph nodes. In some instances, additional inflation might be necessary to solve the problem (see Sect. 8.3.2.2).

The problem of segmental collapse can also be solved by prone-supine imaging (Fig. 8.3).

8.2.1.3
Normal Anatomy and Areas of Danger

Normal anatomy may cause false negative diagnosis in that normal anatomical structures can hide polyps: thickened semilunar folds typical hide polyps in either antegrade or retrograde three-dimensional evaluation (Fig. 8.4). The same holds true for complex folds at the hepatic or splenic flexure, possibly hiding small polyps, impossible to detect using standard antegrade and retrograde three-dimensional views. To overcome the problems of inadequate visualisation of the colonic lumen,

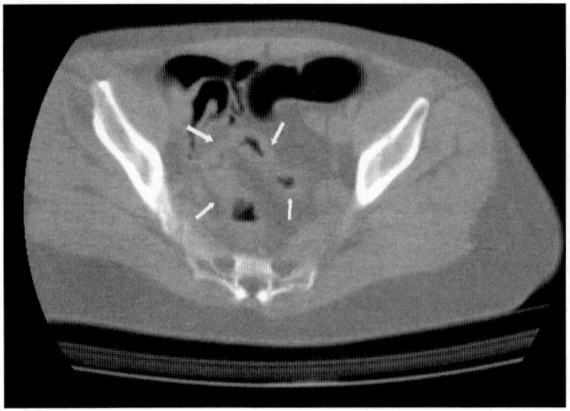
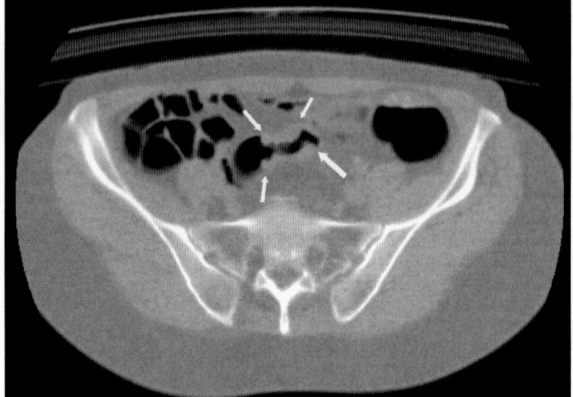
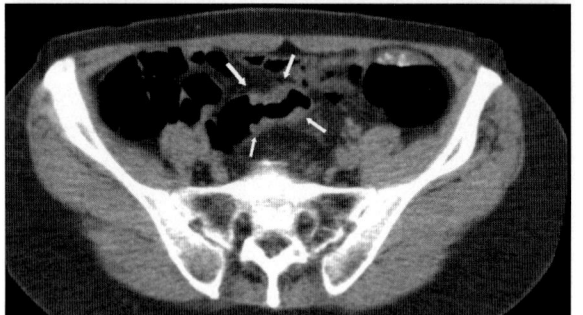

Fig. 8.3-c. False negative diagnosis due to incomplete distension: **a** supine image shows a suboptimal distended sigmoid (*arrows* in a); **b,c** prone image shows a good distension of the sigmoid, revealing the presence of a tumoral lesion (*arrows* in b). The tumoral lesion is better appreciated using abdominal window settings (*arrows* in c), compared to intermediate window settings (*arrows* in b). *Lesson:* Optimal distension is a prerequisite to detect colonic lesions. Optimal distension can be achieved by dual positioning and routine use of butylhyoscine (Buscopan)

different three-dimensional reconstruction methods have been developed, improving the detection of polyps on three-dimensional endoscopic views such as virtual colonic dissection or unfolded cube (HOPPE et al. 2004; VOS et al. 2003; LUO et al. 2004). Each of these different viewing modes aim to display the whole colonic lumen at one view, obviating the need of turning the virtual camera in different angles.

The cecum, hepatic flexure, transverse colon, splenic flexure, and sigmoid colon, are to be considered as "areas of danger" because of the convoluted and mobile nature.

The mobile nature of these segments mimicks positional change of lesions, possibly causing erroneous diagnosis of "mobile" residual stool (Fig. 8.5) (PARK et al. 2005).

Although the rectum is straight and not mobile, one has to take care of not missing rectal lesions. False negative diagnosis of rectal lesions may be caused by "readers fatigue" if one starts at the cecal level, or by rectal balloon catheter hiding rectal lesions (PICKHARDT and CHOI 2005) (Fig. 8.6).

The ileocecal valve is an important "mimicker" of pathology (see below), but one has to keep in mind that the ileocecal valve might hide polyps (Figs. 8.7 and 8.8), or can even be cancerous (Fig. 8.9). Cancers of the ileocecal valve should not be mistaken for lipomatous or papillary transformations. Different window settings are helpful in revealing the cancerous nature of the lesions.

8.2.1.4
Diverticular Disease

In case of diverticular disease, prominent semicircular folds, luminal narrowing and distortion impede good visualisation of the colonic surface resulting in difficult detection of polypoid lesions. In fact, as optimal detection of polyps is only achieved in well-distended segments of the colon, special care has to be taken when examining the involved segments with shortened haustrations and increased luminal tortuosity. In order not to interpret a polyp as a thickened fold, or vice versa, it is important to examine each semicircular fold by scrolling back and forth through the axial images. Imaging in both abdominal and lung window settings is mandatory to detect focal wall thickenings and luminal filling defects, respectively.(LEFERE et al. 2003) Frequent comparison between 2D and 3D images is recommended (MCFARLAND 2002) (Fig. 8.10).

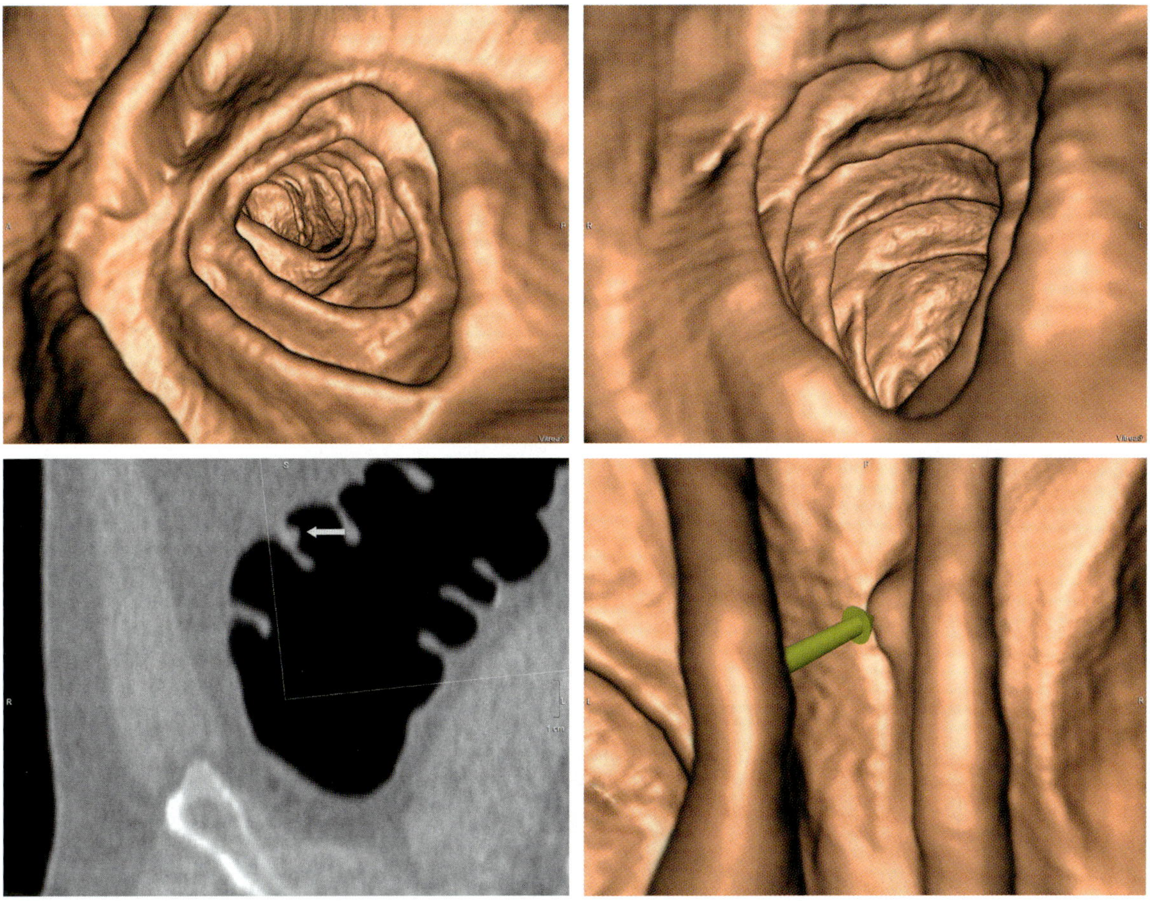

Fig. 8.4a–d. False negative diagnosis: small sessile lesions, located between haustral folds: **a,b** antegrade (a) and retrograde endoluminal views (b) show normal haustral folds in the ascending colon; c corresponding coronal MPR image shows a small sessile lesion, located between two haustral folds (*arrow*); **d** lateral endoluminal 3D image reveals the polyp, located between haustral folds.(*arrow*). *Lesson:* Primary 3D read should include different viewing angles, either by turning the virtual camera, either by using dedicated software, offering different three dimensional reconstruction methods, thus showing the whole colonic wall

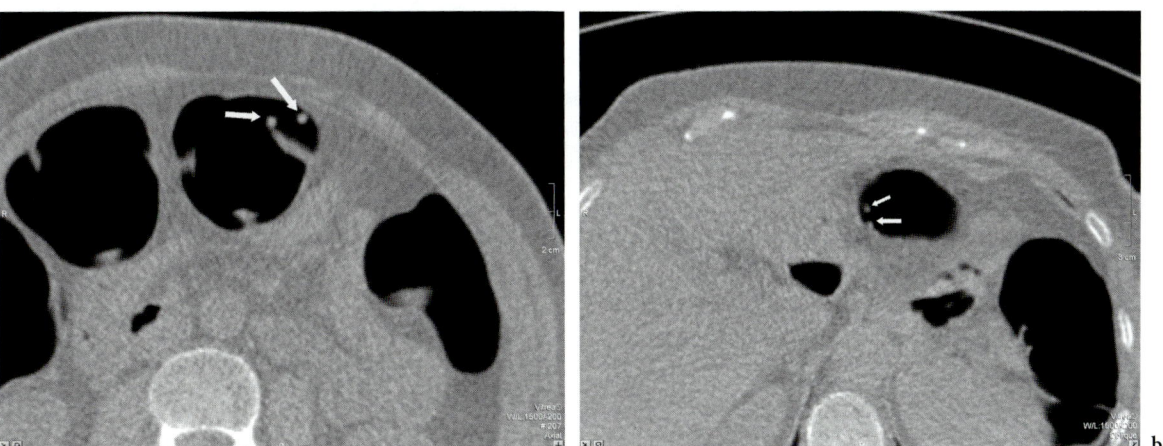

Fig. 8.5a,b. False negative diagnosis: polyps simulating fecal residue in mobile segments. Differential diagnosis of mobile stool or small sessile lesions in a mobile transverse colon: **a** supine scan shows two lesions in the transverse colon. (*arrows*); **b** prone scan shows the lesions in the transverse colon in an apparent different position (*arrows*). Conventional colonoscopy revealed the presence of two small sessile polyps. *Lesson:* Polyps, located in mobile colonic segments such as the transverse colon can cause erroneous diagnosis of "mobile" residual stool

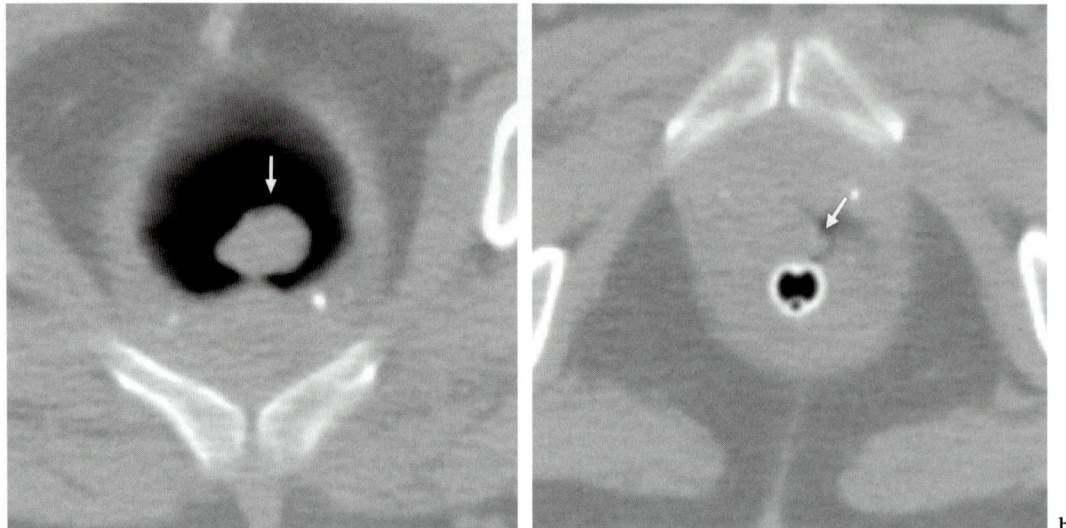

Fig. 8.6a,b. False negative diagnosis: rectal balloon catheter hiding rectal polyp: **a** prone scan after removing the rectal balloon clearly shows a large stalked polyp (*arrow*); **b** the polyp is hidden by the rectal balloon on supine image.(*arrow*). *Lesson:* Thick rectal balloon catheters can hide rectal lesions. Therefore, remove rectal balloon catheter on prone scan

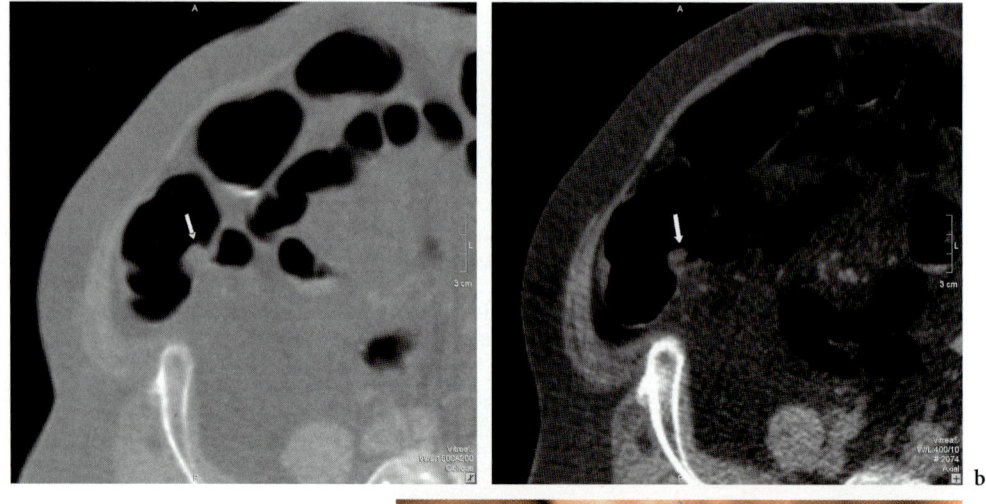

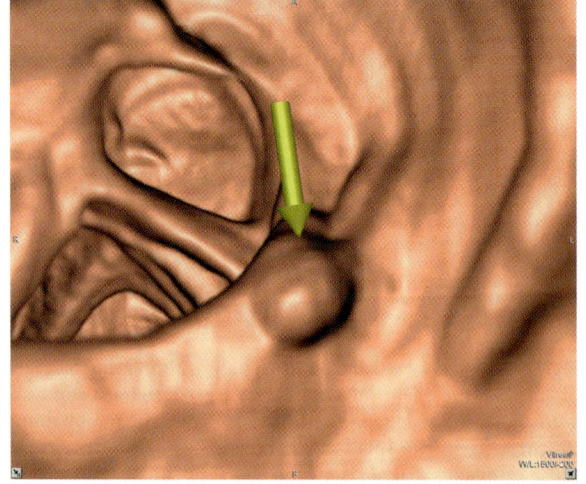

Fig. 8.7a–c. False negative diagnosis: differentiate small sessile polyps located on the ileocecal valve from normal variations of the ileocecal valve. Although the ileocecal valve is an important "mimicker" of pathology, one has to keep in mind that polyps can arise *on* the ileocecal valve (*arrows*). Evaluation in: **a** "intermediate" window setting as well as; **b** "abdominal window setting", combined with: **c** 3D endoluminal view are helpful to differentiate polyps from tumoral (see Fig. 8.9) or lipomatous transformation of the ileocecal valve (see Fig. 8.26). *Lesson:* For the evaluation of pathology of the ileocecal valve, always use different window settings, in combination with endoluminal 3D evaluation

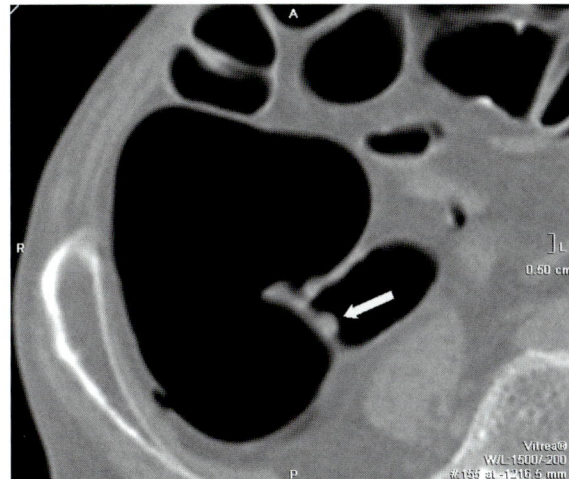

Fig. 8.8. Small sessile polyp located in the ileocecal valve. Although most polyps are located on the ileocecal valve, polyps can also arise *in* the ileocecal valve (*arrow*)

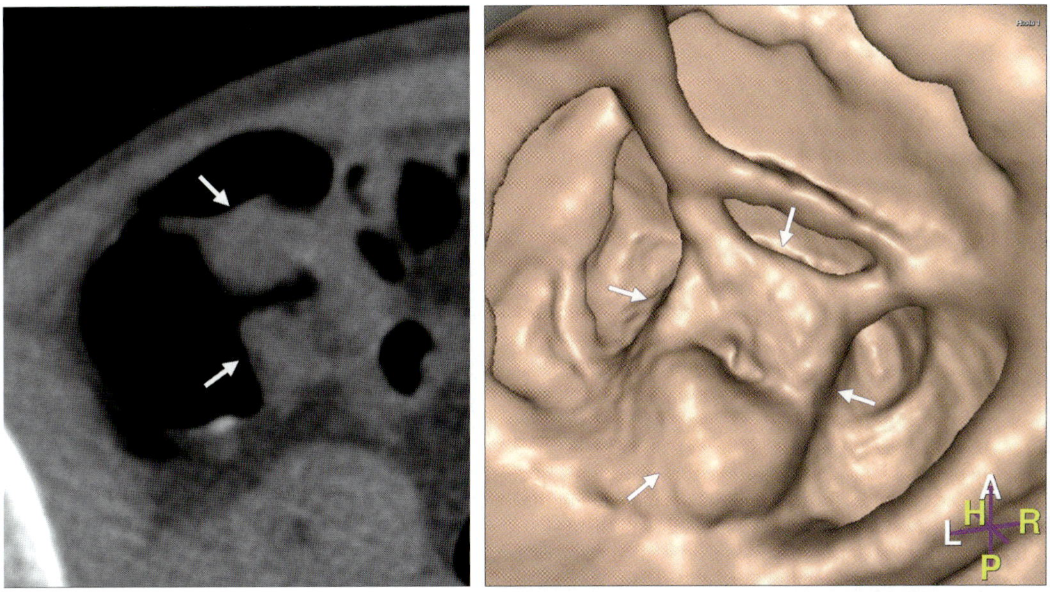

Fig. 8.9a–c. False negative diagnosis: patient with Crohns' disease: tumoral transformation of the ileocecal valve to be differentiated from lipomatous transformation of the valve: **a** axial 2D image shows a dense, extremely enlarged ileocecal valve on abdominal window settings (thus excluding the possibility of lipomatous transformation) (*arrows*); **b** a hypertrophic ileocecal valve is also seen on endoluminal 3D images (*arrows*); **c** corresponding conventional colonoscopic image shows tumoral transformation of the ileocecal valve.(*arrows*). *Lesson:* In case of an extremely enlarged and dense ileocecal valve, keep in mind the possibility of tumoral transformation, to be differentiated from papillary transformation or lipomatous infiltration of the ileocecal valve. (Fig. 8.27). Abdominal window settings are helpful in excluding the possibility of lipomatous transformation of the ileocecal valve

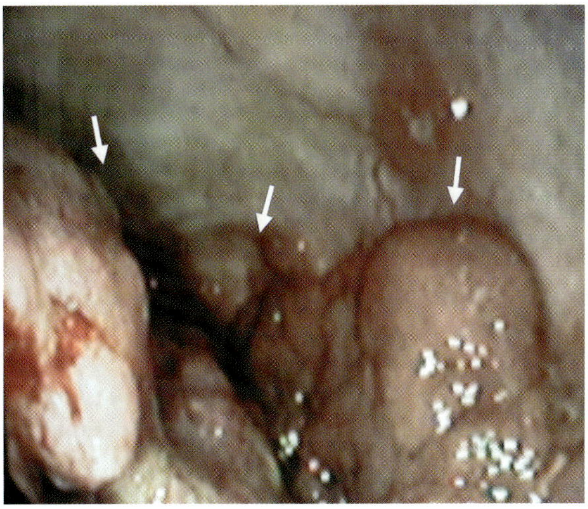

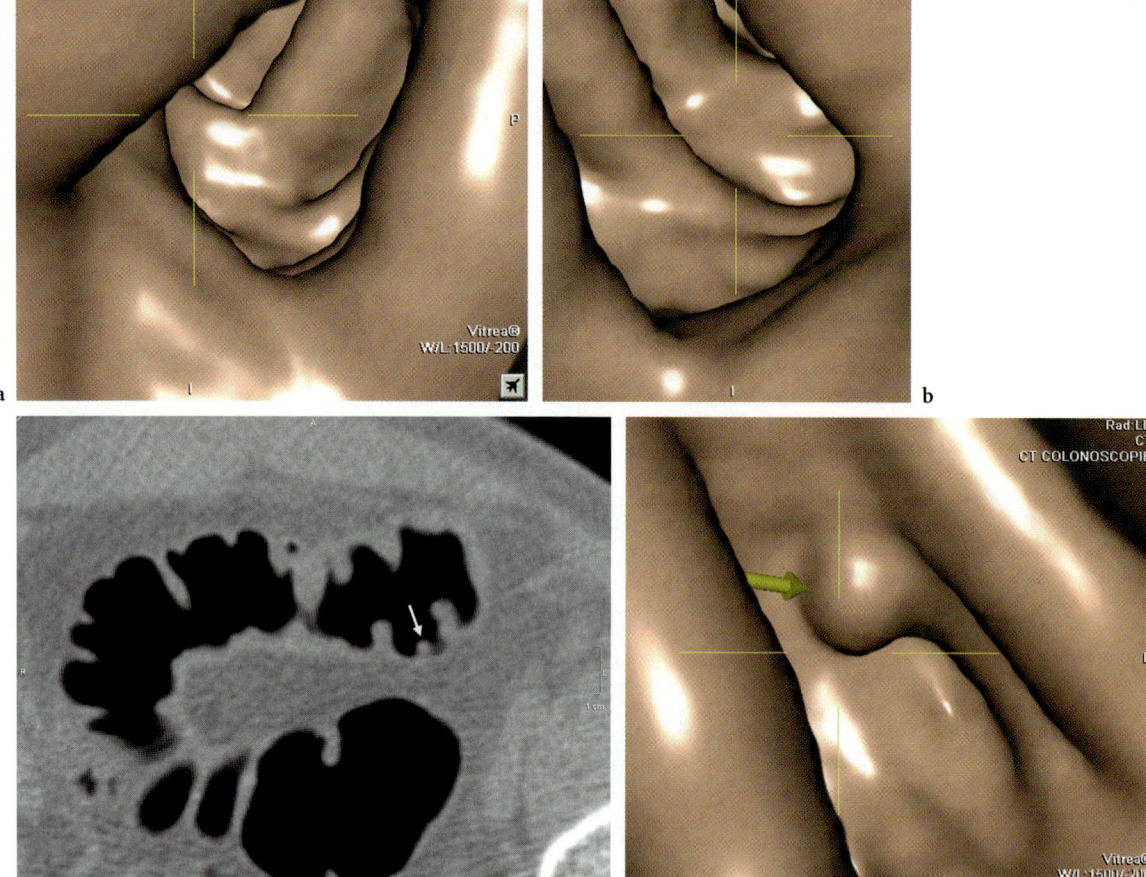

Fig. 8.10a–d. False negative diagnosis: thickened folds in diverticular disease, hiding a small sessile polyp. Diverticular disease is characterised by thickened semilunar folds. The luminal narrowing and the thickened semilunar folds make primary three dimensional evaluation extremely difficult: **a,b** there is a normal antegrade (a) and retrograde view (b) of the narrow lumen with thickened folds in a patient with diverticular disease; **c** corresponding axial 2D image shows a small polyp, interspaced between two thickened semilunar folds. (*arrow*); **d** tailored endoluminal 3D image shows the small polyps (*arrow*) interspaced between thickened haustral folds. *Lesson:* In case of diverticular disease, frequent comparison between 2D and 3D images is necessary, in order not to miss small polyps, interspaced between thickened haustral folds

8.2.1.5
Sessile Polyps

Although sessile polyps have a high conspicuity, if located between folds (Fig. 8.11), those lesions may remain undetected in case the lesions are located on a semilunar fold (Fig. 8.12).

A thickened fold in an otherwise well distended colon might therefore point to the correct diagnosis of a sessile polyp on a haustral fold (FIDLER et al. 2004) (see also Fig. 8.18).

8.2.1.6
Small Lesions and Small Flat Lesions

Park et al. (PARK et al. 2005) found that for the lesions that were not detected for reasons not apparent on retrospective analysis, size of the lesion was the only significant factor associated with lesion detectability. Lesions 5 mm or smaller are more difficult to visualize than those 6 mm or larger. Up to 50% or more of those lesions smaller than 5mm are, however, non-adenomatous, and the need to detect

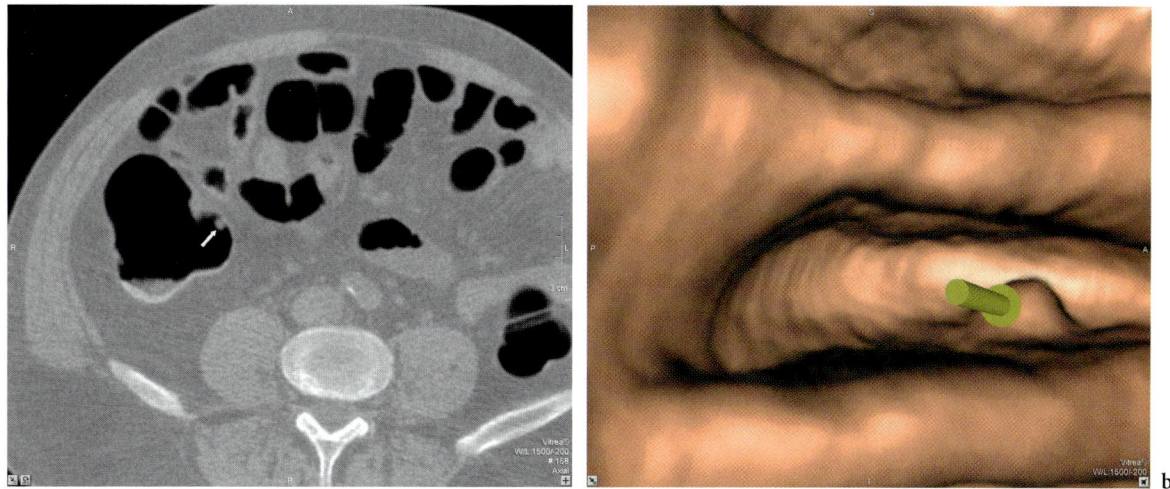

Fig. 8.11a,b. Sessile polyp located between a haustral fold. Polyps located *between* normal haustral folds are easy to detect on: **a** axial 2D image (*arrow*), and; **b** corresponding endoluminal 3D image (*arrow*)

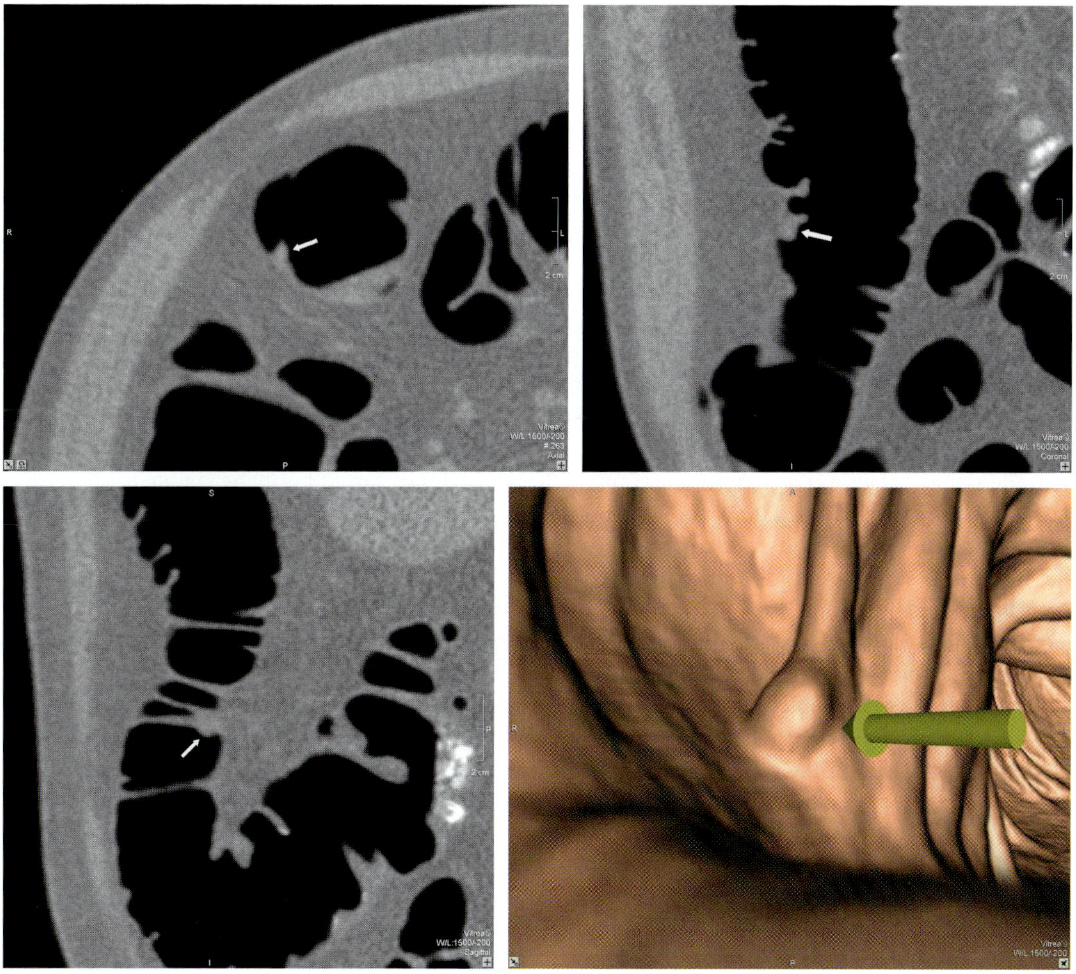

Fig. 8.12a-d. False negative diagnosis : sessile polyp located on a haustral fold. Polyps located *on* a haustral fold are difficult to detect on: **a** axial 2D images (arrow); **b** sagittal 2D images; **c** coronal 2D images, showing a thickened haustral fold in an otherwise well distended segment; **d** corresponding endoluminal 3D image nicely shows a polyp *on* a haustral fold (*arrow*). *Lesson*: A thickened haustral fold in an otherwise well-distended segment is suspicious for a polyp <u>on</u> a haustral fold

those lesions is therefore questionable (Macari et al. 2004; Pickhardt et al. 2004a).

Flat lesions are defined as lesions with a height less than half the lesion diameter (Dachman and Zalis 2004). This definition includes a wide range of flat lesions, including small as well as large lesions.

Small flat lesions will be missed, even on retrospective analysis, for the same reason as small sessile lesions: small lesions are just more difficult to visualise (Macari et al. 2003) (Fig. 8.13).

Larger flat lesions may also cause false negative diagnosis, because of failure to correctly characterise the lesion (see 8.2.2.2).

8.2.2
Failure to Characterise the Lesions

8.2.2.1
Annular Stricturing Lesions

Annular structuring lesions may be misinterpreted as either spasm (Figs. 8.14 and 8.15) or residual fecal material. The use of fecal tagging with an oral contrast agent (Thomeer et al. 2003; Zalis et al. 2003; Pickhardt et al. 2005) seems to help in avoiding interpretive errors caused by residual fecal material.

8.2.2.2
Larger Flat Lesions

Flat lesions can be divided into flat adenomas, flat depressed adenomas, plaque-like carcinomas and carpet lesions (Galdino and Yee 2003).

As discussed, small flat lesions are difficult to detect for the same reason as small sessile lesions: detection is hampered by resolution.

Larger flat lesions however are also difficult to detect and to characterize for several reasons.

First of all, there is the problem of insufficient awareness and familiarity with those lesions: surveillance programs, based on the known adenomacarcinoma sessile or pedunculated lesion, have mainly focused on identifying sessile of pedunculated polyps. This explains why flat lesions are frequently characterised as normal folds. As a rule, a thickened fold in an otherwise well distended colon should raise the question whether or not this lesion could represent a flat lesion.

Second, the plaque-like morphology is likely to be mistaken for residual fecal material (Park et al. 2005): the use of oral contrast media may therefore help in detecting flat lesions. Third, the size and morphology of the lesions explain the necessity of different window settings (Dachman et al. 2004; Fidler et al. 2002): detection of flat lesions is improved by using abdominal window settings, rather than the routinely used intermediate window settings (Fig. 8.16). The necessity to change window settings also explains the low conspicuity of flat lesions, even the larger ones.

Reviewing the literature shows two different morphological characteristics for flat lesions.

If the lesions are located between haustral folds, they appear as a small flat protuberance; if they are located on haustral folds, or near haustral folds, they are associated with minimal fold irregularity; if they arise from a haustral fold, they project into the lumen, creating a cigar-like appearance.

Optimal bowel preparation and distention are therefore prerequisites to detect flat lesions.

Flat adenomas measuring 6 mm or greater are, however, uncommon in a typical Western screening population, and advanced neoplasms are rare. Flat lesions should therefore not be considered a significant drawback for virtual colonoscopy screening (Pickhardt et al. 2004b).

8.2.2.3
Small Sessile Polyps

Small sessile polyps frequently represent hyperplastic polyps. Hyperplastic lesions tend to flatten out in well distended segments, explaining the fact that those lesions might only be visible in somewhat underdistended segments. In that way, those lesions are frequently only recognised on either prone or supine position, and can therefore be mistaken as residual stool.

Hyperplastic lesions however are not to be considered precancerous, and should therefore be considered as "leave-alone" lesions. Misinterpreting those lesions as residual stool is therefore rather beneficial for the patients, avoiding unnecessary conventional colonoscopy (Pickhardt et al. 2004a) (Fig. 8.17).

8.2.2.4
Sessile Cancers

Sessile cancers, if detected, may remain unrecognised by the fact that the lesions are characterised as normal fold; correlating axial 3D images with endoluminal views is helpful in this respect (Fig. 8.18).

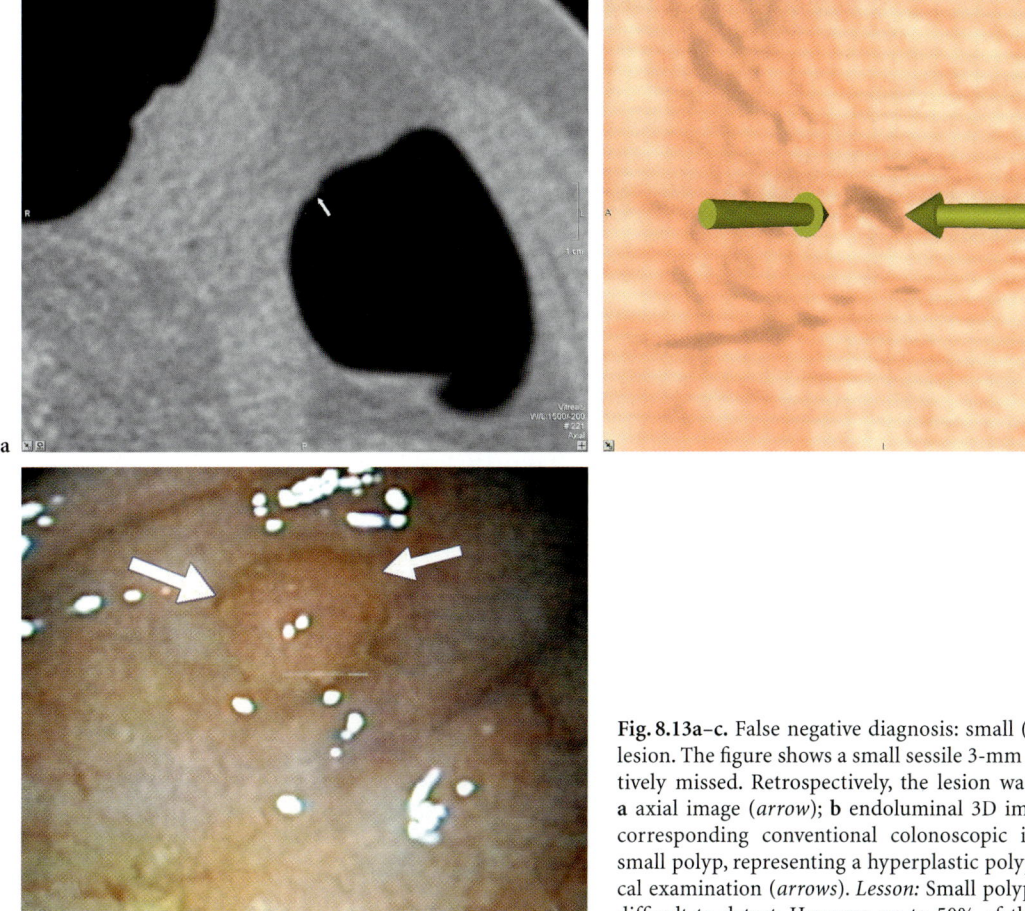

Fig. 8.13a–c. False negative diagnosis: small (<5 mm) sessile lesion. The figure shows a small sessile 3-mm polyp, prospectively missed. Retrospectively, the lesion was identified on: **a** axial image (*arrow*); **b** endoluminal 3D image (*arrows*); **c** corresponding conventional colonoscopic image shows a small polyp, representing a hyperplastic polyp on pathological examination (*arrows*). *Lesson:* Small polyps (<5 mm) are difficult to detect. However, up to 50% of those lesions are non-adenomatous, and the necessity to detect those lesions is therefore questionable

Fig. 8.14a,b. False positive diagnosis: spasm mimicking annular structuring lesion. Spasm can closely resemble annular stricturing lesions (see Fig. 15): **a** a non-distended sigmoid region (*arrow*) in prone position; **b** corresponding supine image shows a normal sigmoid

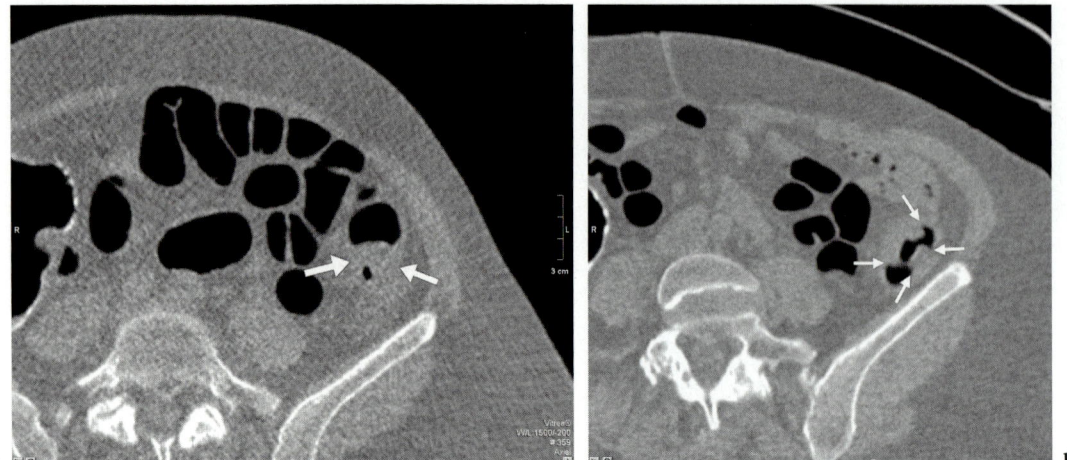

Fig. 8.15a,b. False negative diagnosis – failure to characterise lesions: annular structuring lesions compared to spasm: **a** a non-distended sigmoid region (*arrow*) in supine position; **b** corresponding prone images shows a persistent wall thickening with shoulder forming (*arrows*). Conventional colonoscopy showed a tumoral lesion. *Lesson*: Annular structuring lesions can closely resemble spasm. Dual positioning is mandatory to avoid those pitfalls (compare Figs. 14 and 15)

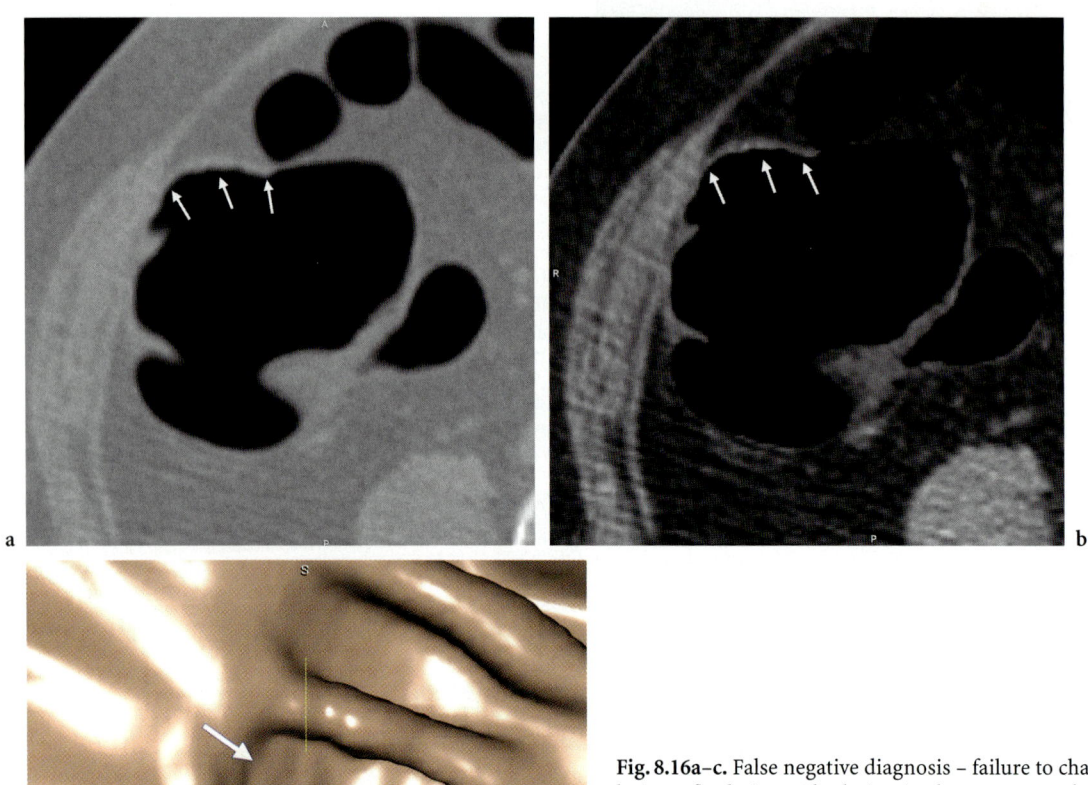

Fig. 8.16a–c. False negative diagnosis – failure to characterise lesions: flat lesions. Flat lesion in the caecum at the level of the ileocecal valve: **a,b** axial image at the level of the ileocecal valve shows subtle wall thickening on intermediate window settings (*arrows* in a), better appreciated on abdominal window settings (*arrows* in b); **c** 3D endo-view image shows subtle wall thickening (*arrows*). Pathology showed a tubular adenoma. *Lesson:* Flat lesions have been defined as lesions with a height less than half the lesion diameter. This nature makes them difficult to recognize. As in this patient, changing the window settings is helpful in diagnosing these lesions

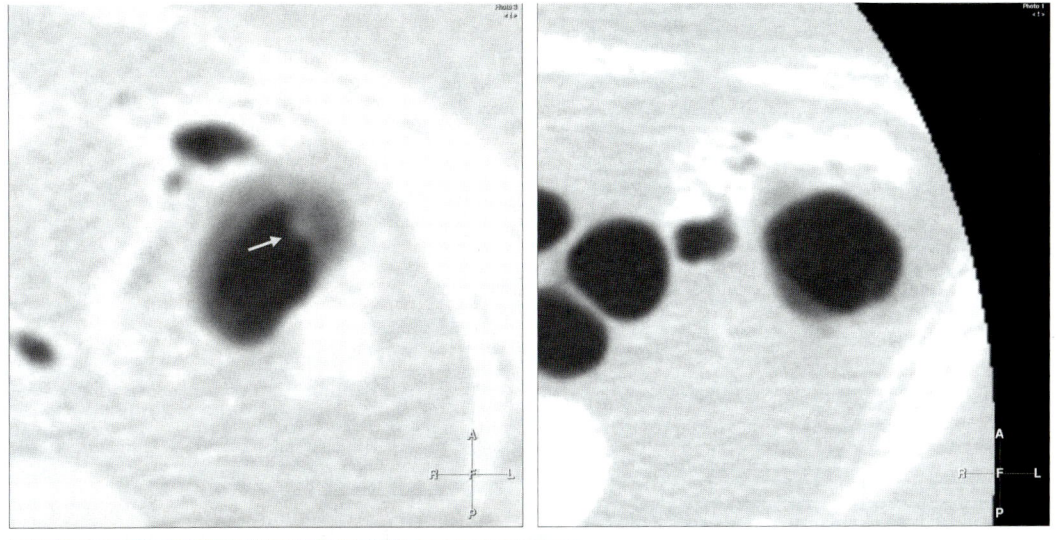

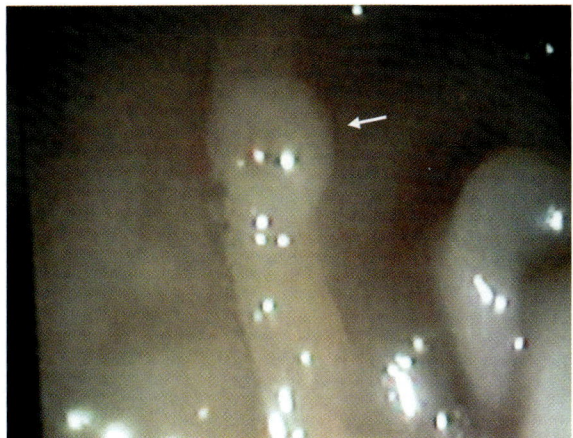

Fig. 8.17a–c. False negative diagnosis – failure to characterise lesions: hyperplastic lesions: a axial, supine 2D image shows a small polyp-like lesion (*arrow*) in a suboptimal distended segment; b corresponding prone scan shows a better distended descending colon, and does not show the lesion anymore. Differential diagnosis was made between hyperplastic polyp and fecal residue; c corresponding conventional colonoscopy reveals a small hyperplastic polyp. *Lesson:* Hyperplastic lesions tend to flatten out in well-distended segments, impeding visualisation in prone or supine position. Therefore, they are frequently misinterpreted as mobile fecal residue

Sessile cancers may also be mistaken for residual stool because of marked surface irregularity, usually attributed to residual stool (GLUECKER et al. 2004).

8.2.2.5
Pedunculated Lesions

Pedunculated lesions may remain undetected because of mischaracterisation as fecal residues or even residual fluid.

Mischaracterisation as fecal residues is caused by the fact that there are three observations that are made to distinguish stool from polyps: presence of gas, morphology (polyps and small cancers have rounded and lobulated smooth borders), and the mobility. In particular, the mobility of the lesions is used in favour of residual stool, analogue to the findings on double contrast barium enema (LAKS et al. 2004).

Pedunculated polyps however change in position between prone and supine images, and may moreover include gas between the stalk and the bowel wall, mimicking residual stool (Fig. 8.19).

A pedunculated polyp can also mimic residual fluid (Fig. 8.20).

8.3
False Positive Diagnosis

8.3.1
Preparation Related False Positive Findings

One of the major reasons why virtual colonoscopy is attractive to the patients is its ability to evaluate the colon without the need for an intensive colon cleansing regimen. Different reduced preparations have been evaluated: reduced amount of PEG in

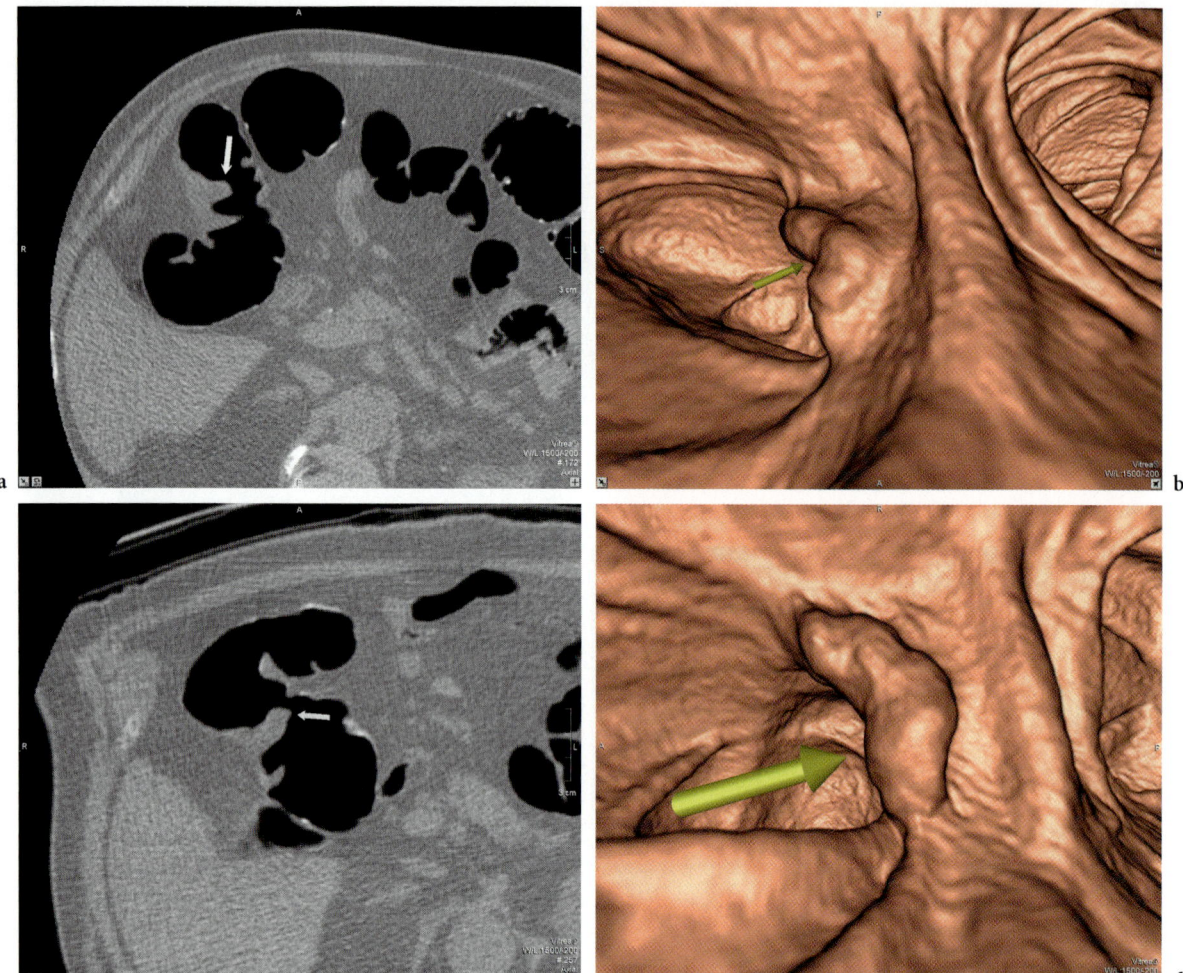

Fig. 8.18a–d. False negative diagnosis – failure to characterise the lesions: sessile cancer: **a,c** broad based thickened haustral fold on supine (*arrows* in a) and prone image (*arrows* in c) at the hepatic flexure. Differential diagnosis: complex haustral fold, normal thickened fold or sessile cancer; **b,d** corresponding endoluminal 3D images show distorted and thickened haustral fold on supine (*arrow* in b) as well as prone scan (*arrow* in d). Conventional colonoscopy showed a flat sessile cancer. *Lesson:* Endoluminal 3D images are useful to differentiate normal thickened folds from sessile cancers. (compare with Fig. 8.29)

combination with bisacodyl, magnesium carbonate with citric acid (Citramag, Pharmaserve LTD, Manchester, UK), a combination of sodium picosulphate with magnesium citrate (Picolax, Ferring Pharmaceuticals Ltd, Berkshire, UK), magnesium citrate combined with bisacodyl tablets and suppository (Losoprep, EZ-EM, Westbury, NY), fleet phosphosoda (YEE 2002; TAYLOR et al. 2003a, b; GRYSPEERDT et al. 2002; MACARI et al. 2001).

Compared to standard colon cleansing regimens, each of these reduced preparations showed fewer side effects and disturbances to daily patients life, while inviting improved patient compliance.

The driest preparations Picolax (TAYLOR et al. 2003a, b), Losoprep (LEFERE et al. 2002) and fleet phosphosoda (MACARI et al. 2001), however, are associated with more retained residue, with subsequent increased risk of false positive findings. False positive findings are mainly related to small fecal residue: larger residues will shift between prone and supine imaging, while smaller residues stick to the wall.

Therefore, there is the need for fecal tagging: fecal tagging reduces false positive diagnosis (LEFERE et al. 2002; GRYSPEERDT et al. 2002) (Figs. 8.21–8.23).

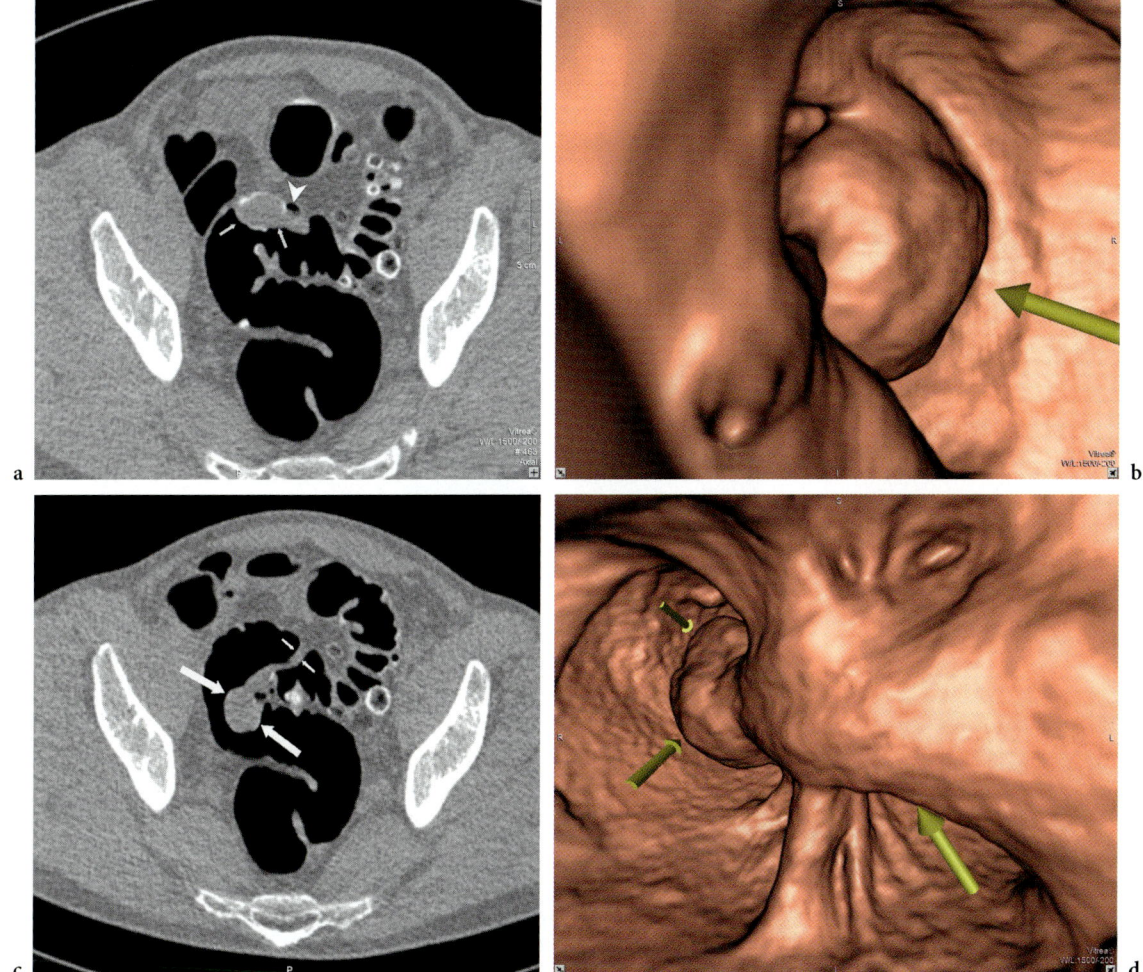

Fig. 8.19a–d. False negative diagnosis – failure to characterise the lesions: pedunculated lesions mimicking residual stool: **a** prone image shows a nodular mass (*arrows*), with air included in the mass (*arrowhead* in a); **b** corresponding endoluminal 3D image shows a nodular lesion (*arrow* in b); **c** supine image shows the lesion is highly mobile (*large arrows*), and suggests the presence of a stalk (*small arrows*); **d** the supine-endoluminal image, clearly shows a pedunculated lesion (*arrows*)

8.3.2
Technical Artefacts Causing False Positive Findings

8.3.2.1
Breathing Artefacts

Most published studies using single slice CT have used a collimation of 3–5 mm and a pitch of 1–2, resulting in breath hold times ranging from 35 to 50 s. Such long breath hold periods were prone to breathing artefacts, simulating polyps. The introduction of multislice CT technology now permits thinner collimation (1–2.5 mm), and reduced breath hold time (15–20 s) (Embleton et al. 2003; Taylor et al. 2003c, d). These reduced breath hold times virtually eliminate severe artefacts. If patients are still unable to maintain a breath hold, left decubitus scanning has been shown a valuable alternative to prone scanning, reducing breathing artefacts if used as the second scan (Gryspeerdt et al. 2004) (Fig. 8.24).

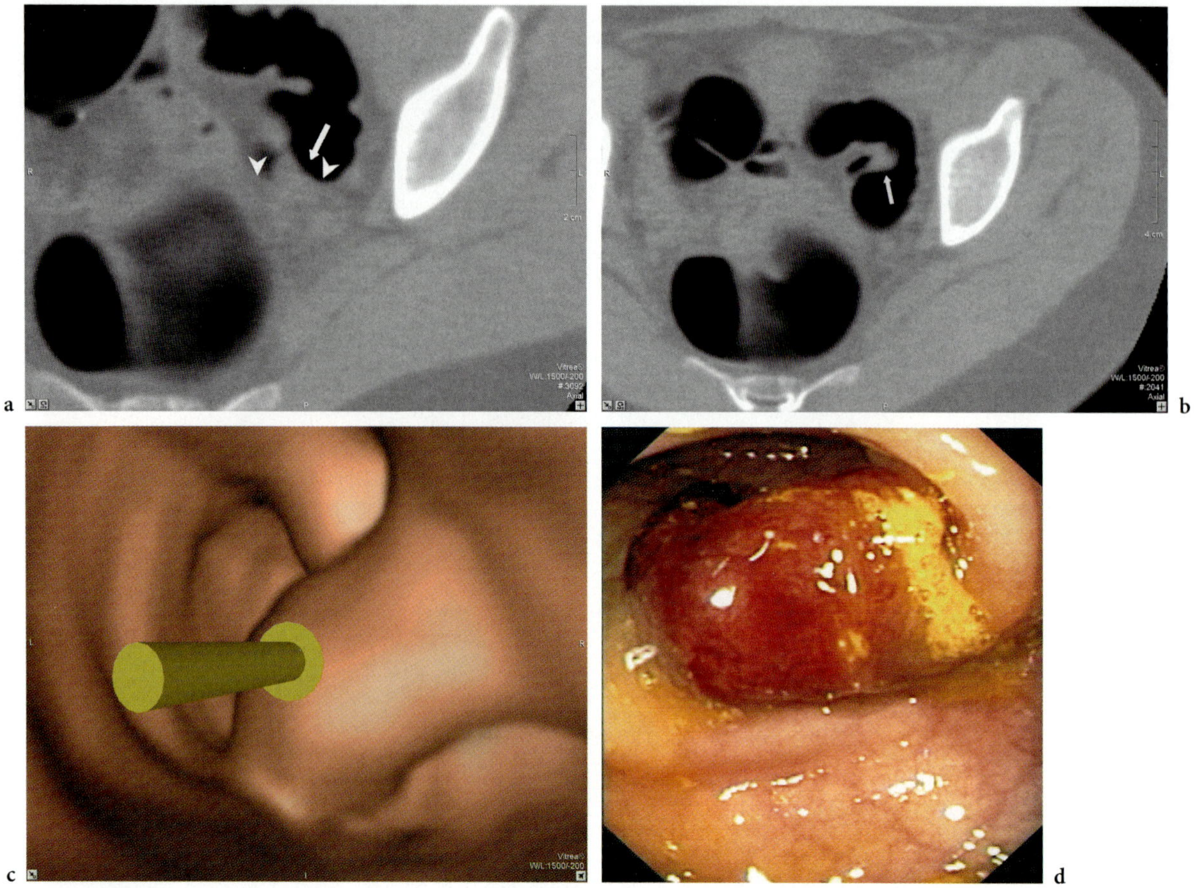

Fig. 8.20a–d. False negative diagnosis – failure to characterise the lesions: pedunculated lesions mimicking residual fluid: **a** supine image shows a thick haustral fold (*arrow*) and suggests the presence of a fluid level.(*arrowheads*); **b–d** corresponding axial (b) and endoluminal 3D image (c) in prone position shows the stalk of a pedunculated lesion (*arrows* in b–d), proven on conventional colonoscopy (d). *Lesson:* Pedunculated lesions may mimick fecal residues (they can include air, due to their stalked nature, and are highly mobile) or fluid levels. Identifying the stalk on 3D endoluminal images points to the diagnosis of a pedunculated lesion

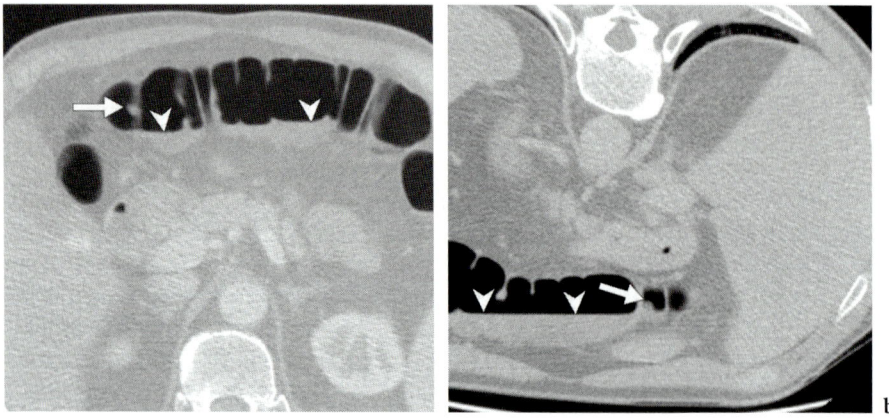

Fig. 8.21a,b. False positive diagnosis: adherent fecal residue. Fecal tagging to facilitate differential diagnosis between fecal residue and polyp. Standard colonoscopic cleansing: false positive diagnosis of polyp due to adherent fecal residue: **a** supine image and; **b** prone image in a patient with incomplete visualisation of the cecum due to redundancy suggested the presence of a 10-mm polypoied lesion in the transverse colon (*arrows* in a and b). Since the transverse colon was reached on repeated conventional colonoscopy, and no lesion was detected, this lesion was interpreted as false positive due to adherent fecal residue. *Arrowheads* in a and b: non-tagged fluid levels, adherent to standard colonoscopic preparation

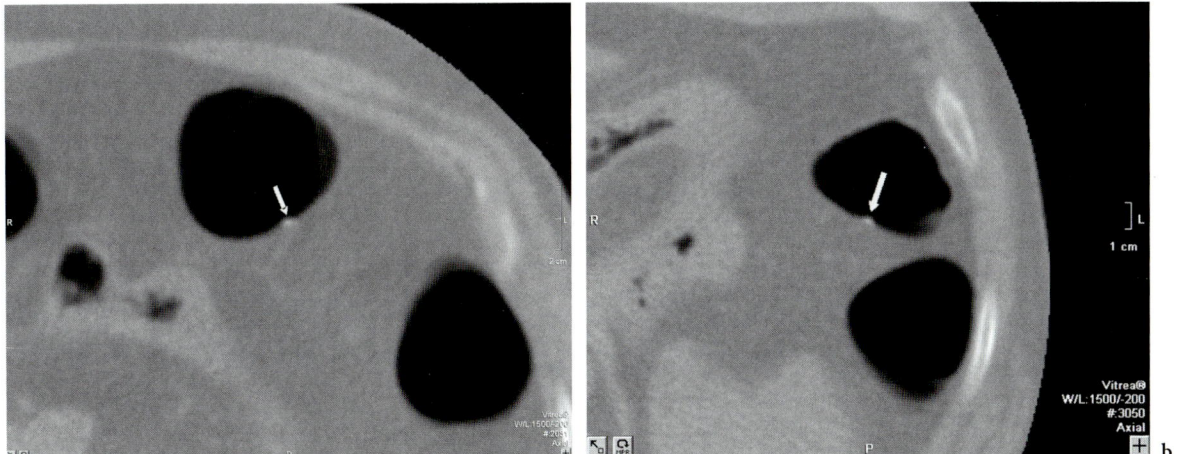

Fig. 8.22a,b. False positive diagnosis: adherent fecal residue. Fecal tagging to facilitate differential diagnosis between fecal residue and polyp.(cont'd). Reduced preparation with fecal tagging using barium as the sole tagging agent. There is a 4-mm lesion on: **a** supine image (*arrow*) and; **b** prone image (*arrow*). The lesion is hyperdense, pointing towards a tagged fecal residue. Conventional colonoscopy did not show any lesions in this patient

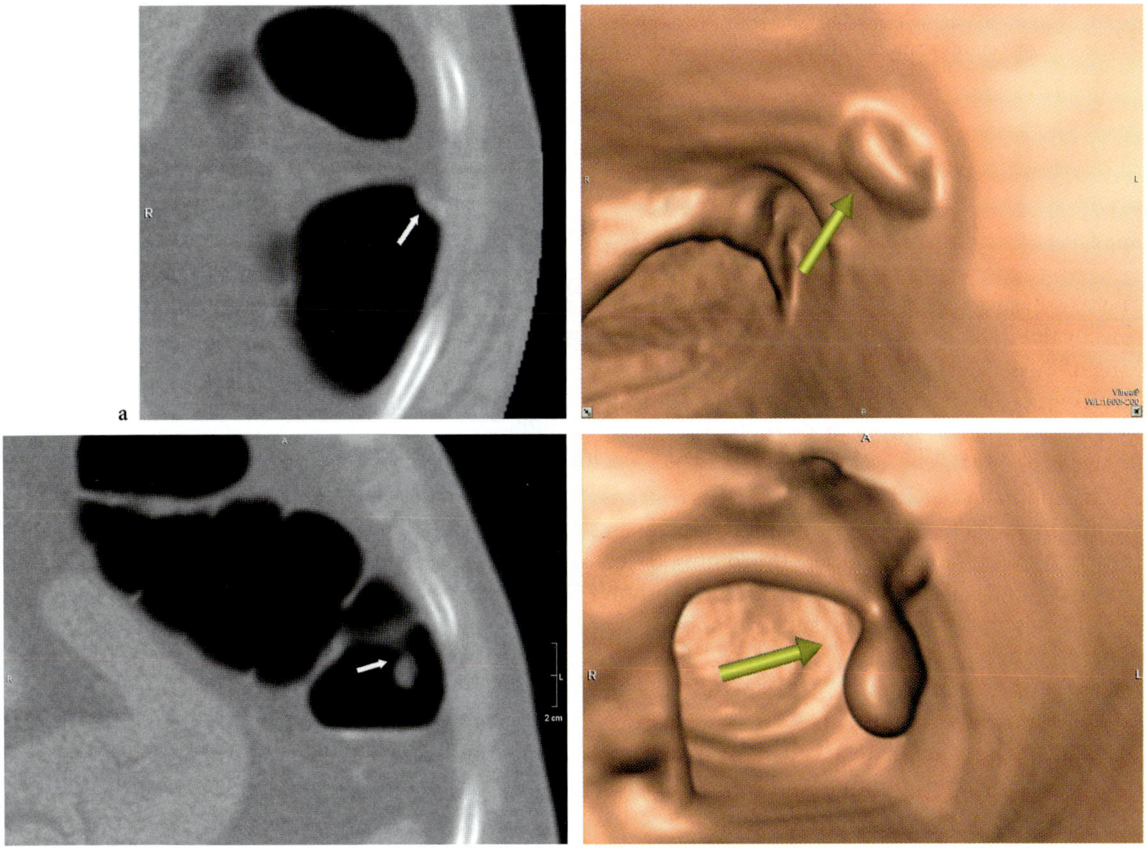

Fig. 8.23a–d. False positive diagnosis: adherent fecal residue. Fecal tagging to facilitate differential diagnosis between fecal residue and polyp (cont'd). Reduced preparation with fecal tagging using barium as the sole tagging agent: **a,b** axial (a) and endoluminal (b) 3D image in prone position: There is a 6-mm non-tagged lesion at the splenic flexure (*arrows*). The non-tagged nature suggests the presence of a polyp; **c,d** correpsonding axial (c) and endoluminal (d) 3D image in supine position. The non-tagged lesion, seen on prone image corresponds to a pedunculated polyp (*arrows*). *Lesson*: Fecal tagging reduces false positive findings due to adherent fecal residue, improves conspicuity of polyps and reduces false positives since the tagged or non-tagged nature of the lesions allows easy differentiation between polyps and fecal residues

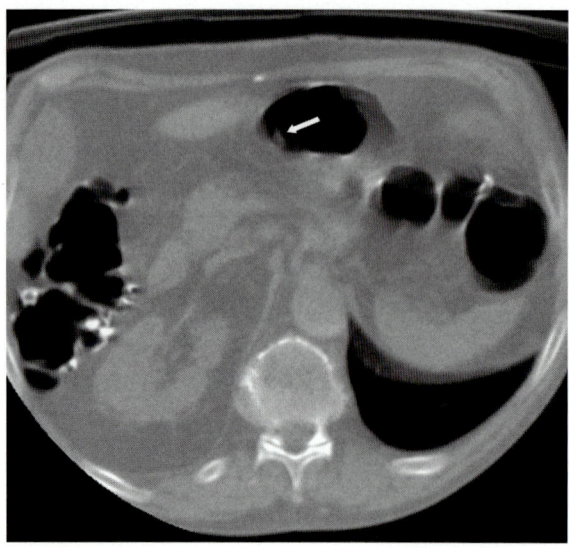 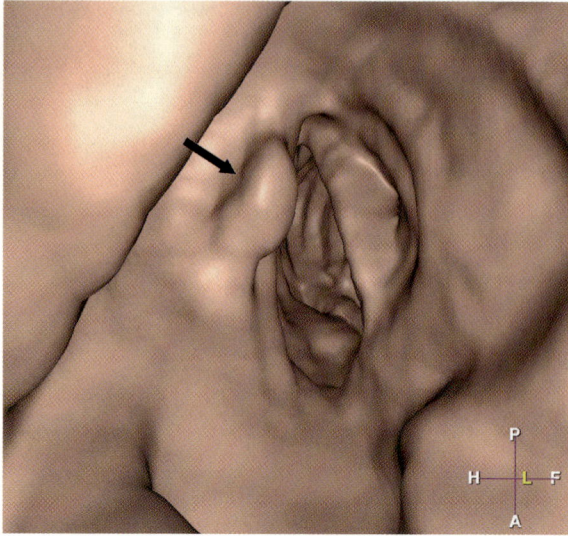

Fig. 8.24a,b. False positive diagnosis: pseudopolyp due to breathing artefacts: **a** axial 2D image obtained in a 66-years-old patient in prone position shows breathing artefacts (*arrow*); **b** corresponding endoluminal 3D image shows pseudopolypoied appearance of the colonic wall, caused by breathing artefact (*arrow*). *Lesson:* In patients who are extremely short of breath, especially prone scanning can be hampered by breathing artefacts, causing pseudo-polypoid appearance on endoluminal 3D images. Left/decubitus scanning instead of prone scanning can be used as an alternative

8.3.2.2
Spasm

There are seven different sphincters (concentric rings; valves), distributed throughout the colon: (1) Ring of Busi, (2) Ring of Hirsh, (3) Ring of Cannon, (4) Ring of Payr-Strauss, (5) Ring of Balli, (6) Ring of Moultier, (7) Ring of Rossi (Reeders and Rosenbush 1994).

The sphincters of Rossi, Balli, and Payr-Strauss are involved in nerve reflexes; the sphincters of Hirsch, Moultier, and Busi are a thickening of longitudinal and circular muscle fibers. Cannon's sphincter is an overlap of the superior and inferior mesenteric nerve plexuses.

Persistent spasm of each of these sfincters can produce tumor-like lesions.

Each of these sphincters can cause persistent spasms, mimicking tumoral disease. To reduce those spasm, butylhyoscine (Buscopan) is used as discussed previously.

Besides the routine use of Buscopan, dual position imaging is also useful, as well as additional inflation in case of doubt (Fig. 8.25).

Spasm can be differentiated from tumoral pathology, based upon the smooth contours of the spasms, in contradiction with circumferential tumors. The presence of surrounding lymph nodes also points towards tumoral pathology.

8.3.3
Pitfalls Related to Normal Anatomy and Non-Tumoral Lesions

8.3.3.1
Ileocecal Valve

The ileocecal valve is located between the large and small bowel, and consists of two segments, the upper and lower lips. The ileocecal valve can appear as a thin slit-like structure, a large intraluminal mass, or is almost invisible. There are three different endoscopic appearances: the labial type, with a slit-like appearance, the papillary type, with a dome shaped appearance, and lipomatous type, with deposits of fat within the lips.

Most visible valves are of the labial type (78%), 21% is of the papillary type and 3% is lipomatous.

Lipomatous and papillary ileocecal valves can mimick neoplasms, and should be differentiated from polyps on the ileocecal valves (Fig. 8.26).

Prolapsing ileocecal valves appear prominent, irrespective of the labial or papillary morphology,

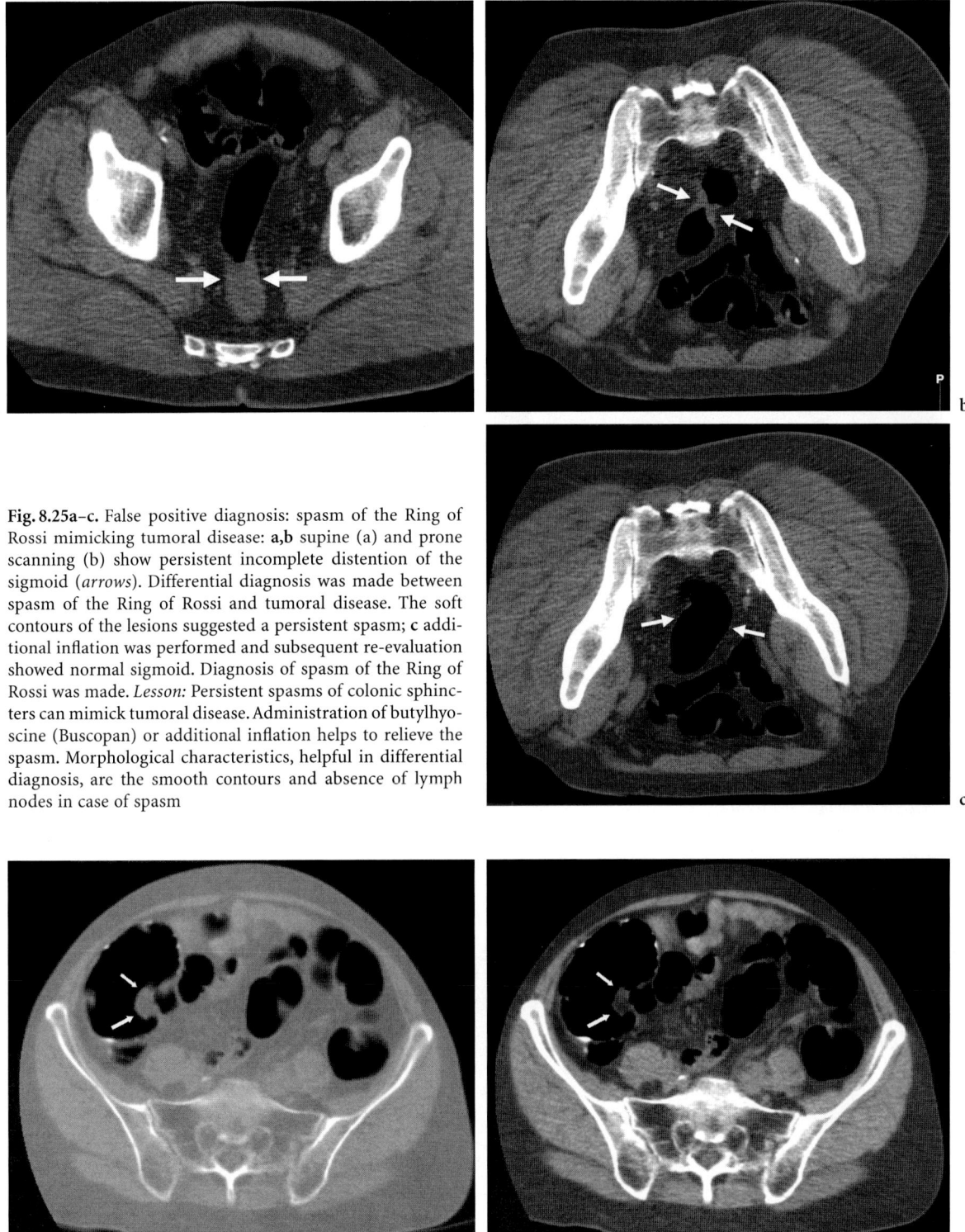

Fig. 8.25a–c. False positive diagnosis: spasm of the Ring of Rossi mimicking tumoral disease: **a,b** supine (a) and prone scanning (b) show persistent incomplete distention of the sigmoid (*arrows*). Differential diagnosis was made between spasm of the Ring of Rossi and tumoral disease. The soft contours of the lesions suggested a persistent spasm; **c** additional inflation was performed and subsequent re-evaluation showed normal sigmoid. Diagnosis of spasm of the Ring of Rossi was made. *Lesson:* Persistent spasms of colonic sphincters can mimick tumoral disease. Administration of butylhyoscine (Buscopan) or additional inflation helps to relieve the spasm. Morphological characteristics, helpful in differential diagnosis, are the smooth contours and absence of lymph nodes in case of spasm

Fig. 8.26a,b. False positive diagnosis: lipomatous transformation of the ileocecal valve: **a** supine image in intermediate window settings shows a hypertrophic nodular ileocecal valve. Differential diagnosis: tumor – lipomatous or papillary transformation of the ileocecal valve; **b** same image as a – abdominal window setting clearly shows the lipomatous transformation of the ileocecal valve. *Lesson:* Lipomatous transformation is a "pseudotumoral" alteration of the ileocecal valve. Use different window settings to reveal the lipomatous nature of the valve. Compare with Figures 8.7, 8.8, and 8.9

and may mimick polyps (Fig. 8.27) (REGGE et al. 2005).

8.3.3.2
Extrinsic Impression

Any organ or structure outside the colon can cause external impression. They compress the colon and may appear as focal neoplasms on 3D endoluminal images. We have noted impressions from the spleen, liver, other bowel loops, spine, psoas muscle, aorta and iliac arteries, as well as uterine fibroids (Fig. 8.28) (MACARI and MEGIBOW 2001).

8.3.3.3
Complex or Thickened Folds

Complex or thickened folds are typically encountered at the splenic and hepatic flexures. Axial CT images might raise the possibility of intraluminal soft tissue masses or tumoral thickened folds. Endoluminal views are frequently helpful in identifying

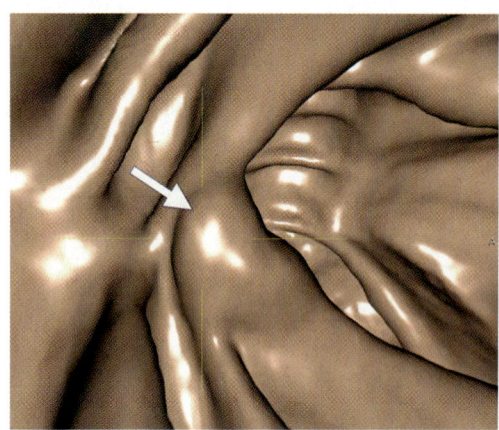 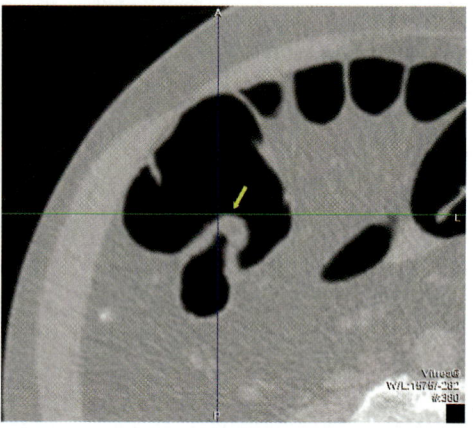

Fig. 8.27a,b. False positive diagnosis: prolapsing ileocecal valve: **a** endoluminal 3D image shows a nodular appearance of the ileocecal valve (*arrow*); **b** corresponding axial image shows that the polypoid appearance is caused by a prolapsing ileocecal valve. *Lesson:* A prolapsing ileocecal valve mimics polypoid pathology on endoluminal 3D image. Comparing with axial 2D correctly points to the diagnosis

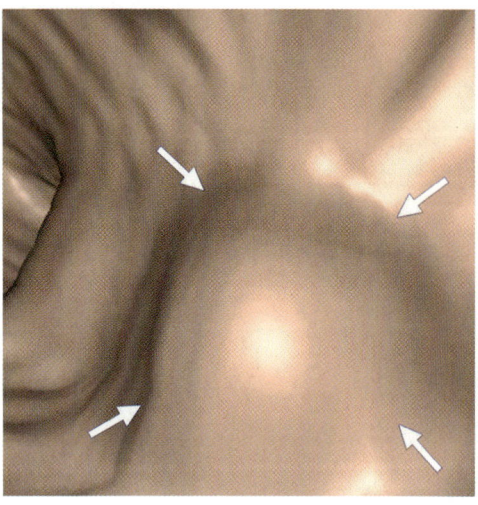 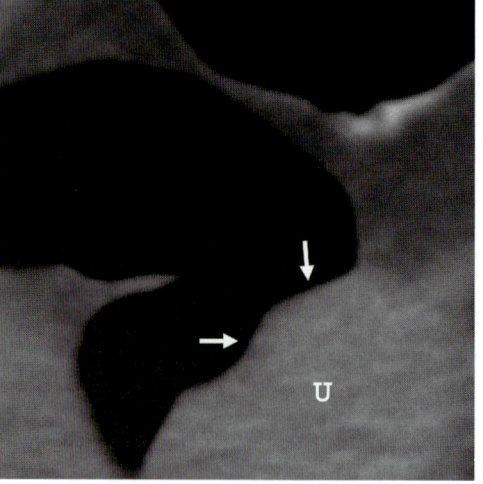

Fig. 8.28a,b. False positive diagnosis: external impression: **a** endoluminal 3D image shows a smoothly delineated nodule in the sigmoid (*arrows*); **b** corresponding axial image shows the nodule is caused by extrinsic uterine impression (*arrows*; *U:* uterus). *Lesson:* Any organ or structure outside the colon can cause external compression. On endoluminal view, these extrinsic impressions simulate tumoral or polypoid disease. Careful correlation of endoluminal 3D image with axial images points towards the diagnosis of external impression

the mass as a complex pattern of normal haustral folds. Endoluminal imaging is also extremely helpful in showing the smooth contours of complex normal folds, as opposed to the irregularity caused by tumoral pathology (Fig. 8.29, compare with Fig. 8.18).

8.3.3.4
Lipoma

Lipomas are rare, but well-recognized "tumors" of the colon. They are more common in the right colon than the left colon. They arise from the submucosa, and may protrude into the lumen as either polypoied or nodular tumor-like lesions. Diagnosis of their lipomatous nature can easily be made by viewing the "tumor" in abdominal window settings (PICKHARDT 2004) (Fig. 8.30).

8.3.3.5
Vascular Lesions

Colonic varices are a complication of portal hypertention, and can be seen in the ano-rectal region, as well as throughout the whole colon. Varices are typically smoothly delineated linear lesions. Identification of afferent venous structures points towards the diagnosis (Fig. 8.31).

Hemorrhoids can be tiny or extremely large, mimicking tumoral pathology. They typically appear as linear, smoothly delineated mucosal irregularities proximal to the ano-rectal margin (Figs. 8.32 and 8.33).

8.3.3.6
Appendiceal Orifice

The normal appearance of appendiceal orifice is a slit-like orifice (Fig. 8.34). The appendiceal orifice can however also protrude, simulating polypoid disease (Fig. 8.35). In case of previous appendectomy, the appendiceal stump can also simulate polypoid disease. The anatomical location, clearly illustrated on coronal or sagital reformats, points to the diagnosis (TAYLOR et al. 2003c).

8.3.3.7
Scar after Polypectomy

After polypectomy, the colonic wall remains edematous, simulating flat or polypoied lesions on virtual CT colonoscopy. Knowledge of the patients history avoids this false positive diagnosis (Fig. 8.36).

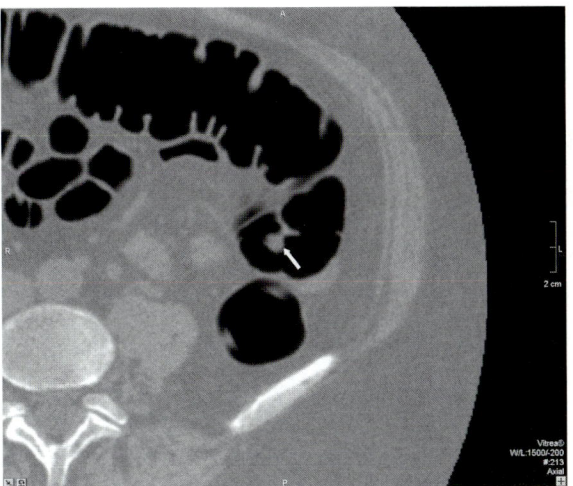
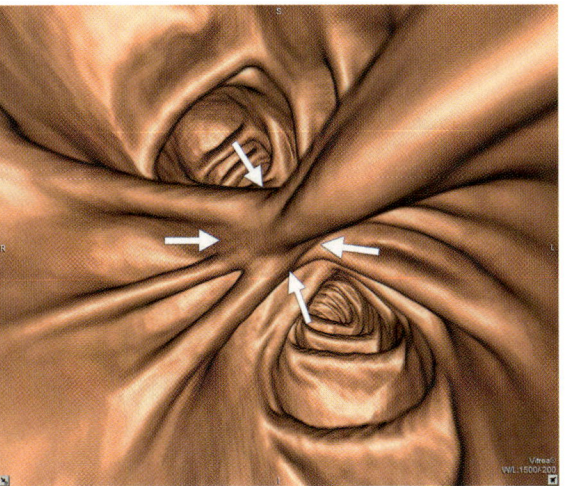

Fig. 8.29a,b. False positive diagnosis: complex folds: **a** axial image shows the splenic flexure, with a thickened nodular-like fold (*arrow*); **b** corresponding endoluminal 3D image clearly shows that the thickened nodular appearance is to be explained by the complexity of the folds at the splenic flexure. *Lesson:* Complex or thickened folds are typically encountered at the splenic and hepatic flexures, and should be differentiated from sessile cancers or polyps. Endoluminal 3D images are extremely helpful for differential diagnosis. Compare with Fig. 8.18

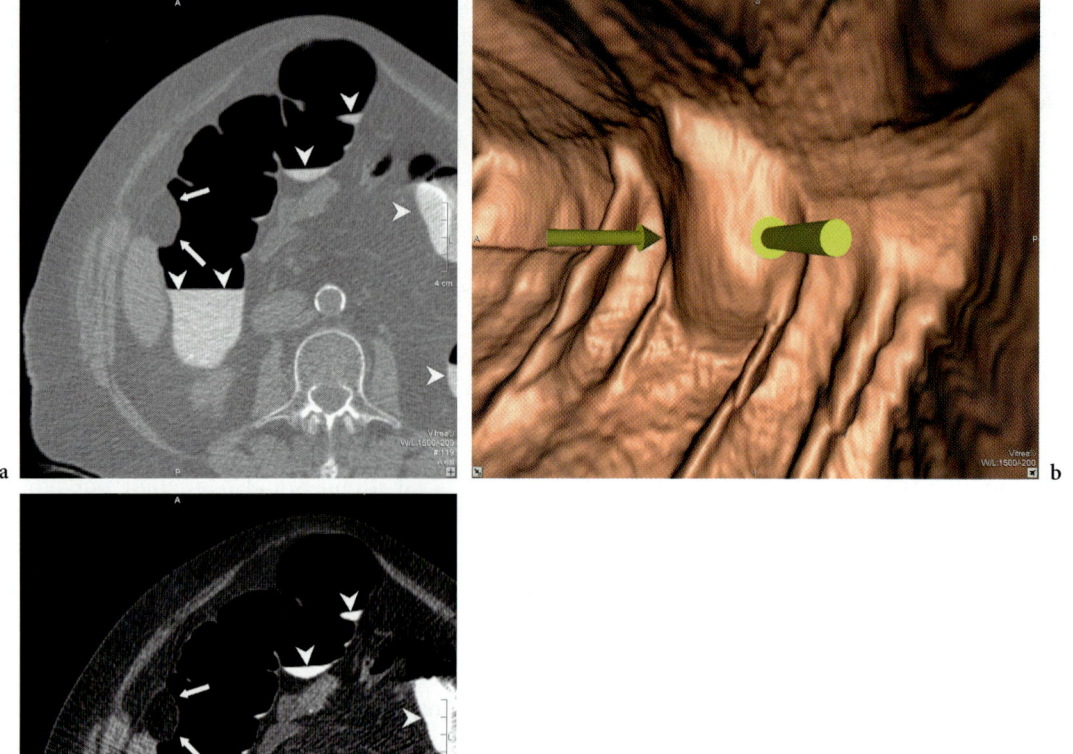

Fig. 8.30a–c. False positive diagnosis: lipoma: **a,b** axial image (a; intermediate window settings) and endoluminal 3D image (b) show a nodular distortion of the colonic wall at the hepatic flexure (*arrows*); **c** corresponding axial image using abdominal window settings shows the lipomatous nature of this lesion. Diagnosis: lipoma. Note: *arrowheads* point towards tagged fluid levels. *Lesson:* Lipomas are submucosal lesions, that are to be considered as "leave-alone" lesions. Correct diagnosis can easily be made by viewing the "tumor" in abdominal window settings

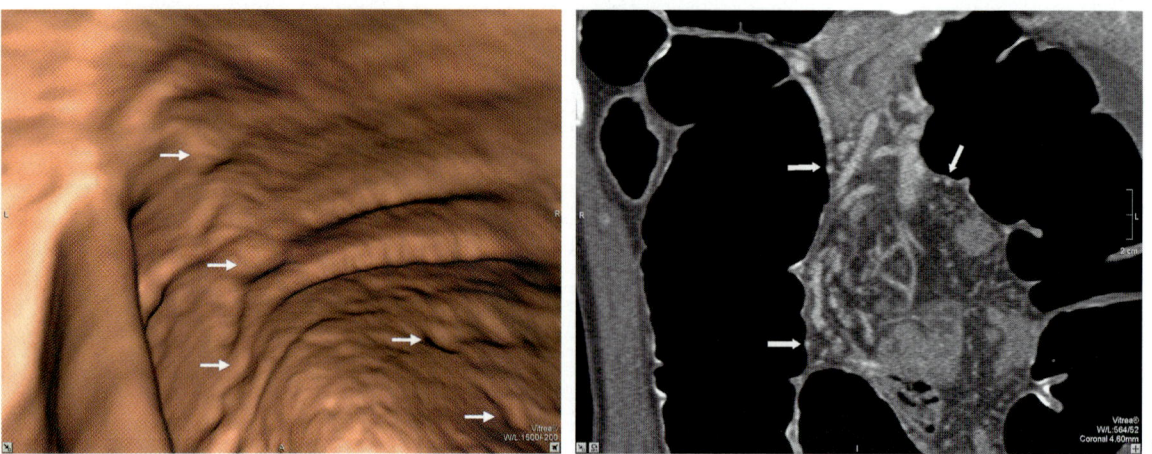

Fig. 8.31a,b. False positive diagnosis: submucosal vascular lesions: **a** endoluminal 3D image in a patient with severe portal hypertention shows multiple tiny polyp-like lesions, distributed throughout the colon. (*arrows*); **b** corresponding contrast enhanced coronal reformatted MPR image shows multiple submucosal veins, explaining the polyp-like lesions on endoluminal 3D images (*arrows*). *Lesson:* In patients with known portal hypertension, think about possible submucosal colonic varices, explaining multiple tiny nodular lesions on endoluminal 3D imaging. Identification of afferent venous structures points towards the diagnosis

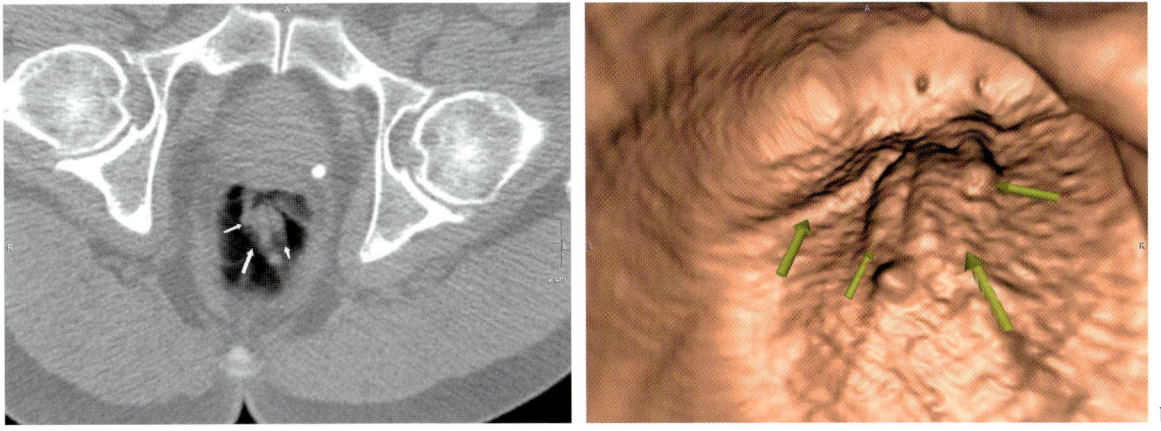

Fig. 8.32a,b. False positive diagnosis: internal haemorrhoids: **a** axial image shows irregular, linear structures at the anorectal region (*arrows*); **b** corresponding endoluminal 3D image shows linear, smoothly delineated structures at the anorectal junction. (*arrows*)

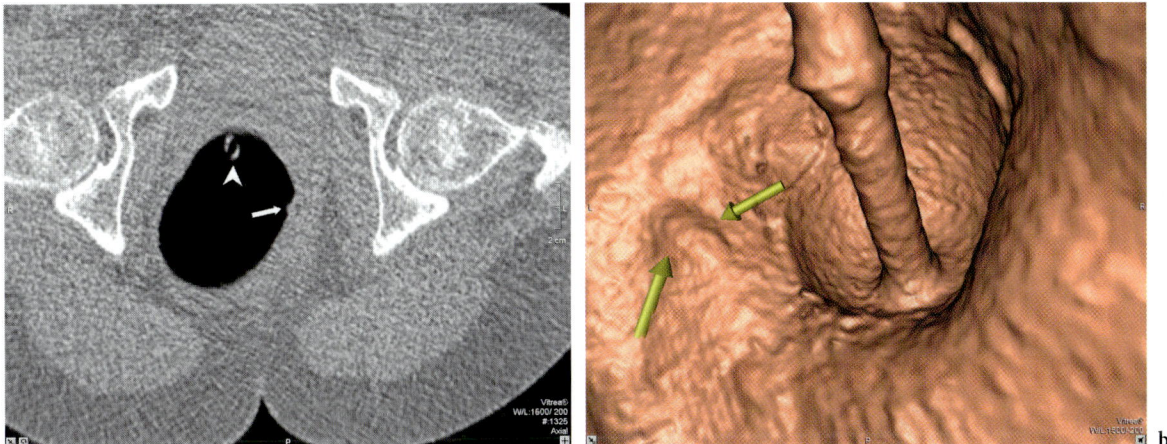

Fig. 8.33a,b. False positive diagnosis: internal haemorrhoids. (cont'd) (note: different patient from Fig. 32): **a** axial image shows a small polyp-like nodule in the anorectal region. (*arrow*). *Arrowhead*: thin rectal tube; **b** corresponding endoluminal 3D image shows a linear, smoothly delineated lesion nearby the anorectal region. (*arrows*). Diagnosis: internal hemorrhoids. *Lesson*: Internal hemorrhoids may mimic polypoid disease. Imaging features pointing towards the diagnosis are the location nearby the anorectal margin, and the tubular-like, smoothly delineated nature on endoluminal 3D images

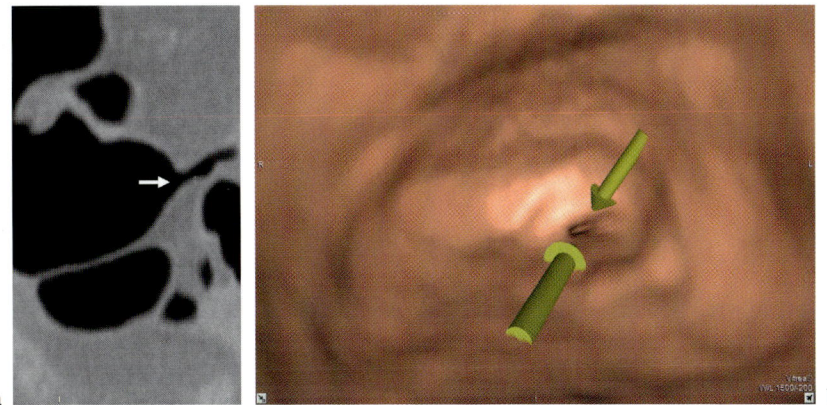

Fig. 8.34a,b. Normal appendiceal orifice. Curved reformatted MPR image shows normal appendiceal orifice (*arrow* in a), appearing as a slit-like orifice on endoluminal 3D images (*arrows* in b)

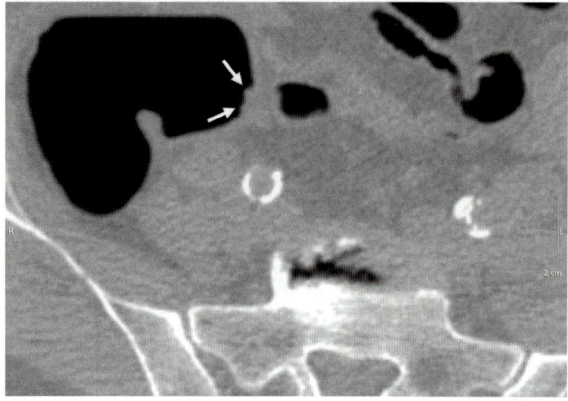 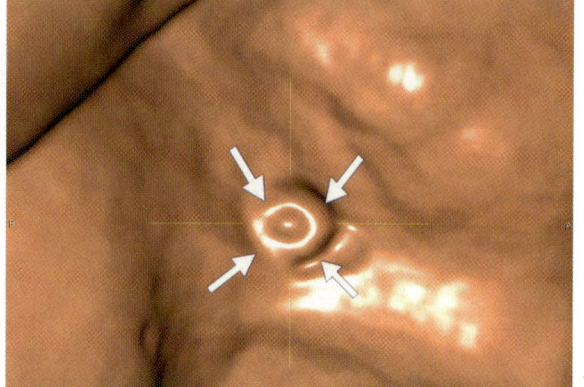

Fig. 8.35a,b. Prolapsing appendiceal orifice, causing false positive diagnosis: **a** axial image at the level of the appendiceal orifice shows a nodular-like lesion (*arrows*); **b** corresponding endoluminal 3D image shows a prolapsing appendiceal orifice (*arrows*). Before making the diagnosis of a polyp in the caecum, closely correlate the lesion with the anatomical landmarks to exclude prolapsing appendiceal orifice or ileal prolapse (Figs. 27 and 35)

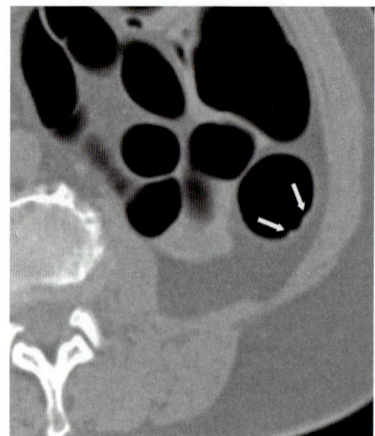 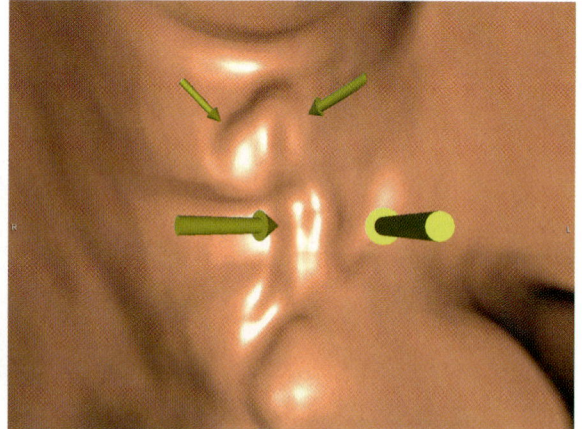

Fig. 8.36a,b. False positive diagnosis: scar after polypectomy: **a** axial image shows a focal mucosal thickening in the descending colon (*arrows*); **b** corresponding endoluminal 3D image confirms the presence of a mucosal lesion, suggesting a flat lesion (*arrows*). This patient had a polypectomy three days prior to the examination. Diagnosis: scar after polypectomy. *Lesson:* The mucosa appears edematous and prominent after polypectomy, closely resembling flat lesions

8.3.3.8
Spasm of the Internal Sphincter

Spasm of the internal sphincter causes a smoothly delineated contour irregularity at the anorectal junction and should not be mistaken for a flat lesion (Fig. 8.37).

8.3.3.9
Intermittently Prolapsing Rectal Mucosa

Intermittently prolapsing rectal mucosa appears as a low rectal mass, causing a smooth soft tissue defect. Sigmoidoscopy shows edematous mucosa due to rectal prolapse (Taylor 2003c) (Fig. 8.38).

8.3.3.10
Diverticular Disease

8.3.3.10.1
The Diverticular Fecalith

A pseudopolypoid lesion occurs when a diverticulum becomes inspissated with fecal matter. As the diverticulum lacks the muscularis propria, the fecal material easily remains in the diverticulum and hardens into a fecalith. Imaging findings are unequivocal when it presents as a hyperdense ring with a hypodense centre on the axial images. The corresponding endoluminal 3D images shows a polypoid lesion. On conventional colonoscopy they are recognised as fecal balls falling into the lumen. Confusion with polyps has been

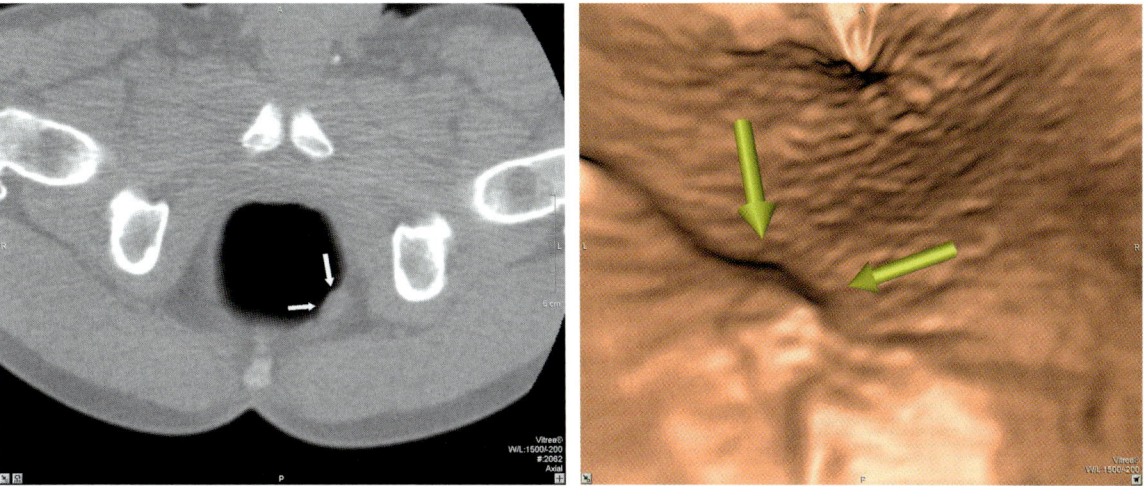

Fig. 8.37a,b. False positive diagnosis: spasm of the internal sphincter: **a** axial image shows a smoothly delineated (sub)mucosal irregularity, located at the region of the internal sphincter (*arrows*); **b** corresponding endoluminal 3D image shows a wall thickening of the rectal mucosa at the anorectal region. (*arrows*). Conventional colonoscopy was normal. Diagnosis: Spasm of the internal sphincter. *Lesson:* Submucosal contracted muscle layers may mimick pathology

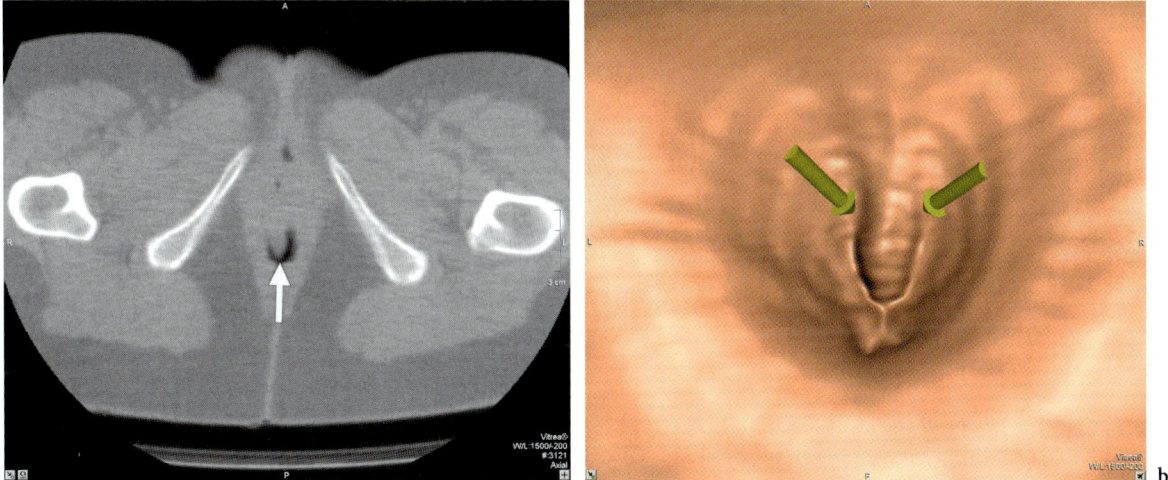

Fig. 8.38a,b. False positive diagnosis: intermittently prolapsing rectal mucosa: **a** axial image shows a smooth soft tissue filling defect at the anorectal region (*arrow*); **b** endoluminal 3D image shows an apparent low rectal "mass" (*arrows*). Conventional colonoscopy showed edematous mucosa due to rectal prolapse. *Lesson:* Rectal mucosa can appear very prominent, particularly in case of mucosal prolapse, simulating low rectal masses

described. Some controversy exists over the origin of these imaging findings. Fletcher et al. (Fletcher et al. 1999) described the hyperdensity as being caused by barium remnants in the diverticulum mixed with a fecalith rather than by the fecalith itself. However, Lefere et al. (Lefere et al. 2003) reported that anatomopathological examination of a surgical specimen of a divericulum with a fecalith showed that the contents of the diverticulum corresponded to fecal material. No barium was detected in the diverticulum.

A thrombus filling the diverticulum after an intra-diverticular bleeding has been described as a possible pseudolesion by Keller et al. (Keller et al. 1984) (Fig. 8.39).

8.3.3.10.2
Inverted Diverticulum

A diverticulum may occasionally invert into the colonic lumen and produce a pseudopolypoid lesion.

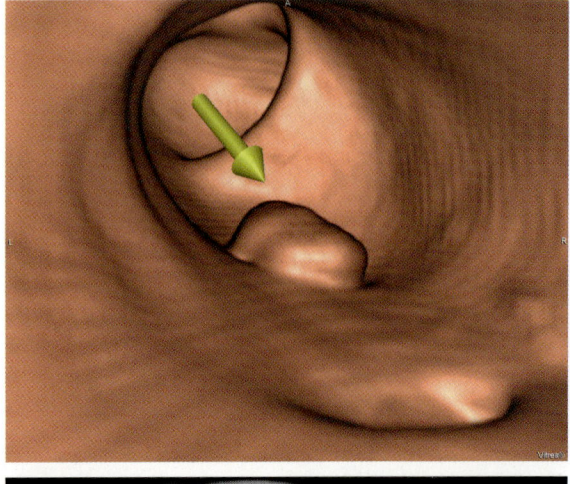
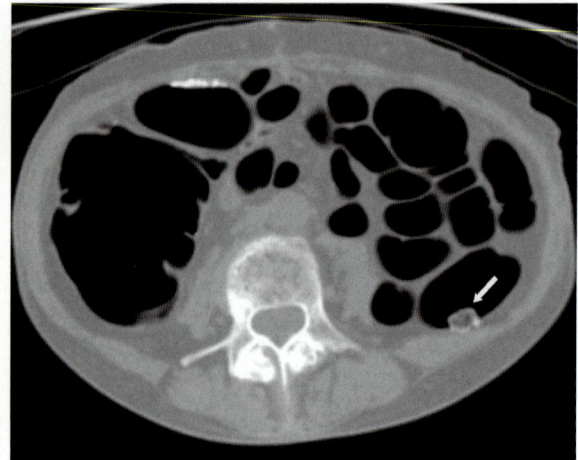
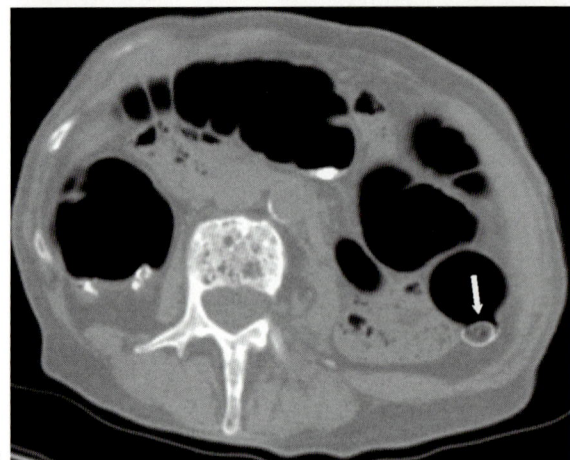

Fig. 8.39a–c. False positive diagnosis: diverticular fecalith: **a** endoluminal 3D image in prone position shows a polyp-like lesion in the descending colon (*arrow*); **b** corresponding axial image shows the lesion has a hyperdense ring and a hypodense centre (*arrow*b); **c** corresponding axial image in supine position shows the lesion is incorporated in a diverticulum (*arrow*). Diagnosis: diverticular fecalith. *Lesson:* A polypoid lesion with a hyperdense ring and hypodense centre corresponds to a diverticular fecalith

It can be the source of colonic bleeding (Silverstein and Tytgat 1997). In a series of six patients, Glick (Glick 1991) described the lesion as a 1.5- to 2-cm lesion with a central umbilication on double-contrast barium enema. Imaging findings are unequivocal when on the axial images a sessile polypoid lesion contains some air due to a central umbilication in the inverted part of the diverticulum (Posner and Solomon 1995) (Fig. 8.40) or when it presents with a fat attenuation due to an inclusion of perisigmoidal fat (Fenlon 2002). The corresponding endoluminal 3D image invariably has a polypoid aspect and does not help in making the correct diagnosis. Sometimes imaging findings are equivocal when the inverted diverticulum presents without air or fat. In CC inverted diverticula have been described to cause inadvertent diverticulectomy because of their pseudopolypoid appearance (Fenlon 2002; Yusuf and Grant 2000); thus it is important in case of an additional conventional colonoscopy to inform the endoscopist of this finding.

8.3.3.10.3
Polyp-Simulating Mucosal Prolapse Syndrome

When diverticular disease progresses, further shortening, thickening and contraction of the muscular layer and taeniae cause an excess of mucosa, prolapsing into the colonic lumen as a redundant fold. This gives rise to a pseudopolypoid or non-neoplastic lesion (Yoshida et al. 1996). These polypoid lesions usually present with a broad base (Kelly 1991).

Oedema and erythema are possible due to repetitive trapping of the mucosa in a contraction of the colonic wall. These lesions can be the cause of recurrent bleeding. Imaging findings are equivocal. As on the axial and endoluminal 3D images, they present as a polypoid lesion, and the polyp-

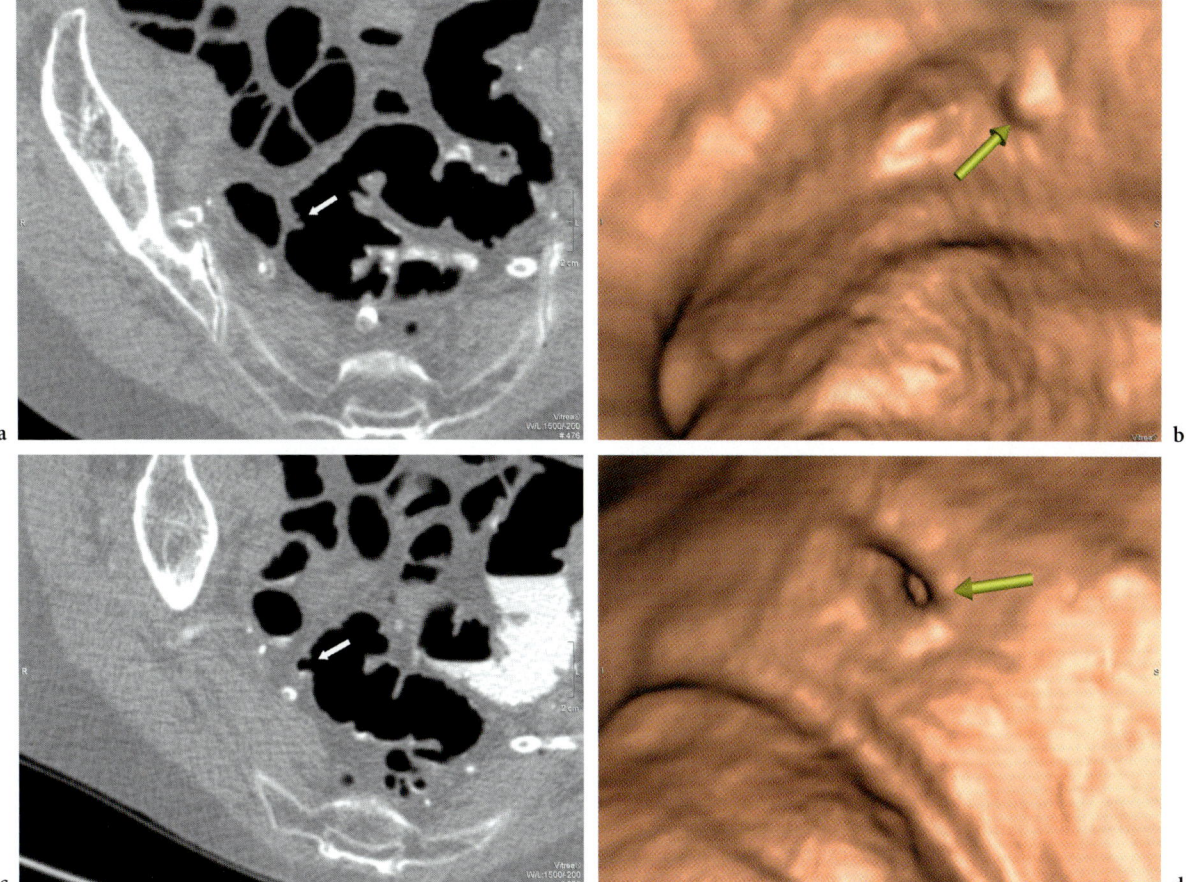

Fig. 8.40a–d. False positive diagnosis: inverted diverticulum: **a,b** prone image in a patient with severe diverticular disease shows an endoluminal protruding structure with air inclusion (*arrow* in a), resulting in a polyp-like structure on axial (*arrow* in a) and endoluminal 3D view (*arrow* in b); **c,d** supine image in the same patient shows the presence of a diverticulum at the same level, seen on axial (*arrow* in c) and endoluminal 3D image (*arrow* in d). Diagnosis: inverted diverticulum. *Lesson:* Diverticulae may invert, resulting in pseudopolypoid lesions. The clue to the diagnosis is the presence of air, as in this patient, or fat, included in the lesion

simulating mucosal prolapse syndrome is indistinguishable from actual polyps. On conventional colonoscopy these lesions, appearing as a hyperaemic mass, are also difficult to distinguish from adenomatous polyps. Sometimes these ambiguous lesions are only diagnosed after biopsy with histology showing hemosiderin-laden macrophages, capillary thrombi and congestion with telangiectasia (MATHUS-VLIEGEN and TYTGAT 1986).

Kelly (KELLY 1991) suggested that these lesions were quite common in the population as they were detected in 8 of a series of 118 resected colonic specimens. The polyp-simulating mucosal prolapse syndrome is histologically similar to the prolapse described in the solitary rectal ulcer syndrome, inflammatory cloacogenic polyps and gastric antral vascular ectasia (TENDLER et al. 2002) (Fig. 8.41).

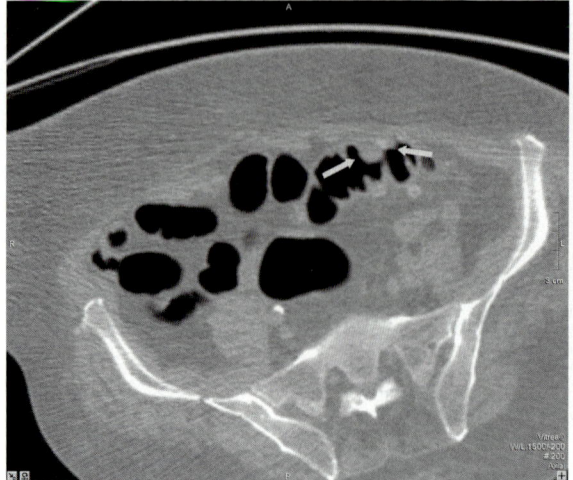 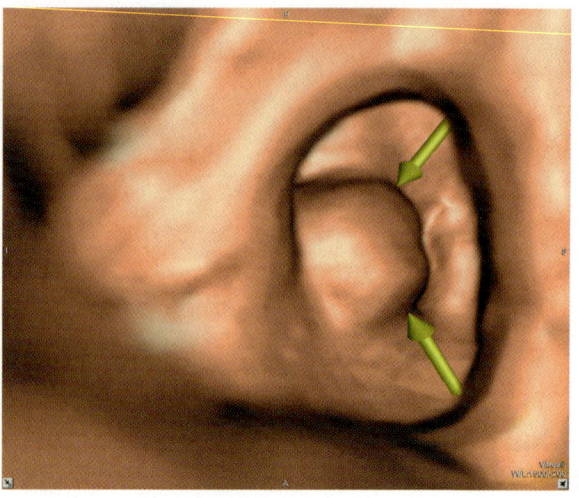

Fig. 8.41a,b. False positive diagnosis: mucosal prolapse syndrome: **a,b** prone image in a patient with severe diverticular disease shows a focal nodular wall thickening on axial image (*arrows* in a) and endoluminal 3D images (*arrows* in b). Biopsy showed hemosiderin-laden macrophages, capillary trombi and congestion with telangiectasia. Diagnosis of mucosal prolapse syndrome was made. *Lesson:* When diverticular disease progresses, shortening, thickening and contraction of the muscle layer cause an excess of mucosa, prolapsing into the colonic lumen as a redundant fold. Imaging features are equivocal since on 2D and 3D images mucosal prolapse presents as a polypoied lesion

References

Bielen D, Thomeer M, Vanbeckevoort D, Kiss G, Maes F, Marchal G, Rutgeerts P (2003) Dry preparation for virtual CT colonography with fecal tagging using water-soluble contrast medium: initial results. Eur Radiol 13(3):453–458

Bova JG, Bhattacharjee N, Jurdi R, Bennett WF (1999) Comparison of no medication, placebo, and hyoscyamine for reducing pain during a barium enema. Am J Roentgenol 172(5):1285–1287

Bruzzi JF, Moss AC, Brennan DD, MacMathuna P, Fenlon HM (2003) Efficacy of IV Buscopan as a muscle relaxant in CT colonography. Eur Radiol 13(10):2264–2270

Callstrom MR, Johnson CD, Fletcher JG, Reed JE, Ahlquist DA, Harmsen WS, Tait K, Wilson LA, Corcoran KE (2001) CT colonography without cathartic preparation: feasibility study. Radiology 219(3):693–698

Dachman AH, Zalis ME (2004) Quality and consistency in CT colonography and research reporting. Radiology 230(2):319–323

Dachman AH, Schumm P, Heckel B, Yoshida H, LaRiviere P (2004) The effect of reconstruction algorithm on conspicuity of polyps in CT colonography. Am J Roentgenol 183(5):1349–1353

Embleton KV, Nicholson DA, Hufton AP, Jackson A (2003) Optimization of scanning parameters for multi-slice CT colonography: experiments with synthetic and animal phantoms. Clin Radiol 58(12):955–963

Fenlon M (2002) CT colonography: pitfalls and interpretation. Abdom Imaging 27:284–291

Fidler JL, Johnson CD, MacCarty RL, Welch TJ, Hara AK, Harmsen WS (2002) Detection of flat lesions in the colon with CT colonography. Abdom Imaging 27(3):292–300

Fidler JL, Fletcher JG, Johnson CD, Huprich JE, Barlow JM, Earnest F IV, Bartholmai BJ (2004) Understanding interpretive errors in radiologists learning computed tomography colonography. Acad Radiol 11(7):750–756

Fletcher JG, Johnson CD, MacCarty RL, Welch TJ, Reed JE, Hara AK (1999) CT colonography: potential pitfalls and problem-solving techniques. Am J Roentgenol 172(5):1271–1278

Fletcher JG, Booya F, Johnson CD, Ahlquist D (2005) CT colonography: unraveling the twists and turns. Curr Opin Gastroenterol 21(1):90–98

Galdino GM, Yee J (2003) Carpet lesion on CT colonography: a potential pitfall. Am J Roentgenol 180(5):1332–1334

Glick SN (1991) Inverted colonic diverticulum: air contrast barium enema findings in six cases. Am J Roentgenol 156:961–964

Gluecker T, Meuwly JY, Pescatore P, Schnyder P, Delarive J, Jornod P, Meuli R, Dorta G (2002) Effect of investigator experience in CT colonography. Eur Radiol 12(6):1405–1409

Gluecker TM, Fletcher JG, Welch TJ, MacCarty RL, Harmsen WS, Harrington JR, Ilstrup D, Wilson LA, Corcoran KE, Johnson CD (2004) Characterization of lesions missed on interpretation of CT colonography using a 2D search method. Am J Roentgenol 182(4):881–889

Gryspeerdt S, Lefere P, Dewyspelaere J, Baekelandt M, van Holsbeeck B (2002) Optimisation of colon cleansing prior to computed tomographic colonography. JBR-BTR 85(6):289–296

Gryspeerdt SS, Herman MJ, Baekelandt MA, van Holsbeeck BG, Lefere PA (2004) Supine/left decubitus scanning: a valuable alternative to supine/prone scanning in CT colonography. Eur Radiol 14(5):768–777

Goei R, Nix M, Kessels AH, Ten Tusscher MP (1995) Use of antispasmodic drugs in double contrast barium enema examination: glucagon or buscopan? Clin Radiol 50(8):553–557

Hoppe H, Quattropani C, Spreng A, Mattich J, Netzer P, Dinkel HP (2004) Virtual colon dissection with CT colonography compared with axial interpretation and conventional colonoscopy: preliminary results. Am J Roentgenol 182(5):1151–1158

Hwang I, Wong RK (2005) Limitations of virtual colonoscopy. Ann Intern Med 142(2):154–155; author reply 155

Johnson CD, Harmsen WS, Wilson LA, Maccarty RL, Welch TJ, Ilstrup DM, Ahlquist DA (2003) Prospective blinded evaluation of computed tomographic colonography for screen detection of colorectal polyps. Gastroenterology 125(2):311–319

Keller CE, Halpert RD, Fecsko PJ, Simms SM (1984) Radiologic recognition of colonic diverticula simulating polyps. Am J Roentgenol 143:93–97

Kelly JK (1991) Polypoid prolapsing mucosal folds in diverticular disease. Am J Surg Pathol 15:871–878

Laks S, Macari M, Bini EJ (2004) Positional change in colon polyps at CT colonography. Radiology 231(3):761–766

Lefere PA, Gryspeerdt SS, Dewyspelaere J, Baekelandt M, Van Holsbeeck BG (2002) Dietary fecal tagging as a cleansing method before CT colonography: initial results polyp detection and patient acceptance. Radiology 224(2):393–403

Lefere P, Gryspeerdt S, Baekelandt M, Dewyspelaere J, van Holsbeeck B (2003) Diverticular disease in CT colonography. Eur Radiol 13 Suppl 4:L62–74

Lefere P, Gryspeerdt S, Baekelandt M, Van Holsbeeck B (2004) Laxative-free CT colonography. Am J Roentgenol 183(4):945–948

Luo MY, Shan H, Yao LQ, Zhou KR, Liang WW (2004) Post-processing techniques of CT colonography in detection of colorectal carcinoma. World J Gastroenterol 1 10(11):1574–1577

Macari M, Megibow AJ (2001) Pitfalls of using three-dimensional CT colonography with two-dimensional imaging correlation. Am J Roentgenol 176(1):137–143

Macari M, Lavelle M, Pedrosa I, Milano A, Dicker M, Megibow AJ, Xue X (2001) Effect of different bowel preparations on residual fluid at CT colonography. Radiology 218(1):274–277

Macari M, Bini EJ, Jacobs SL, Lange N, Lui YW (2003) Filling defects at CT colonography: pseudo- and diminutive lesions (the good), polyps (the bad), flat lesions, masses, and carcinomas (the ugly). Radiographics 23(5):1073–1091

Macari M, Bini EJ, Jacobs SL, Lui YW, Laks S, Milano A, Babb J (2004) Significance of missed polyps at CT colonography. Am J Roentgenol 183(1):127–134

Mathus-Vliegen EMH, Tytgat GNJ (1986) Polyp-simulating mucosal prolapse syndrome in (pre-) diverticular disease. Endoscopy 18:84–86

McFarland EG (2002) Reader strategies for CT colonography. Abdom Imaging 27(3):275–283

McFarland EG, Zalis ME (2004) CT colonography: progress toward colorectal evaluation without catharsis. Gastroenterology 127(5):1623–1626

Morrin MM, Farrell RJ, Keogan MT, Kruskal JB, Yam CS, Raptopoulos V (2002) CT colonography: colonic distention improved by dual positioning but not intravenous glucagon. Eur Radiol 12(3):525–530

Park SH, Ha HK, Kim MJ, Kim KW, Kim AY, Yang DH, Lee MG, Kim PN, Shin YM, Yang SK, Myung SJ, Min YI (2005) False-negative results at multi-detector row CT colonography: multivariate analysis of causes for missed lesions. Radiology 235(2):495–502

Pickhardt PJ (2004) Differential diagnosis of polypoid lesions seen at CT colonography (virtual colonoscopy). Radiographics 24(6):1535–1556; discussion 1557–1559

Pickhardt PJ (2005) CT colonography (virtual colonoscopy) for primary colorectal screening: challenges facing clinical implementation. Abdom Imaging 30(1):1–4

Pickhardt PJ, Choi JR (2005) Adenomatous polyp obscured by small-caliber rectal catheter at low-dose CT colonography: a rare diagnostic pitfall. Am J Roentgenol 184(5):1581–1583

Pickhardt PJ, Choi JR, Hwang I, Butler JA, Puckett ML, Hildebrandt HA, Wong RK, Nugent PA, Mysliwiec PA, Schindler WR (2003) Computed tomographic virtual colonoscopy to screen for colorectal neoplasia in asymptomatic adults. N Engl J Med 349(23):2191–2200

Pickhardt PJ, Choi JR, Hwang I, Schindler WR (2004a) Nonadenomatous polyps at CT colonography: prevalence, size distribution, and detection rates. Radiology 232(3):784–790

Pickhardt PJ, Nugent PA, Choi JR, Schindler WR (2004b) Flat colorectal lesions in asymptomatic adults: implications for screening with CT virtual colonoscopy. Am J Roentgenol 183(5):1343–1347

Pickhardt PJ, Taylor AJ, Johnson GL, Fleming LA, Jones DA, Pfau PR, Reichelderfer M (2005) Building a CT colonography program: necessary ingredients for reimbursement and clinical success. Radiology 235(1):17–20

Pineau BC, Paskett ED, Chen GJ, Espeland MA, Phillips K, Han JP, Mikulaninec C, Vining DJ (2003) Virtual colonoscopy using oral contrast compared with colonoscopy for the detection of patients with colorectal polyps. Gastroenterology 125(2):304–310

Posner R, Solomon A (1995) Dilemma of an inverted cecal diverticulum simulating a pedunculated polyp: CT appearance. Abdom Imaging 20:440–441

Reeders J, Rosenbush G (1994) Clinical radiology and endoscopy of the colon. Thieme Medical Publishers, New York

Regge D, Gallo TM, Nieddu G, Galatola G, Fracchia M, Neri E, Vagli P, Bartolozzi C (2005) Ileocecal valve imaging on computed tomographic colonography. Abdom Imaging 30(1):20–25

Silverstein FE, Tytgat GNJ (1997) Gastrointestinal endoscopy, 3rd edn. Mosby, London

Spinzi G, Belloni G, Martegani A, Sangiovanni A, Del Favero C, Minoli G (2001) Computed tomographic colonography and conventional colonoscopy for colon diseases: a prospective, blinded study. Am J Gastroenterol 96(2):394–400

Taylor SA, Halligan S, Bartram CI (2003c) CT colonography: methods, pathology and pitfalls. Clin Radiol 58(3):179–190

Taylor SA, Halligan S, Bartram CI, Morgan PR, Talbot IC, Fry N, Saunders BP, Khosraviani K, Atkin W (2003d) Multi-detector row CT colonography: effect of collimation, pitch, and orientation on polyp detection in a human colectomy specimen. Radiology 229(1):109–118

Taylor SA, Halligan S, Goh V, Morley S, Atkin W, Bartram CI (2003b) Optimizing bowel preparation for multidetector row CT colonography: effect of Citramag and Picolax. Clin Radiol 58(9):723–732

Taylor SA, Halligan S, Goh V, Morley S, Bassett P, Atkin W,

Bartram CI (2003a) Optimizing colonic distention for multi-detector row CT colonography: effect of hyoscine butylbromide and rectal balloon catheter. Radiology 229(1):99–108

Taylor SA, Halligan S, Burling D, Morley S, Bassett P, Atkin W, Bartram CI (2004) CT colonography: effect of experience and training on reader performance. Eur Radiol 14(6):1025–1033

Tendler DA, Aboudola S, Zacks JF, O'Brien MJ, Kelly CP (2002) Prolapsing mucosal polyps: an underrecognized form of colonic polyp–a clinopathological study of 15 cases. Am J Gastroenterol 97:370–376

Thomeer M, Carbone I, Bosmans H, Kiss G, Bielen D, Vanbeckevoort D, Van Cutsem E, Rutgeerts P, Marchal G (2003) Stool tagging applied in thin-slice multidetector computed tomography colonography. J Comput Assist Tomogr 27(2):132–139

Vos FM, van Gelder RE, Serlie IW, Florie J, Nio CY, Glas AS, Post FH, Truyen R, Gerritsen FA, Stoker J (2003) Three-dimensional display modes for CT colonography: conventional 3D virtual colonoscopy versus unfolded cube projection. Radiology 228(3):878–885

Yee J (2002) CT colonography: examination prerequisites. Abdom Imaging 27(3):244–252

Yee J, Hung RK, Akerkar GA, Wall SD (1999) The usefulness of glucagon hydrochloride for colonic distention in CT colonography. Am J Roentgenol 173(1):169–172

Yoshida M, Kawabata K, Kutsumi H, Fujita T, Soga T, Nishimura K, Kawanami C, Kinoshita Y, Chiba T, Fujimoto S (1996) Polypoid prolapsing mucosal folds associated with diverticular disease in the sigmoid colon: usefulness of colonoscopy and endoscopic ultrasonography for the diagnosis. Gastrointest Endosc 44:489–491

Yusuf SI, Grant C (2000) Inverted colonic diverticulum: a rare finding in a common condition? Gastrointest Endosc 52:111–115

Zalis ME, Perumpillichira J, Del Frate C, Hahn PF (2003) CT colonography: digital subtraction bowel cleansing with mucosal reconstruction initial observations. Radiology 226(3):911–917

9 3D Imaging: Invaluable for the Correct Diagnosis?

Ayso H. de Vries, Rogier E. van Gelder, and Jaap Stoker

CONTENTS

9.1 Introduction 117
9.2 Three-dimensional Reconstruction 117
9.3 Three-dimensional Display Methods 118
9.3.1 Conventional 3D Display 118
9.3.2 Alternative 3D Display Methods 119
9.4 2D and 3D Reading are Complementary 120
9.5 Fecal Tagging and Electronic Cleansing 123
9.6 Primary 2D and Primary 3D: Difference in Accuracy? 123
9.6.1 High Prevalence Population 123
9.6.1.1 Two-dimensional Methods 123
9.6.1.2 2D vs 3D 123
9.6.2 Low Prevalence Population 124
9.6.2.1 3D Methods 124
9.6.2.2 2D Methods 124
9.6.2.3 2D vs 3D Methods 124
9.6.2.4 Discussion 125
9.7 Review Time 125
9.8 Conclusion and Future Development 126
References 127

9.1
Introduction

In evaluation of computed tomography (CT) colonography (virtual colonoscopy) examinations there are basically two principles of reviewing: it can be done two-dimensionally (2D) or three-dimensionally (3D) (Fig. 9.1).

The simplest 2D approach is to view the axial helical CT images without any additional processing, although in general this will be performed with multi planar reformatting (MPR), or a combination of both MPR and 3D display. The method is named *primary* 2D if 3D is used for problem solving.

A. H. de Vries MD; R. E. van Gelder, MD; J. Stoker, MD, Professor of Radiology
Department of Radiology, Academic Medical Center, University of Amsterdam, Meibergdreef 9, 1105 AZ G1-226, Amsterdam, The Netherlands

Alternatively, evaluation of CT-colonography examinations can be done in a primary 3D approach, in which an (endo)luminal view of the colon is combined with a requisite 2D method.

In this chapter the pros and cons of 3D reviewing of colonography examinations are discussed. This discussion will be based on data of CT colonography only since no comparative studies have been published on MR-colonography yet.

9.2
Three-dimensional Reconstruction

Currently there are two rendering techniques used to produce virtual colonoscopy; surface rendering and volume rendering.

Surface rendering uses a specific attenuation coefficient to define the air-lumen interface. This is done by attaching an opacity value of 0 (complete transparency) to voxels that have an attenuation coefficient under a certain threshold and an opacity value of 1 (no transparency at all) for voxels above this threshold. Consequently, surface rendering assigns all structures either into luminal air or colonic wall, depending on the attenuation coefficient selected. By raising the threshold, more voxels of the colonic mucosa will be assigned to the lumen since the attenuation coefficient in transition zone (mucosa) typically lies between that of air and soft tissue.

Unfortunately, the attenuation coefficient varies within patients as well as with pathologic findings, which decreases the detail seen on the image. A second drawback is the method's sensitivity to noise and artifacts (Hopper et al. 2000).

The second method is volume rendering. This method categorizes voxels into multiple groups on the basis of their attenuation coefficient. Unlike surface rendering, volume rendering allows the transition voxels (colonic mucosa) between air and bowel wall to be reconstructed as a separate, specific structure. Although this method requires more computer

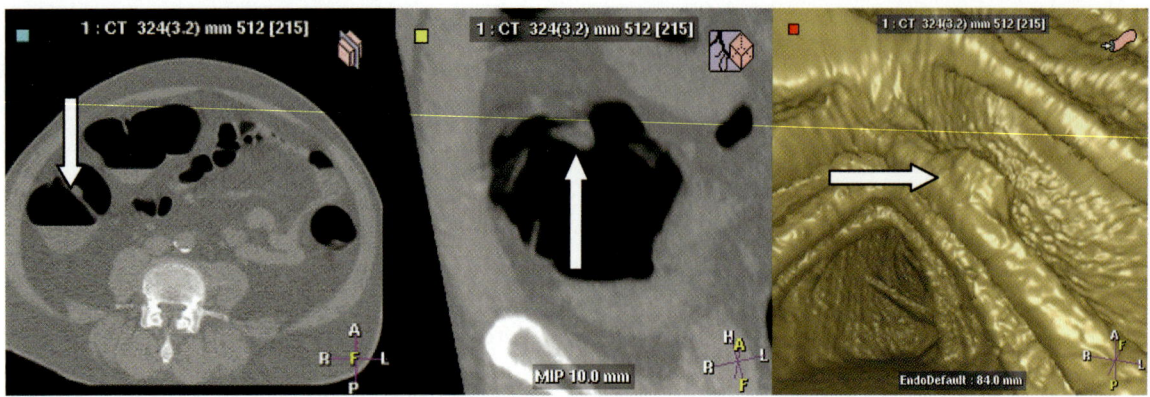

Fig. 9.1. Image of a 14 mm polyp in the cecum displayed at axial 2D (*left*), MPR (*middle*) and 3D (*right*)

power, it provides smoother rendering and provides the possibility to peer into the colon wall (HOPPER et al. 2000). Most of the commercially available software is based on this method.

Until recently most implementations of both rendering methods did not allow for interactive visualization but now interactive visualization has been introduced. In contrast to real time rendering, image sequences are generated off-line for later diagnostic examination by the physician. Viewing positions are generated at regular intervals along the central path which generates the illusion of flying through the lumen of the colon (virtual colonoscopy). This central path is generated in a (semi) automatic way through the lumen of the colon. Several different methods for the calculation of the centerline are used, though comparative studies are lacking. If the colon is discontinuous because a segment is collapsed or entirely filled with fecal material or fluid, the centerline may need to be manually adjusted.

9.3
Three-dimensional Display Methods

9.3.1
Conventional 3D Display

The first 3D visualization method for CT colonography was adopted from conventional endoscopy, and has a similar disadvantage: areas behind haustral folds are not easily visualized. As a consequence, in *conventional* 3D methods the colon needs to be evaluated in both antegrade and retrograde directions in order to visualize sufficient colonic surface. With a fly-through in one direction substantial parts of the colonic wall and therefore polyps will be obscured by haustral folds, as happens in optical colonoscopy (Fig. 9.2). Two-directional fly-through evaluation reduces these unseen colonic areas considerably (PAIK et al. 2000; Vos et al. 2003). However, even with a two-directional fly-through, substantial parts of the colonic wall that potentially harbor polyps remain non-visualized. Interactive evaluation can overcome this problem at the expense of an additional, and often substantial, increase in reading time.

An other solution to this problem is to use an algorithm that identifies areas that are not visualized during bidirectional evaluation. These areas, indicated for example by color, are presented to the observer after completing the bidirectional evaluation (Fig. 9.3). For practical purposes, the areas can be presented in descending order of size. The observer can then decide whether to skip small-sizes areas as these will not hide clinical relevant polyps.

An alternative approach to reduce unseen areas is to increase the viewing angle of the virtual camera. Consequently more colonic surface is displayed. A major drawback is the resulting distortion, especially at the edges, that prevents the use of these large viewing angles (Fig. 9.4).

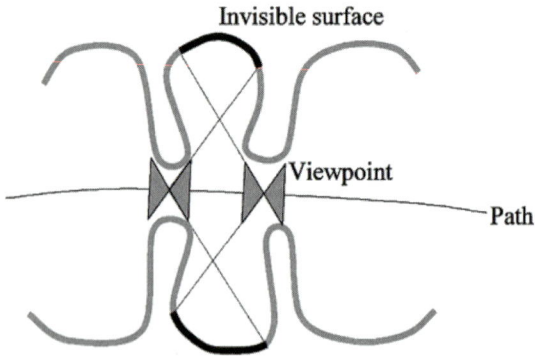

Fig. 9.2. Schematic shows areas in black that are missed in conventional 3D view. Reprinted with permission of Vos et al.

3D Imaging: Invaluable for the Correct Diagnosis?

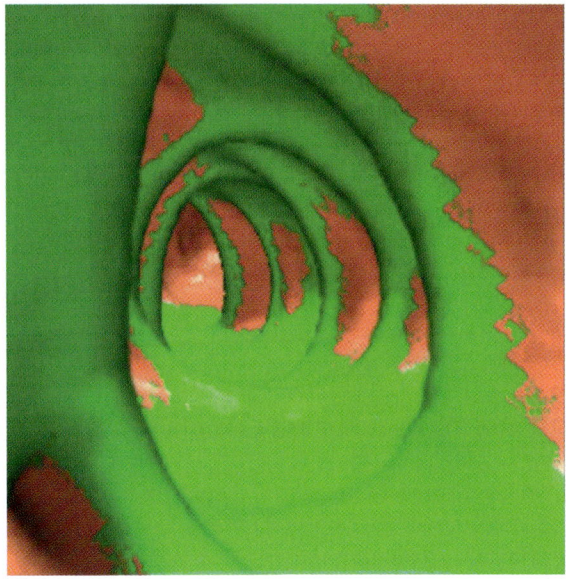

Fig. 9.3. Endoluminal view with "Missed Region Tool." This feature allows the reader to investigate areas (*indicated in pink*) that were not previously viewed during conventional fly through. (Figure courtesy of Viatronix, Stony Brook, NY)

9.3.2
Alternative 3D Display Methods

The ideal 3D display mode shows the complete colonic surface (so in theory no polyps can be missed) in a time efficient way and without image distortion (so polyps can be recognized as such).

Several groups have studied alternative 3D methods, which all have in common a less 'colonoscopy'-like representation of the colonic surface than the conventional fly-through.

A so-called "flattening method" can be used to straighten and flatten the colon mathematically. BEAULIEU et al. (1999) evaluated a method called "Panoramic endoscopy" (Fig. 9.5). With this method the inner colonic surface is depicted as a flattened structure. The camera is rotated around the path in 60° increments, which generated six image panels at an interval of 3 mm along the central path. When these image panels are displayed side by side, they depict a panoramic view of the colonic wall.

In a comparative study of display methods for CT colonography with the use of *simulated* polyps of different size and morphology, panoramic endoscopy had a significantly higher sensitivity (90%) than bidirectional virtual endoscopy (68%) for polyps 7 mm or larger. Part of the difference could be explained by the invisibility of some lesions during bidirectional virtual endoscopy since this method does not visualize the complete colonic surface.

"Virtual colon dissection" is an improvement of the "Panoramic endoscopy" method evaluated by HOPPE et al. (2004). In this method the virtual camera captures one quarter of the circumference of the complete colon length at each viewing position with a 90° camera field of view that can be rotated in 45° increments. Eight contiguous panels displaying the colonic circumference are generated by rotating the virtual camera in 45° increments around the path.

In a study of 20 patients (31 colonic lesions of which 9 were 10 mm or larger) reviewed by 2 radiologists, Hoppe et al. reported a sensitivity of 67% and 89% for virtual colon dissection and 89% and 100% for axial 2D interpretation. The authors concluded that although virtual colon dissection may facilitate detection of colonic polyps in isolated cased, its detection rate is not superior to axial 2D interpretation. This can mainly be attributed to failed rendering of a high number of insufficiently distended colonic segments or regions with residual feces in this series.

Virtual dissection, as depicted in Fig. 9.6, is an image display method that is another improvement of the "flattening method". Virtual dissection is a method that has recently become available and has, according to our knowledge, not been evaluated yet. It opens and straightens the entire lumen of the colon along the longitudinal axis with a 45° overlap

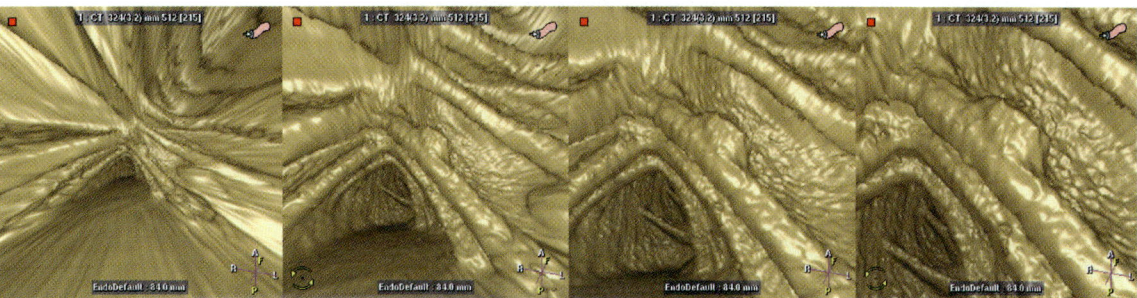

Fig. 9.4. Distortion illustrated of a polyp at four different endoluminal views of 160°, 120°, 90° and 60°

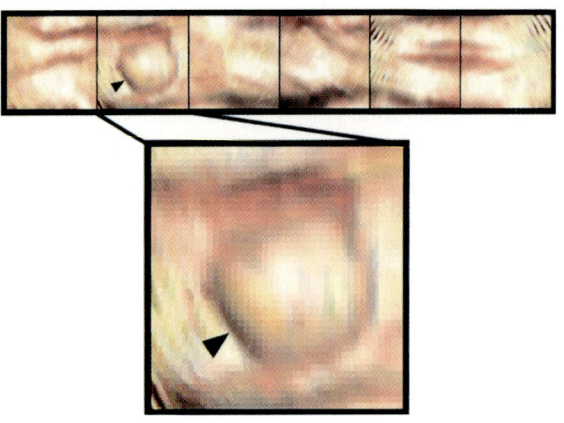

Fig. 9.5. "Panoramic endoscopy" display. Reprinted with permission of BEAULIEU et al.

on each side. The potential advantages of this "flattening method" include the easy overview over a substantial part of the colonic surface and complete visualization of the entire mucosal surface. This may lead to a reduction in interpretation time.

A drawback of the method is that straightening of a curved structure like the colon results in distortion of the colonic surface. Moreover it does not display the forward and backward viewing directions. Consequently, the frontal site and back site of structures are not visible. This problem can be overcome by combining the method with a conventional 3D method.

The "unfolded cube" method (Fig. 9.7) is a solution that tackled the problem of colon coverage in a different way. It was published by SERLIE et al. (2001). In this method the colonic surface is projected on a cube. On the cube faces, 90° views are projected. By folding out the six images onto a single plane (unfolded cube display) the complete field of view is rendered.

In a comparative series 99.5% of the colonic surface was displayed with this technique (Vos et al. 2003) as compared to 93.8% with antegrade and retrograde reviewing with a conventional 3D (120°) endoluminal view. Bidirectional reviewing is not mandatory with this method and therefore the additional evaluation time compared to 2D reviewing is less compared to the additional evaluation time of *conventional* 3D reviewing (VAN GELDER et al. 2004c).

9.4
2D and 3D Reading are Complementary

Two- and three-dimensional display methods must be considered as complementary instruments to evaluate CT colonography.

If a suspicious area is detected when using a primary 2D review method, a 3D snapshot can be used to obtain more information about the nature of the abnormality (e.g. folds and ileocecal valves) (Figs. 9.8 and 9.9).

On the other hand, a 3D method needs to be complemented by a method that can assess the heterogeneity and level of the attenuation values within an area of interest. Information about the attenuation values of a suspected lesion is mandatory for an accurate differentiation between a polyp and fecal material (Fig. 9.10). In practice this means that the method is combined with an axial or MPR 2D method (Fig. 9.11) or a method that demonstrates attenuation values in a 3D view (PICKHARDT 2004) (Fig. 9.12).

Obviously 2D and 3D methods are complementary, and a combination of both methods is essential for review of CT colonography. The question that remains, however, is which method is preferable for the primary review?

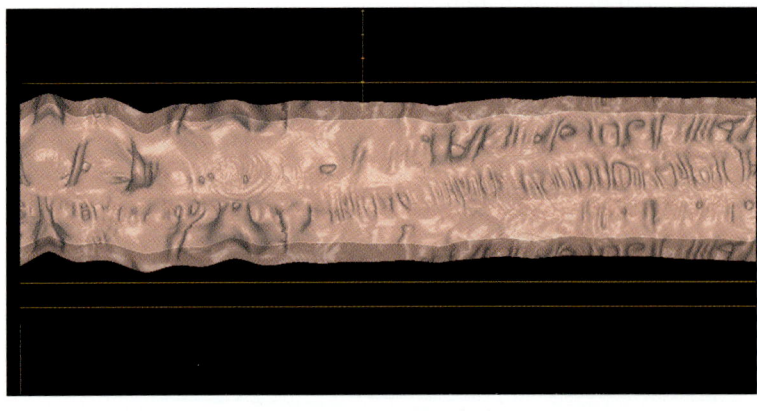

Fig. 9.6. Virtual dissected colon. (Courtesy of GE Medical Systems, Milwaukee, USA)

3D Imaging: Invaluable for the Correct Diagnosis?

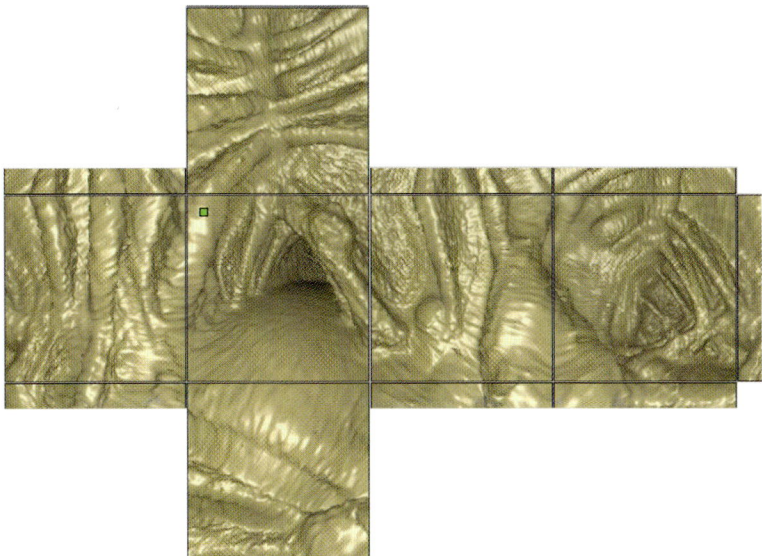

Fig. 9.7. Unfolded cube display of the colon. (Figure courtesy of Philips Medical Systems, Best, the Netherlands)

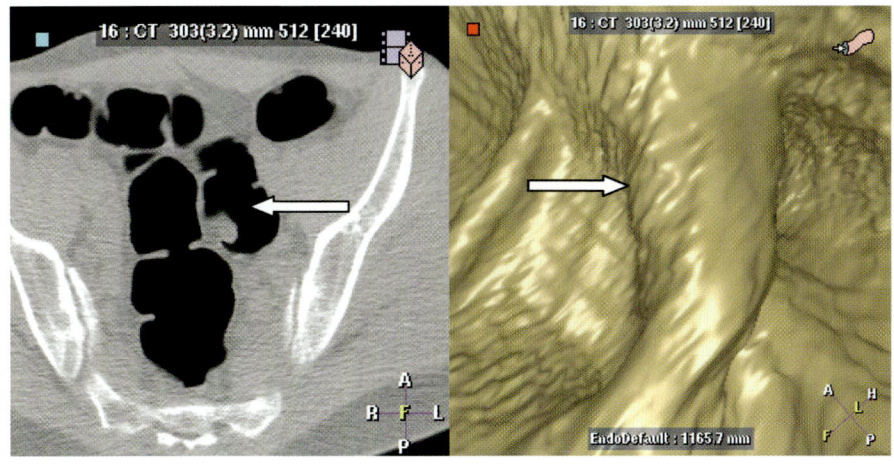

Fig. 9.8. Complex fold that resembles a polyp in the sigmoid colon in axial 2D (*left*), but is not in a conventional 3D view (*right*)

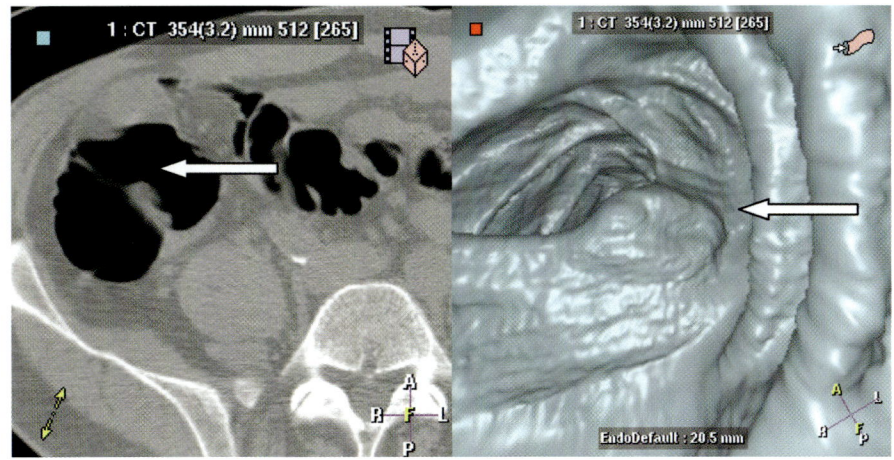

Fig. 9.9. Protruding ileocecal valve seen on axial 2D (*left*) and well recognizable on 3D (*right*)

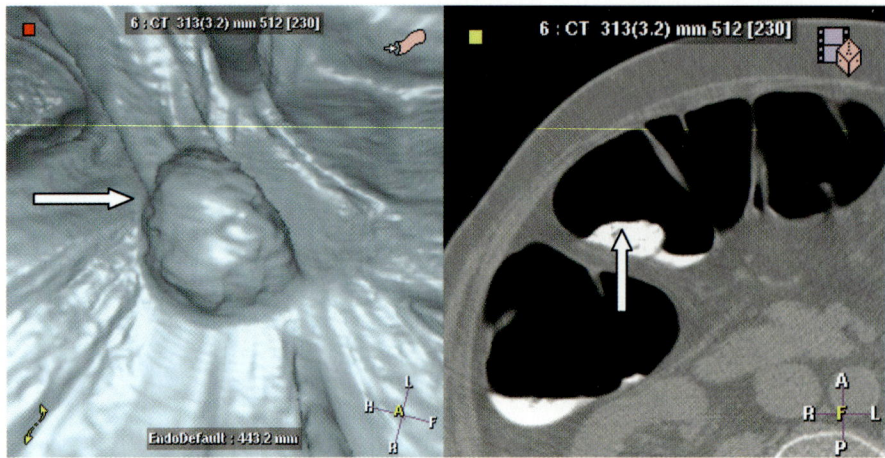

Fig. 9.10. Polyp in the transverse colon, seen on 3D (*left*) proves to be tagged fecal material in a 2D axial view (*right*)

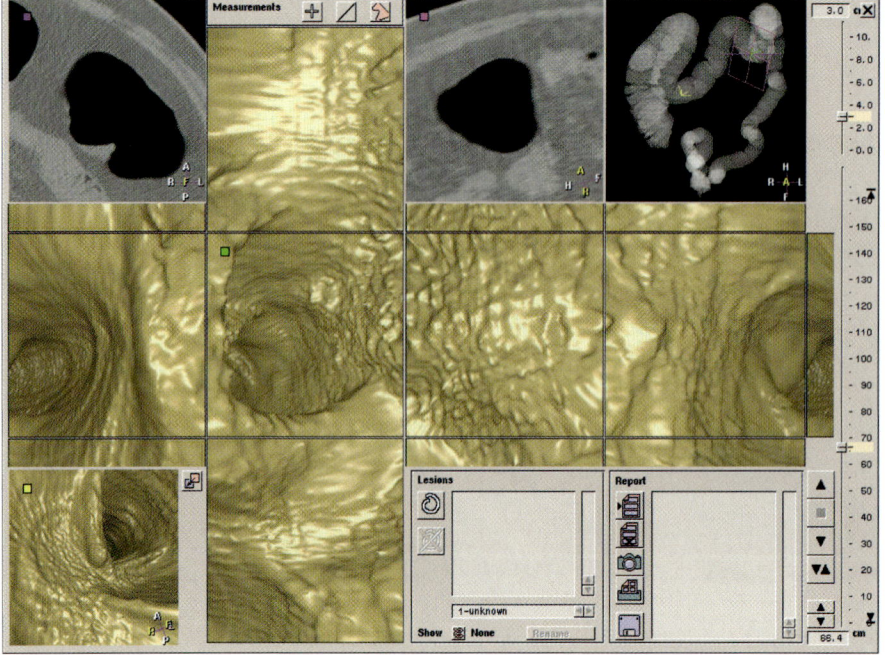

Fig. 9.11. Screen panel that combines a conventional endoluminal view (*bottom left*), an unfolded cube display (*center*), an axial 2D display (*top left*), a 2D MPR display (*top center*) and an overview of the colon (*top right*)

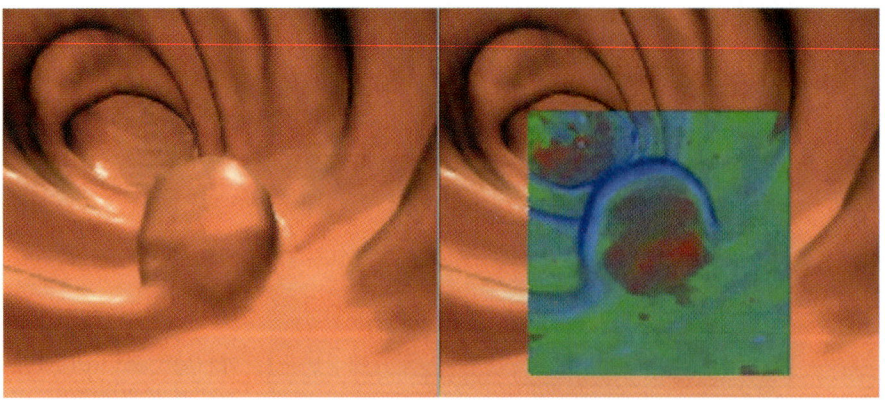

Fig. 9.12. Translucency rendering applied to a 3D image (*right*). The polyp shows a red interior which is indicative of soft tissue attenuation

9.5
Fecal Tagging and Electronic Cleansing

A 3D evaluation will be less time-consuming and labor-intensive if the colon is empty; colonic contents can hamper an efficient review as fecal material can resemble a polyp and fluid levels can hamper polyp detection. In principle an empty colon can be achieved in two different ways. The colon can be cathartically prepared with a laxative agent or its contents can be tagged after which it can be electronically cleansed.

In the latter method patients are asked to ingest a contrast agent approximately two days before the actual colonography examination. The tagged contents of the colon can be digitally subtracted after the data acquisition with the use of specialized software. This results in theory in a virtual clean colon that can be evaluated three-dimensionally, in which polyps are still in situ.

Tagging will probably add to the patient's compliance since laxative preparation is often experienced as a heavy burden (Lefere et al. 2002; Iannaccone et al. 2004a; van Gelder et al. 2004a).

9.6
Primary 2D and Primary 3D: Difference in Accuracy?

The accuracy of a diagnostic tool can vary with the prevalence of a disease or disorder. This may apply for the accuracy of both display methods as well. As a consequence a differentiation between high and low prevalence studies is made in this paragraph.

The sensitivity per polyp is used as a criterion for the functioning of the review methods different diagnostic modes, since it is a more precise way to measure the visibility of a polyp. However, in a screening setting the sensitivity per patient is a more important outcome parameter since the consequence of a positive colonography will be a referral for colonoscopy.

In this paragraph both *primary* 2D and *primary* 3D are described. It is likely that in primary 2D the combination with 3D problem solving will reduce the amount of false positive findings compared to 2D reviewing only; Cotton et al. (2004) who used a 2D method combined with 3D for problem solving in only a part of the patients described an increase in correct lesion identifications when the 3D method was used, McFarland et al. (2001) stated that in individual cases the added value of 3D was anecdotal.

9.6.1
High Prevalence Population

Several clinical studies have used primary 2D evaluation in high prevalence populations. Primary 3D evaluation, however, has only been performed in comparative studies of 2D and 3D, not in clinical studies.

9.6.1.1
Two-dimensional Methods

Pineau et al. (2003) conducted a comparative study with optic colonoscopy assessing the diagnostic accuracy of virtual colonoscopy using oral contrast. The colonography examination was done with a primary 2D method with 3D problem solving. In a population of 205 patients the sensitivity for large (≥10 mm) colorectal polyps was 78%. The reported specificity was higher (95%). This decreased for medium-sized (6–9 mm) polyps to 75 and 83% respectively.

Johnson et al. (2003b) conducted a multi-center accuracy study (18 radiologists) with a primary axial 2D method with MPR and 3D for problem solving. The average sensitivity for large polyps was 75% with a corresponding specificity of 73%, for polyps ≥6 mm these figures were 54 and 72% respectively. Experienced readers performed better.

Iannaccone et al. (2004b) used a primary axial 2D method for detection of colorectal polyps in a partly symptomatic population of 203 patients. Patients had not been cathartically prepared but oral contrast was added to a low fiber diet, two days prior to the colonography examination. The average sensitivity per polyp for three observers was 100% for large polyps and 86% for polyps ≥6 mm. Specificity per patient was 100% for large polyps and 94% for polyps ≥6 mm.

These studies show that in a high prevalence population, primary 2D studies report good results for large polyps.

9.6.1.2
2D vs 3D

McFarland et al. (2001) compared three specific 2D and 3D image-display techniques. First a 2D MPR image display, secondly a 3D MPR image display (10 mm slab) and thirdly a 3D endoscopic view display. This was done in 30 colon segments. McFarland et al. concluded that among experienced abdominal radiologists, similar diagnostic performance in polyp detection was found among 2D MPR and the two 3D display techniques, although individual cases showed improved characterization with 3D display techniques. Overall no statistically significant differences were seen in the three different image display techniques.

Macari et al. (2004) compared two review methods in 30 selected patients. The datasets were examined primary 2D with 3D problem solving and primary 3D and randomly predetermined with at least a one week-interval. The overall sensitivity for primary 2D for medium polyps and large polyps was 50 and 81%. The overall sensitivity for primary 3D was 67 and 81%, respectively. This difference was not statistically significant. The specificity was similar for the 2D and 3D evaluations: 93.3%.

Iannaccone et al. (2004b) compared the diagnostic performance of primary 2D and primary 3D display techniques in a selected population of 50 patients. Mean polyp sensitivity for all lesions and false positive rate were 73.3 and 21.4% for primary 2D, and 76.6 and 23.3% for primary 3D. As McFarland and Macari, Iannaccone concluded that for polyps measuring >6 mm in size, there was no difference in the sensitivity between a primary 2D or 3D technique.

In summary, these studies in high prevalence populations report a good sensitivity for primary 2D review methods with 3D problem solving, and second, in none of the comparative studies of 2D and 3D was a significant difference detected.

9.6.2
Low Prevalence Population

9.6.2.1
3D Methods

Pickhardt et al. (2003) studied the accuracy of CT colonography in an asymptomatic population of 1233 patients of average risk for colorectal cancer. A primary 3D endoluminal bidirectional fly-through was used for detection of polyps, after electronic cleansing. Non-visualized areas were presented to the observers after the fly-through (Fig. 9.3). Pickhardt reported a sensitivity and specificity for large adenomatous polyps of respectively 92 and 96%. For adenomatous polyps larger than 6 mm the results were respectively 86 and 80%. The authors concluded that CT virtual colonoscopy with the use of a 3D approach is an accurate screening method for the detection of colorectal neoplasia. It even compared *favorably* with optical colonoscopy.

van Gelder et al. (2004b) evaluated CT-colonography with a primary 3D approach, using an unfolded cube display method (Fig. 9.4). The study included 249 surveillance patients, 20 patients having a history of mild symptoms. CT colonography reported a sensitivity and specificity of 76 and 92% for large polyps and of both 70% for medium polyps (between 6 and 9 mm). Van Gelder et al. concluded that CT colonography and colonoscopy have a *similar* ability to identify individuals with large polyps in patients at increased risk for colorectal cancer.

9.6.2.2
2D Methods

Less favorable results were reported in studies performed by Johnson et al. and Cotton et al.

Johnson et al. (2003a) studied the accuracy of CT colonography in a population of 703 asymptomatic patients. CT colonography was reviewed, in contrary to the latter two studies, with a primary axial 2D method combined with 2D MPR and 3D for problem solving. This was done by three reviewers. The sensitivity reported for detection of large colorectal polyps was between 32 and 73%, depending on the reader. The specificity ranged from 97 to 98%. For medium sized polyps the sensitivity ranged from 29 to 57%, the specificity from 88 to 95%. The author concluded that in this low prevalence population, the detection rates of CT colonography were *inferior* to colonoscopy.

Cotton et al. (2004) reported a sensitivity of 52% for large polyps and 32% for medium-sized polyps in a population of 615 patients. The specificity was 96 and 93% respectively. As in the study performed by Johnson, the detection rates of CT colonography were *inferior* to colonoscopy.

9.6.2.3
2D vs 3D Methods

Macari et al. (2000) compared the findings of two review methods and conventional colonoscopy in detecting colorectal polyps in 42 patients. In method 1, axial 2D datasets were examined in a cine mode using 3D review for problem solving. In method 2, datasets were examined exactly as in method 1, and subsequent to that review, datasets were examined with simultaneous 3D fly-through and MPR images. Using method 1, three of five medium-sized polyps and one large polyp were detected. With method 2, the same polyps were seen as with method 1. No additional polyps were detected. Macari concluded that primary axial 2D CT colonography with 3D problem solving was comparable to complete 2D and 3D CT colonography in detecting colorectal polyps.

van Gelder et al. (2004c) compared primary 2D evaluation with a primary 3D evaluation method (unfolded cube projection) in a series of 77 patients. Mean sensitivity for large polyps for the primary 3D and 2D review methods were 83 and 72%, respectively. The specificity was 92 and 94% respectively. Fewer perceptive errors, although not statistically significant ($p=0.06$), were made with the primary 3D method than with the primary 2D method although at expense of a slight increase of the number of false positives.

In contrast to Macari, Van Gelder at al. concluded that 3D review of CT colonography seems to improve polyp detection as fewer perceptive errors are made.

9.6.2.4
Discussion

In this section on accuracy, a distinction between high and low prevalence has been made. The difference that is made in this spectrum is of course arbitrary and is not absolute. However by drawing this line, a difference in performance of both methods is apparent.

In studies with a high prevalence for colorectal polyps or cancer, primary 2D reviewing performed well (Pineau et al. 2003; Johnson et al. 2003b; Iannaccone et al. 2004a) and in comparative studies (primary 2D vs primary 3D) (McFarland et al. 2001; Macari et al. 2004; Iannaccone et al. 2004a) no difference in sensitivity was detected between primary 2D and primary 3D review methods. It is noteworthy that in these comparative series most likely conventional 3D methods with suboptimal surface visualization were used. This may have underestimated the diagnostic value of 3D.

In the low prevalence group a discrepancy can be seen between studies with good results (Pickhardt et al. 2003; van Gelder et al. 2004b) and moderate outcomes (Johnson et al. 2003a; Cotton et al. 2004). These controversial results have resulted in speculations about its cause: the review method (primary 2D or primary 3D), the bowel preparation (with or without oral contrast), scanning parameters (5 mm vs thinner), the role of reviewer experience, etc.

Although we cannot determine the definite cause for the differences in the mentioned papers, it is striking that the two studies that reported the highest sensitivity used primary 3D review methods with improved surface visualization to detect polyps, whereas the two studies with the lower sensitivity used a primary 2D review method.

In all direct comparative studies there was no statistical difference between both methods, although the differences between both methods described by van Gelder were very close to significance ($p=0,06$).

It is widely known that polyp size is a major determinant of detection. Comparing visualization methods in populations with large polyps that are detected easily, may obscure difference that emerge in average risk patients with generally smaller polyps. The differences between primary 2D and primary 3D must be assessed in the situation to which it most likely applies: patients with a low prevalence of polyps.

The potentially superior performance of 3D is most likely based on the more intuitive presentation (Fig. 9.13) and the longer exposure time to polyps (Lee and Pickhardt, 2004). Lee and Pickhardt compared exposure time of 20 polyps in an axial 2D method with a conventional endoluminal 3D method. Lee concluded that the opportunity of polyp detection, including both exposure time and distance of polyp visualization, is significantly greater for the 3D endoluminal display. A consequence may be that less perceptive errors are made by the reviewer.

9.7
Review Time

Although exposure fold characterization is easier (Fig. 9.11) when using the 3D display, the barriers to 3D evaluation as the primary strategy for review have been its time-consuming and labor-intensive nature (Macari et al. 2000; McFarland et al. 2001).

Two matters underlie its time consuming nature. First, additional processing time is needed in order to create a 3D rendered view. In order to create a 3D view the CT-data files need additional processing by a computer. The speed of this process is dependent on the calculation speed of the used computers, RAM capacity, 3D rendering-interval (increment) along the central path and the resolution of both the raw CT data and the display-method. Improvements in

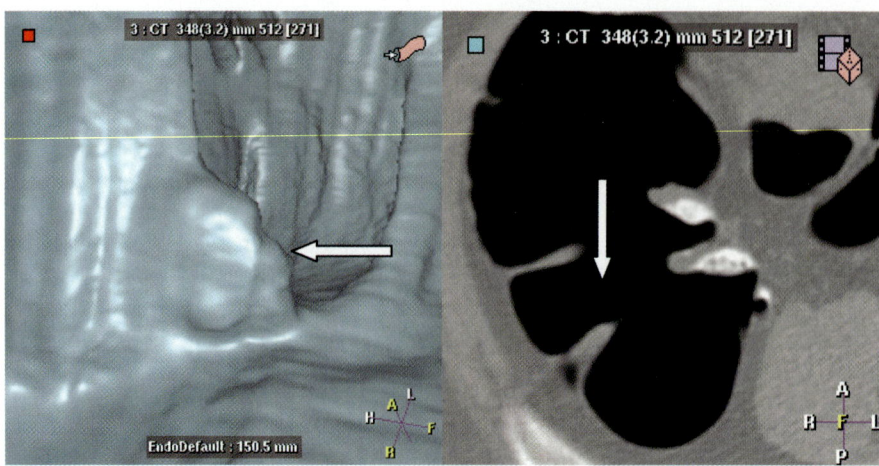

Fig. 9.13. Polyp in cecum, initially missed with an axial 2D method (*right*), but well detectable with 3D (*left*)

processing speed have reduced the time needed for this process and in future this process will reduce even further.

Although this processing time is not part of the reviewing time, it results in waiting time before the examination can be evaluated. With 3D methods, processing may not be fully automated and require interaction, which is a disadvantage as compared to 2D methods. Recent data on processing time are sparse; Hoppe et al. (2004) published processing times for the dissected colon method varying from 4.5 to 42 min with an average of nearly 16 min.

Fenlon et al. (1999) reported an average time of 30 min for endoluminal reconstruction. Although the computer details were not specified, it is likely that at least part of this time difference with Hoppe et al. can be attributed to the improved increase of computer power in the more recent study. Introduction of real time image rendering will probably even further reduce this time.

The second cause of its time consuming nature is the extra time needed to examine a colon compared to the 2D method. The cause of this problem lies within the fact that to cover as much colonic surface as possible with conventional 3D methods, evaluation in both antegrade and retrograde direction is mandatory. Consequently, in comparative studies primary conventional 3D evaluation requires an extra 50 to 70% in interpretation time compared to 2D evaluation (McFarland et al. 2001; Iannaccone et al. 2004b).

Studies that used display modes that did not require bidirectional fly-through demanded less extra time or were even faster compared to 2D evaluation. Van Gelder et al. who used an unfolded cube display only used an additional 15% evaluation time compared to 2D evaluation. Hoppe et al. reported an examination time of 20.9 minutes for virtual dissection display, compared to a 2D examination time of 29.2 minutes. Although in this study virtual colon dissection was not feasible in both prone and supine position in 30% of segments, the method did not require bi-directional viewing.

9.8
Conclusion and Future Development

Three-dimensional display is an integral part of reviewing of CT-colonography examinations and most likely a prerequisite for good sensitivity. The method can be used either primary or as adjunct to 2D evaluation. In populations with a high polyp prevalence the use of primary 3D does not seem advantageous compared to primary 2D, although comparative data are sparse and no optimized 3D methods have been used. The use of the later methods might prove to be valuable. The question which review method should be used as a screening method for colorectal cancer (low polyp prevalence) is a major issue. At the time of writing of this chapter no strong evidence for either primary 2D or primary 3D is available. Though, a higher sensitivity in polyp detection with primary 3D may make this review technique for the purpose of screening more appropriate. This question will be one of the main topics of research in CT colonography in the next couple of years.

An important topic in CT colonography is the reduction of ionizing radiation in CT colonography. This topic becomes of particular interest when CT colonography is used as a potential screening tool in the prevention of colorectal cancer. Although the imaging of structures with a high contrast difference (polyps vs air or tagged stool) allows a higher noise level (resulting from lower radiation exposure), noise related artifacts arise. This noise in the data can be counteracted by smoothing the images by using a smooth reconstruction filter. Although the benefit of these filters is reduction of the noise level, this is at the expense of image resolution.

Two-dimensional images seem less affected by this noise than 3D images since noise on a 3D endoluminal image appears as floating endoluminal debris that obscures the intraluminal anatomy and as coarsened mucosal texture that makes the detection of small or flat polyps difficult (JOHNSON and DACHMAN, 2000). However, in a experimental setting the radiation dose in a 3D setting can be reduced to very low levels without negative effect on sensitivity for large polyps (VAN GELDER et al. 2004d).

An important matter that may influence the discussion of 2D vs 3D is the use of computer aided diagnosis (CAD), as discussed in the following chapter. Currently, CAD is still in an experimental stage, but it most likely becomes implemented in the coming years. CAD has the potential to increase diagnostic performance, to reduce inter-reader variability and/or reduce reader time. At present it is not known which role CAD will play, e.g. as first reader or as second reader. The place of the CAD algorithm in the reading of CT-colonography examinations most likely will influence the use of either primary 2D or primary 3D. One can envision that a CAD algorithm will present polyp candidates in a 3D display with either 2D (axial or MPR) or attenuation display in color for verification of heterogeneity.

Acknowledgements
Frans M. Vos is acknowledged for his comments.

References

Beaulieu CF, Jeffrey RB, Karadi C, Paik DS, Napel S (1999) Display modes for CT colonography - part II. Blinded comparison of axial CT and virtual endoscopic and panoramic endoscopic volume-rendered studies. Radiology 212:203–212

Cotton PB, Durkalski VL, Benoit PC, Palesch YY, Mauldin PD, Hoffman B, Vining DJ, Small WC, Affronti J, Rex D, Kopecky KK, Ackerman S, Burdick JS, Brewington C, Turner MA, Zfass A, Wright AR, Iyer RB, Lynch P, Sivak MV, Butler H (2004) Computed tomographic colonography (virtual colonoscopy) – a multicenter comparison with standard colonoscopy for detection of colorectal neoplasia. J Am Med Assoc 291:1713–1719

Fenlon HM, Nunes DP, Schroy PC, Barish MA, Clarke PD, Ferrucci JT (1999) A comparison of virtual and conventional colonoscopy for the detection of colorectal polyps. N Engl J Med 341:1496–1503

Hoppe H, Quattropani C, Spreng A, Mattich J, Netzer P, Dinkel HP (2004) Virtual colon dissection with CT colonography compared with axial interpretation and conventional colonoscopy: preliminary results. Am J Roentgenol 182:1151–1158

Hopper KD, Iyriboz AT, Wise SW, Neuman JD, Mauger DT, Kasales CJ (2000) Mucosal detail at CT virtual reality: surface versus volume rendering. Radiology 214:517–522

Iannaccone R, Laghi A, Catalano C, Mangiapane F, Lamazza A, Schillaci A, Sinibaldi G, Murakami T, Sammartino P, Hori M, Piacentini F, Nofroni I, Stipa V, Passariello R (2004a) Computed tomographic colonography without cathartic preparation for the detection of colorectal polyps. Gastroenterology 127:1300–1311

Iannaccone R, Laghi A, Catalano C, Mangiapane F, Marin D, Passariello R (2004b) Interpretation methods at CT colonography: two-dimensional (2D) versus three-dimensional (3D) reading. Proc 90th Scientific Assembly and Annual Meeting of the Radiological Society of North America, Chicago, 30-11-2004

Johnson CD, Dachman AH (2000) CT colonography: the next colon screening examination? Radiology 216:331–341

Johnson CD, Harmsen WS, Wilson LA, MacCarty RL, Welch TJ, Ilstrup DM, Ahlquist DA (2003a) Prospective blinded evaluation of computed tomographic colonography for screen detection of colorectal polyps. Gastroenterology 125:311–319

Johnson CD, Toledano AY, Herman BA, Dachman AH, McFarland EG, Barish MA, Brink JA, Ernst RD, Fletcher JG, Halvorsen RA Jr, Hara AK, Hopper KD, Koehler RE, Lu DS, Macari M, MacCarty RL, Miller FH, Morrin M, Paulson EK, Yee J, Zalis M (2003b) Computerized tomographic colonography: performance evaluation in a retrospective multicenter setting. Gastroenterology 125:688–695

Lee A, Pickhardt P (2004) Polyp visualization at CT colonography: comparison of 2D axial and 3D endoluminal displays. Proc 90th Scientific Assembly and Annual Meeting of the Radiological Society of North America, Chicago, 30-11-2004

Lefere PA, Gryspeerdt SS, Dewyspelaere J, Baekelandt M, Van Holsbeeck BG (2002) Dietary fecal tagging as a cleansing method before CT colonography: initial results – polyp detection and patient acceptance. Radiology 224:393–403

Macari M, Milano A, Lavelle M, Berman P, Megibow AJ (2000) Comparison of time-efficient CT colonography with two- and three-dimensional colonic evaluation for detecting colorectal polyps. Am J Roentgenol 174:1543–1549

Macari M, Lee J, Garcia Figueiras R, Megibow A, Bennett G, Babb J (2004) Primary 2D versus 3D interpretation techniques using thin section multi-detector row CT colonography (CTC). Proc 90th Scientific Assembly and Annual Meeting of the Radiological Society of North America, Chicago, 30-11-2004. Ref Type: Conference Proceeding

McFarland EG, Brink JA, Pilgram TK, Heiken JP, Balfe DM, Hirselj DA, Weinstock L, Littenberg B (2001) Spiral CT colonography: reader agreement and diagnostic performance with two- and three-dimensional image-display techniques. Radiology 218:375–383

Paik DS, Beaulieu CF, Jeffrey RB, Karadi CA, Napel S (2000) Visualization modes for CT colonography using cylindrical and planar map projections. J Comput Assist Tomogr 24:179–188

Pickhardt PJ (2004) Translucency rendering in 3D endoluminal CT colonography: a useful tool for increasing polyp specificity and decreasing interpretation time. Am J Roentgenol 183:429–436

Pickhardt PJ, Choi JR, Hwang I, Butler JA, Puckett ML, Hildebrandt HA, Wong RK, Nugent PA, Mysliwiec PA, Schindler WR (2003) Computed tomographic virtual colonoscopy to screen for colorectal neoplasia in asymptomatic adults. N Engl J Med 349:2191–2200

Pineau BC, Paskett ED, Chen GJ, Espeland MA, Phillips K, Han JP, Mikulaninec C, Vining DJ (2003) Virtual colonoscopy using oral contrast compared with colonoscopy for the detection of patients with colorectal polyps. Gastroenterology 125:304–310

Serlie I, Vos FM, van Gelder RE, Stoker J, Truyen R, Gerritsen F, Nio Y, Post F (2001) Improved visualization in virtual colonoscopy using image-based rendering. Proceedings of the Joint Eurographics and IEEE TCVG Symposium on Visualization, pp 137–146

van Gelder RE, Birnie E, Florie J, Schutter MP, Bartelsman JF, Snel P, Lameris JS, Bonsel GJ, Stoker J (2004a) CT colonography and colonoscopy: assessment of patient preference in a 5-week follow-up study. Radiology 233:328–337

van Gelder RE, Nio CY, Florie J, Bartelsman JF, Snel P, de Jager SW, Van Deventer SJ, Lameris JS, Bossuyt PM, Stoker J (2004b) Computed tomographic colonography compared with colonoscopy in patients at increased risk for colorectal cancer. Gastroenterology 127:41–48

van Gelder RE, Florie J, Yung C, Jensch S, de Jager SW, Vos FM, Venema HW, Bartelsman JF, Reitsma H, Bossuyt PMM, Lameris JS, Stoker J (2004c) A comparison of primary 2D and 3D methods to review CT colonography. Proc 90th Scientific Assembly and Annual Meeting of the Radiological Society of North America, Chicago, 30-11-2004

van Gelder RE, Venema HW, Florie J, Nio CY, Serlie IW, Schutter MP, van Rijn JC, Vos FM, Glas AS, Bossuyt PM, Bartelsman JF, Lameris JS, Stoker J (2004d) CT Colonography: feasibility of substantial dose reduction – comparison of medium to very low doses in identical patients. Radiology 232:611–620

Vos FM, van Gelder RE, Serlie IWO, Florie J, Nio CY, Glas AS, Post FH, Truyen R, Gerritsen FA, Stoker J (2003) Three-dimensional display modes for CT colonography: conventional 3D virtual colonoscopy versus unfolded cube projection. Radiology 228:878–885

10 Extracolonic Findings in CT Colonography

STEFAAN GRYSPEERDT and PHILIPPE LEFERE

CONTENTS

10.1 Introduction 129
10.2 Definitions 129
10.3 Frequency and Importance of Extracolonic Findings 130
10.4 Nature of Extracolonic Findings 132
10.5 Does Patient Population Affect Extracolonic Findings 132
10.6 Does the Scanning Technique Influence Extra-Colonic Findings? 132
10.7 False Positive and False Negative Diagnosis 134
10.8 Economical Impact 134
10.9 Impact on Patient Care and Well-Being and Ethical Impact 135
10.10 Conclusion 135
References 135

10.1 Introduction

A unique capability of CT colonography over other colorectal examinations is its capability of examining the entire abdominal and pelvic content. This offers the possibility of detecting extracolonic pathology.

Detection of incidental extracolonic findings has many possible advantages, such as early detection of malignant disease or of an unruptured abdominal aortic aneurysm. Early treatment can improve a patient's prognosis and decrease costs owing to less complicated surgical procedures and shorter hospital stays.

On the other hand, extracolonic findings leading to further workup may cause unnecessary patient anxiety, entailing higher costs and superfluous exposure to radiation.

Detection and evaluation of extracolonic findings therefore balances between potential benefits and potential harm.

S. GRYSPEERDT, MD; P. LEFERE, MD
Stedelijk Ziekenhuis, Bruggesteenweg 90, 8800 Roeselare, Belgium

This chapter gives a review of the current literature and some reflections upon ethical and medicolegal aspects of detection and evaluation of extracolonic findings.

10.2 Definitions

Extracolonic findings are categorised by most authors as highly important, moderately important or of low importance.

Highly important lesions are usually defined as lesions that require surgical treatment, medical intervention, and/or further investigation during that patient care visit. Examples include indeterminate solid organ masses, previously unknown abdominal aortic aneurysms 3 cm or larger, aneurysms of the splenic or renal arteries, indeterminate chest nodule, adenopathy, and pancreatic masses.

Moderately important lesions include conditions that do not require immediate treatment but would likely require investigation, recognition or treatment at a later time. Examples of moderate importance include calculi of various organs, previously known abdominal aneurysms, adrenal masses, pancreatic pseudo cysts, indeterminate cysts of various organs, uterine enlargement in post-menopausal women, and coronary artery calcifications.

Findings of low importance are considered benign and unlikely to require further medical treatment or additional work-up. Examples include vascular calcifications, granulomas, diverticulosis, simple solid organ cysts, small to medium-sized hiatal hernias, and abdominal wall hernias containing fat.

When evaluating and comparing the results of the different studies, however, one has to keep in mind that size-definitions concerning significant pathology related to aortic aneurysms, adrenal gland, adenopathy, etc., differ from one study to another, thus influencing results.

10.3
Frequency and Importance of Extracolonic Findings

The results of the major studies published after 2000, and reporting upon extracolonic findings and their follow-up, are tabulated in Tables 10.1–10.3 and Figs. 10.1 and 10.2.

The reported percentages of incidental lesions is high, but shows a rather high inter-study variability, with a median of 68.9% of patients with incidental extracolonic findings.

The reported percentages of highly important lesions also show great inter-study variability, but is also high, with a median of 12.5% of patients, and 11.7% of lesions.

Table 10.1. Extracolonic findings on CT colonography from primary papers published since 2000 reporting details upon further follow-up. Overall evaluation

	IV contrast?	Dose	Screening or diagnostic	No. of patients	Avg age	Extracolonic findings			
						Lesions	Lesions/ patient	Patients	% patients
Edwards JT et al. 2001	No	70 mAs	Diagnostic	100	65	16	0.2	15	15.0
Ginnerup Pederson et al. 2003	No	70 mAs	Diagnostic	75	61	68	0.9	49	65.3
Gluecker et al. 2003	No	70 mAs	Screening	681	64	858	1.3	469	68.9
Hara et al. 2000	No	70 mAs	Screening	264	64	151	0.6	109	41.3
Hellstrom et al. 2004	No	125 mAs	Diagnostic	111	66	232	2.1	94	84.7
Pickhard PJ et al. 2003	No	100 mAs	Screening	1233	58	?	?	?	?
Spreng A et al. 2005	No	200 mAs	Diagnostic	30	66	88	2.9	23	76.7
Spreng A et al. 2005	Yes	200 mAs	Diagnostic	72	66	215	3.0	68	94.4

Table 10.2. Extracolonic findings on CT colonography from primary papers published since 2000 reporting details upon further follow-up. Evaluation according to importance and outcome. Per patient analysis

	IV contrast?	Total number of patients	% Low importance	% Moderate importance	% High importance (A)[a]	% Immediate treatment	% Cancers
Edwards JT et al. 2001	No	100	?	?	11	2.0	1
Ginnerup Pederson et al. 2003	No	75	?	?	12	2.7	1.3
Gluecker et al. 2003	No	681	50	26.9	10.4	1.3	1
Hara et al. 2000	No	264	20.8	24.2	12.9	2.3	0.7
Hellstrom et al. 2004	No	111	26.1	52.3	23.4	0.9	3.6
Pickhard PJ et al. 2003	No	1233	?	?	4.5	0.1	0.4
Spreng A et al.2005	No	30	?	?	13.3	6.7	6.6
Spreng A et al. 2005	Yes	72	?	?	30.6	18.1	6.9

[a] As defined by author

Table 10.3. Nature of extracolonic findings on CT colonography from primary papers published since 2000 reporting details upon further follow-up. Evaluation according to importance and outcome. Per lesion analysis

	IV contrast?	Total number of lesions	% Low importance	% Moderate importance	% High importance (A)[a]
Edwards JT et al. 2001	No	15	?	?	73.3
Ginnerup Pederson et al. 2003	No	68	?	?	11.7
Gluecker et al. 2003	No	858	66.9	22.8	10.3
Hara et al. 2000	No	151	45	32.4	22.5
Hellstrom et al. 2004	No	166	27.7	50	22.3
Pickhard PJ et al. 2003	No	?	?	?	?
Spreng A et al. 2005	No	88	?	?	4.5
Spreng et al. 2005	Yes	215	?	?	10.2

[a] As defined by author

The reported percentages of patients with immediate treatment is much lower, as is the same looking at patients with extracolonic cancers: median of 2.15% of patients with immediate treatment and 1.3% of patients with cancer.

A total of 2566 patients are included in those 7 studies, with 233 patients (9%) having extracolonic findings of high importance, 31 patients having immediate treatment (1.2%), and 27 patients having cancer (1%).

Thus, the total incidence of lesions is high, the number of lesions requiring further investigation is also high, but the incidence of serious disease is low, relative to the total number of lesions found. This is in conjunction with the findings of Xiong et al. (Xiong et al. 2005).

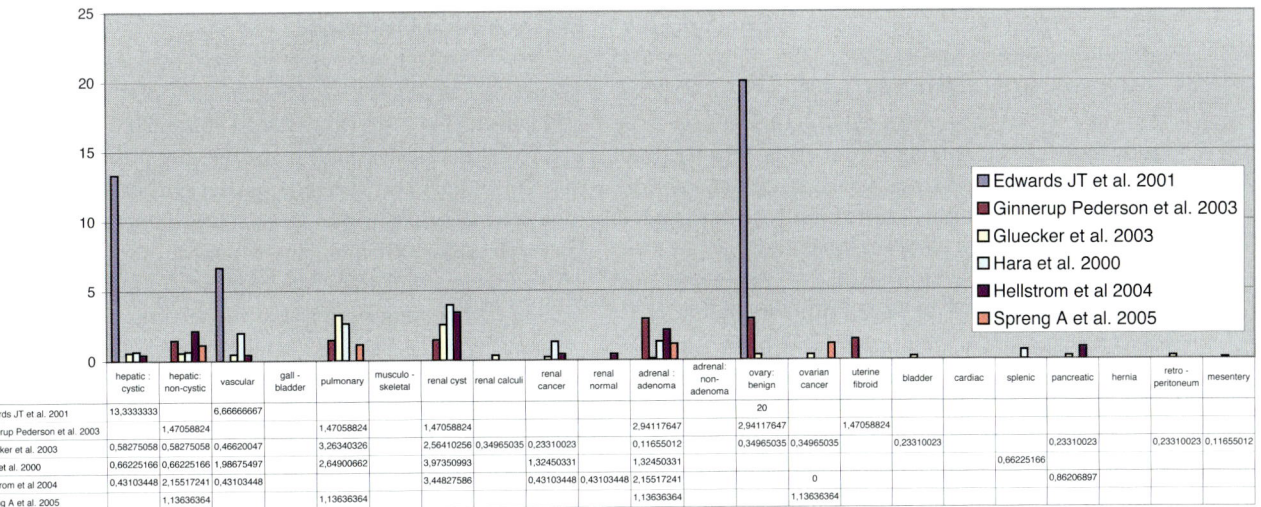

Fig. 10.1. CTC without IV contrast: nature and percentage of total number of lesions causing additional investigations

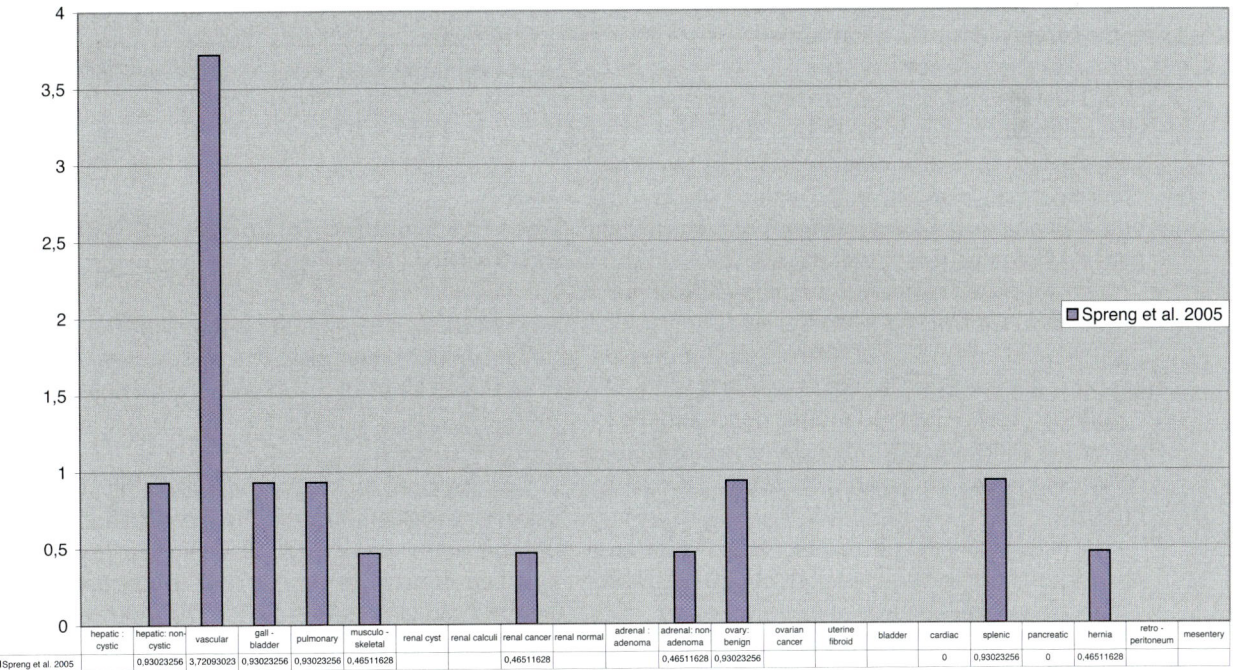

Fig. 10.2. CTC with IV contrast: nature and percentage of total number of lesions causing additional investigations

10.4
Nature of Extracolonic Findings

When we look at the nature of the lesions causing additional investigations, hepatic lesions, renal lesions, adrenal lesions, ovarian and pulmonary lesions constitute the majority in all six studies where this detailed information is available.

This is in conjunction with the findings of HOMMA et al. (HOMMA et al. 1995), who found that, in 1985, 13% of all renal cell carcinomas were found incidentally, increasing to 73% in 1993.

MIHARA et al. (MIHARA et al. 1999) reported that the incidence of renal cell carcinoma in a large study was 0.09%. It is moreover important to note that the stage and prognosis of renal cell carcinoma are significantly better when tumour is detected at an asymptomatic stage (TSUI et al. 2000).

CHERVU et al. (CHERVU et al. 1995) reported that aortic aneurysms (AAA) are found incidentally in 62%. Similar prevalence rates have been reported among urology patients referred for ultrasound (US). KYRIAKIDES et al. (KYRIAKIDES et al. 2000) reported that, in ultrasound screening program for abdominal aortic aneurysm, 4.9% of men aged 65 years have an asymptomatic AAA. Screening for AAAs has been shown to reduce the incidence of AAAs by 49% (WILMINK et al. 1999) and pilot population screening studies are underway (JAMROZIK et al. 2000). As for renal cell carcinoma, early detection is beneficial: mortality rate is much lower for elective early surgery (5%) than for surgery after rupture (85–95%) (NEVITT et al. 1989).

KLOOS et al. (KLOOS et al. 1997) reported that adrenal incidentalomas are found in up to 5% of patients having CT for other reasons. In the series reported here, however, none of the patients had non-adenomatous adrenal disease, so none of the patients had benefit of this diagnosis.

Ovarian cystic lesions are common (26% of postmenopausal women) (VAN NAGELL et al. 1990). The positive predictive value of such lesions for ovarian cancer is however low (JACOBS et al. 1993).

Taking these findings into account, and looking at Figs. 10.1 and 10.2, one could conclude that renal lesions and aortic aneurysms are "not to be missed".

The axial scans should also be evaluated for pulmonary or liver lesions, possibly indicating metastatic primary malignancy.

Adrenal lesions and lesions of the ovaries should be regarded with care, both because of the low positive predictive value.

Finally, the different nature of possibly important extracolonic findings necessitates the evaluation of the axial images in different window settings, e.g. abdominal window settings, lung window settings and bone window settings (Fig. 10.3).

10.5
Does Patient Population Affect Extracolonic Findings

The studies of GLUECKER et al. (GLUECKER et al. 2003) and PICKHARD et al. (PICKHARD et al. 2003) are the only two studies evaluating a screening population, and are remarkably the two studies with the lowest incidence of highly important extracolonic findings, findings with additional investigation, or cancers. This indicates that significant extracolonic findings are lower in screening population settings.

Looking at the age of patients, again, the study of PICKHARD et al. (PICKHARD et al. 2003), has the youngest patient population, indicating that extracolonic findings increase with age.

This is in conjunction with the findings of NG et al. (NG et al. 2004) who reported upon extracolonic findings in the frail and elderly undergoing abdomino-pelvic CT for suspected colorectal carcinoma. In this patient population, previously undiagnosed malignancies were found twice as common (2%), indicating that with an aging population and an increased use of cross-sectional imaging, an increased number of incidental findings will occur.

10.6
Does the Scanning Technique Influence Extra-Colonic Findings?

Most studies use a low dose technique, without additional use of IV contrast. The reasons are the care of radiation dose in a technique requiring prone-supine imaging, and the fear of adverse reaction using IV contrast.

The low dose technique capitalizes on the high contrast that exists between the air-filled lumen and the soft tissue density wall. Polyps protruding into air-filled lumen can be detected using these low-dose technique.

Solid organ contrast however requires higher radiation dose and correct diagnosis frequently necessitates IV contrast. As a result, it is likely that

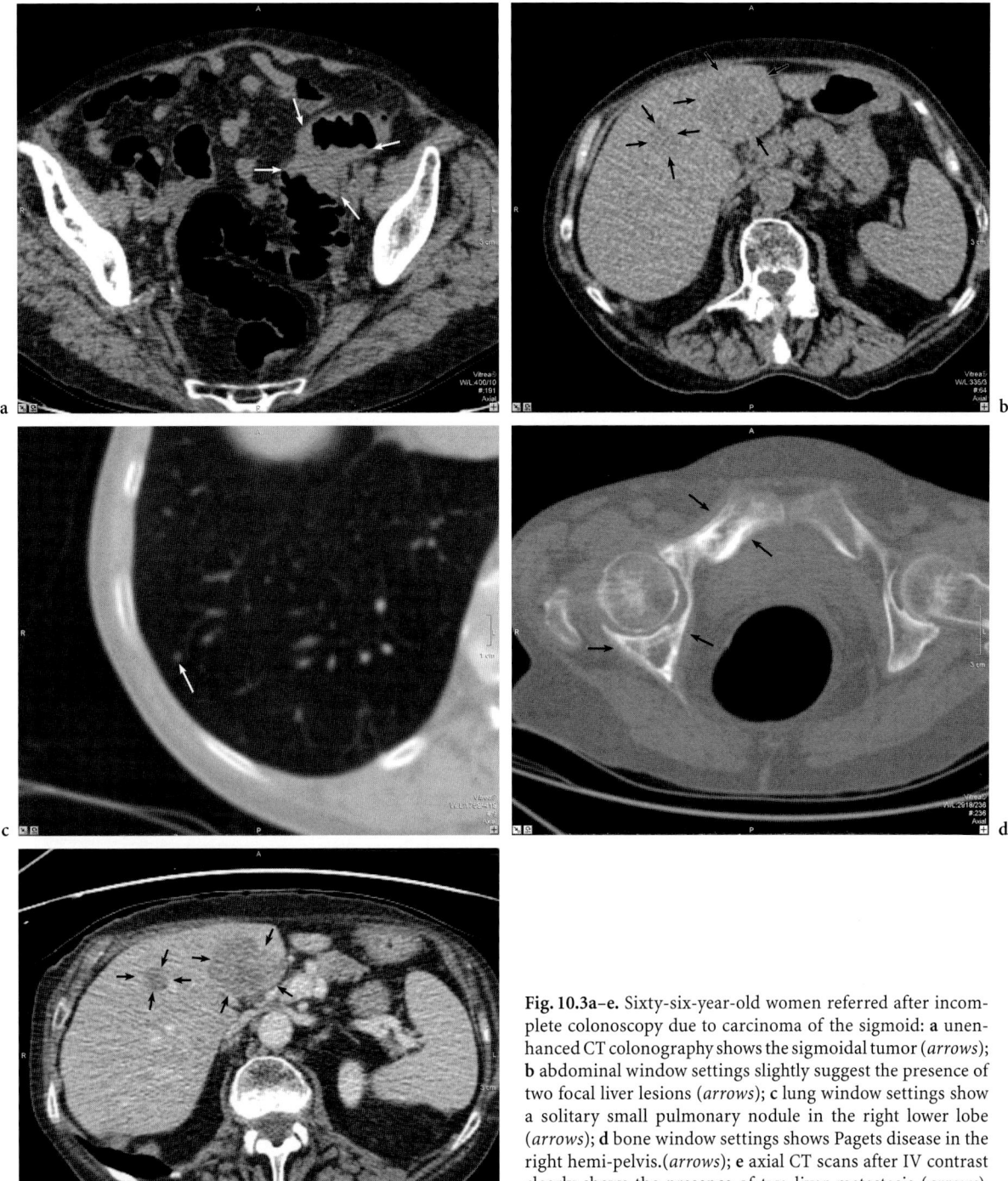

Fig. 10.3a–e. Sixty-six-year-old women referred after incomplete colonoscopy due to carcinoma of the sigmoid: a unenhanced CT colonography shows the sigmoidal tumor (*arrows*); b abdominal window settings slightly suggest the presence of two focal liver lesions (*arrows*); c lung window settings show a solitary small pulmonary nodule in the right lower lobe (*arrows*); d bone window settings shows Pagets disease in the right hemi-pelvis.(*arrows*); e axial CT scans after IV contrast clearly shows the presence of two liver metastasis (*arrows*). This case clearly illustrates the need for different window settings, and the difficulty of recognizing solid liver lesions using low dose unenhanced CT scans

solid organ lesions will remain undetected using low dose CTC without IV contrast (Fig. 10.3). This is nicely reflected when we compare the results of the population evaluated in the study by SPRENG et al., using high dose and IV contrast (SPRENG et al. 2005): compared with other studies, this study has the highest number of patients with extracolonic findings.

In our institution, we use a low dose technique (140 KV, with 10 mAs for supine, and 30 mAs for prone scanning), without IV contrast. For the evaluation of the colon, 0.6-mm slices are reconstructed at every 0.3 mm; for the evaluation of extracolonic findings, 3 mm thick slices are reconstructed at every 1.5 mm. The latter reduces noise, enabling visualisation of solid organ lesions (Fig. 10.4).

Since the use of IV contrast and normal dose might influence diagnosis of extracolonic findings, an active online physician monitoring could be considered to identify immediately patients who need IV contrast (Hara et al. 2000).

same holds true for focal fatty infiltration or normal variants in renal or pancreatic morphology.

Low dose scanning without IV contrast also causes false negatives, as reported by Hara et al. (Hara et al. 2000), and Gluecker et al. (Gluecker et al. 2003). Hara reported one missed gastric carcinoma, one psoas metastasis, and one invasive transitional cell carcinoma of the bladder. Gluecker reported one missed adenocarcinoma of the pancreas, one splenic and one ovarian mass.

It can thus be concluded that low dose technique without IV contrast results in possible, but low (<1.5%) false negative diagnosis (Hara 2005).

10.7
False Positive and False Negative Diagnosis

Most studies using low dose CT without IV contrast report upon hepatic or renal cysts that were further evaluated. False positives are thus caused by a low dose technique without IV contrast. For example, in the study of Hellstrom et al. (Hellstrom et al. 2004), there were four false positives: two cases of renal cysts, one normal pancreas, and one case of focal fatty infiltration. The contrary is reflected in the results of the study of Spreng et al. (Spreng et al. 2005), and focus on the group of patients with normal dose CT after IV contrast: in this single study no false positives were caused by renal or hepatic cysts. The

10.8
Economical Impact

Hara et al. (Hara et al. 2000) reported that the additional and recommended work-up added $28 to the examination cost per patient. If all highly important lesions would be further investigated, the added costs would be $36 per patient.

Gluecker (Gluecker et al. 2003) reported an added costs of $34 to the average cost.

Given the fact that in truly screening patient populations the total number of highly suspected findings is expected to be lower, as shown by Pickhard (Pickhard et al. 2003), both authors conclude that the added costs are more than acceptable.

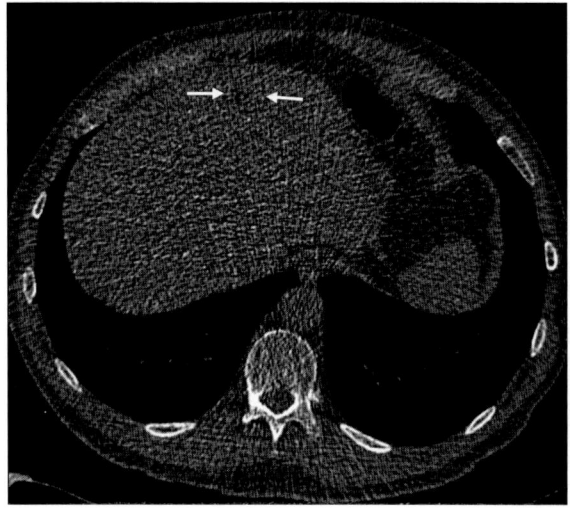 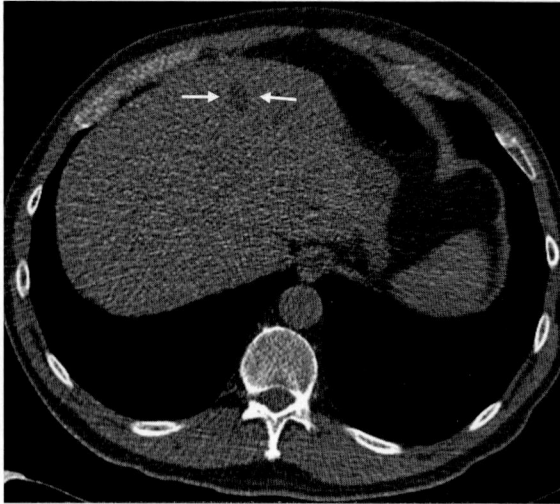

Fig. 10.4a,b. Fifty-five-year-old women referred for screening CTC. Low dose (10 mAs) unenhanced CT scan with 3 mm slice thickness reconstructed with a 1.5 mm reconstruction interval clearly shows the presence of biliary cyst: **a** the cyst is extremely difficult to detect on 0.6 mm slice thickness with a 0.3 mm reconstruction interval; **b** this case illustrates the use of thicker slice thickness to reduce noise and increase lesion conspicuity

10.9
Impact on Patient Care and Well-Being and Ethical Impact

It is clear that in case of true positive findings, such as the early diagnosis of abdominal aortic aneurysm or renal cell carcinoma, patients will benefit from incidental extracolonic findings.

Moreover, Westbrook et al. (Westbrook et al. 1998) reported that even untreatable patients may appreciate a warning to organize their lives.

The converse is, however, also true: the awareness of findings, even of medium or low importance, might create distress for patients, such that the referring physician must initiate further work-up for those findings.

Lerman et al. (Lerman et al. 1991) reported on psychological side effects of breast cancer screening. This study showed that women with suspicious mammography findings showed significantly elevated mammography-related anxiety, despite the fact that malignancy was ruled out.

As already pointed out, we are not only confronted with possible false positive diagnosis, but also false negative diagnosis. Therefore, the patient cannot be sure of "not being ill".

One could thus argue, in view of possible false negative and false positive diagnosis, in relation to low dose scanning without IV contrast, not to look for possible extracolonic findings. To do so, radiologists could blind themselves by only looking at 3D reconstructed images, or axial images in lung window settings.

However, data for axial images showing extracolonic findings have still been obtained.

The question therefore remains whether it is appropriate – and ethically as well as legally feasible – to ignore these data, since life-saving data might remain hidden.

10.10
Conclusion

1. The incidence of extracolonic findings is high, but the majority of patients will have benign disease.
2. Older and symptomatic patients are more likely to have significant extra-colonic findings compared to a younger screening population.
3. A minority of patients will undergo medical or surgical treatment for previously undiagnosed extracolonic findings.
4. The technique of CTC, using low dose and no IV contrast, however results in possible false negative as well false positive diagnosis.
5. And finally, further studies are needed to evaluate the influence on mortality, morbidity, patients well-being, as well as economic impact, related to incidentally diagnosed extra-colonic findings.

References

Chervu A, Clagett GP, Valentine RJ, Myers SI, Rossi PJ (1995) Role of physical examination in detection of abdominal aortic aneurysms. Surgery 117(4):454–457

Edwards JT, Wood CJ, Mendelson RM, Forbes GM (2001) Extracolonic findings at virtual colonoscopy: implications for screening programs. Am J Gastroenterol 96(10):3009–3012

Ginnerup Pedersen B, Rosenkilde M, Christiansen TE, Laurberg S (2003) Extracolonic findings at computed tomography colonography are a challenge. Gut 52(12):1744–1747

Gluecker TM, Johnson CD, Wilson LA, Maccarty RL, Welch TJ, Vanness DJ, Ahlquist DA (2003) Extracolonic findings at CT colonography: evaluation of prevalence and cost in a screening population. Gastroenterology 124(4):911–916

Hara AK, Johnson CD, MacCarty RL, Welch TJ (2000) Incidental extracolonic findings at CT colonography. Radiology 215(2):353–357

Hara AK (2005) Extracolonic findings at CT colonography. Semin Ultrasound CT MR 26(1):24–27

Hellstrom M, Svensson MH, Lasson A (2004) Extracolonic and incidental findings on CT colonography (virtual colonoscopy). Am J Roentgenol 182(3):631–638

Homma Y, Kawabe K, Kitamura T, Nishimura Y, Shinohara M, Kondo Y, Saito I, Minowada S, Asakage Y (1995) Increased incidental detection and reduced mortality in renal cancer-recent retrospective analysis at eight institutions. Int J Urol 2(2):77–80

Jacobs I, Davies AP, Bridges J, Stabile I, Fay T, Lower A, Grudzinskas JG, Oram D (1993) Prevalence screening for ovarian cancer in postmenopausal women by CA 125 measurement and ultrasonography. BMJ 306:1030–1034

Jamrozik K, Norman PE, Spencer CA, Parsons RW, Tuohy R, Lawrence-Brown MM, Dickinson JA (2000) Screening for abdominal aortic aneurysm: lessons from a population-based study. Med J Aust 173(7):345–350

Kloos RT, Korobkin M, Thompson NW, Francis IR, Shapiro B, Gross MD (1997) Incidentally discovered adrenal masses. Cancer Treat Res 89:263–292

Kyriakides C, Byrne J, Green S, Hulton NR (2000) Screening of abdominal aortic aneurysm: a pragmatic approach. Ann R Coll Surg Engl 82(1):59–63

Lerman C, Trock B, Rimer BK, Jepson C, Brody D, Boyce A (1991) Psychological side effects of breast cancer screening. Health Psychol 10(4):259–267

Mihara S, Kuroda K, Yoshioka R, Koyama W (1999) Early detection of renal cell carcinoma by ultrasonographic screening-based on the results of 13 years screening in Japan. Ultrasound Med Biol 25(7):1033–1039

Nevitt MP, Ballard DJ, Hallett JW Jr (1989) Prognosis of

abdominal aortic aneurysms. A population-based study. N Engl J Med 321(15):1009–1014

Ng CS, Doyle TC, Courtney HM, Campbell GA, Freeman AH, Dixon AK (2004) Extracolonic findings in patients undergoing abdomino-pelvic CT for suspected colorectal carcinoma in the frail and disabled patient. Clin Radiol 59(5):421–430

Pickhardt PJ, Choi JR, Hwang I, Butler JA, Puckett ML, Hildebrandt HA, Wong RK, Nugent PA, Mysliwiec PA, Schindler WR (2003) Computed tomographic virtual colonoscopy to screen for colorectal neoplasia in asymptomatic adults. N Engl J Med 349(23):2191–2200

Spreng A, Netzer P, Mattich J, Dinkel HP, Vock P, Hoppe H (2005) Importance of extracolonic findings at IV contrast medium-enhanced CT colonography versus those at non-enhanced CT colonography. Eur Radiol Jun 18 [Epub ahead of print]

Tsui KH, Shvarts O, Smith RB, Figlin RA, deKernion JB, Belldegrun A (2000) Prognostic indicators for renal cell carcinoma: a multivariate analysis of 643 patients using the revised 1997 TNM staging criteria. J Urol 163(4):1090–1095; quiz 1295

van Nagell JR Jr, Higgins RV, Donaldson ES, Gallion HH, Powell DE, Pavlik EJ, Woods CH, Thompson EA (1990) Transvaginal sonography as a screening method for ovarian cancer. A report of the first 1000 cases screened. Cancer 65(3):573–577

Westbrook JI, Braithwaite J, McIntosh JH (1998) The outcomes for patients with incidental lesions: serendipitous or iatrogenic? Am J Roentgenol 171(5):1193–1196

Wilmink TB, Quick CR, Hubbard CS, Day NE (1999) The influence of screening on the incidence of ruptured abdominal aortic aneurysms. J Vasc Surg 30(2):203–208

Xiong T, Richardson M, Woodroffe R, Halligan S, Morton D, Lilford RJ (2005) Incidental lesions found on CT colonography: their nature and frequency. Br J Radiol 78(925):22–29

11 The Future: Computer-Aided Detection

Hiroyuki Yoshida

CONTENTS

11.1 Introduction 137
11.2 Why CAD? 138
11.3 CAD Techniques for Detection of Polyps 139
11.4 Performance in the Detection of Polyps 140
11.4.1 Performance of CAD 140
11.4.2 Improvement of Radiologists' Detection Performance 142
11.5 CAD Pitfalls 142
11.5.1 CAD False Negatives 142
11.5.2 CAD False Positives 143
11.6 Current and Future Challenges 145
11.6.1 Detection and Extraction of Colorectal Masses 145
11.6.2 Use of Correspondence Between Supine and Prone Views 145
11.6.3 Effect of Fecal Tagging and Digital Bowel Cleansing 146
11.6.4 CAD for Rapid Interpretation: First Reader Paradigm 148
11.7 Conclusion 148
References 149

11.1 Introduction

During the past decade, computer-aided diagnosis (CAD) has been shown to be of clinical benefit in fields such as detection of microcalcifications and classification of masses in mammograms (Astley and Gilbert 2004). The concept of CAD is not unique to these fields; indeed, it is more important and beneficial for examinations in which a large quantity of images need to be interpreted rapidly for finding a lesion with low incidence, such as the detection of polyps in CT colonography (CTC) and the detection of lung nodules in thoracic CT scans. In its most general form, CAD can be defined as a diagnosis made by a radiologist who uses the output of a computerized scheme for automated image analysis as a diagnostic aid (Doi 2004). Conventionally, CAD acts as a "second reader," pointing out abnormalities to the radiologist that otherwise might have been missed. The final diagnosis is made by the radiologist. This definition emphasizes the intent of CAD to support rather than substitute for the human reader in the detection of polyps.

CAD for CTC typically refers to a computerized scheme for automated detection of polyps and masses in CTC data. It provides the locations of suspicious polyps and masses to radiologists. This offers a second opinion that has the potential to improve radiologists' detection performance and to reduce variability of the diagnostic accuracy among radiologists, without significantly increasing the reading time. Such a CAD scheme should be distinguished from semi-automated computer applications in radiology that automate only one of these components and depend on user interaction for the remaining tasks. A typical example is the 3D visualization of semi-automatically segmented organs (e.g., segmentation of the liver, endoluminal visualization of the colon and bronchus), or image processing of a part of an organ for generation of an image that is more easily interpreted by human readers (e.g., peripheral equalization of the breast in mammograms, digital subtraction bowel cleansing in virtual colonoscopy).

Despite its relatively short history, CAD is becoming a major area of investigation and developments in CTC. Rapid technical developments have established the fundamental CAD scheme for the detection of polyps during the last several years. Prototype CAD systems have been demonstrated at conferences (Näppi et al. 2005b; Yoshida et al. 2004b) (Fig. 11.1) and commercial systems that implement the full CAD scheme or a part of it are becoming available in the market with names such as the Poly Enhanced View (Siemens Medical Solutions) and Colon Computer-Assisted Rader (MedicSight Inc.).

In the colon CAD workstation shown in Fig. 11.1, for example, the left and right images show the 2D

H. Yoshida, PhD
Associate Professor, Department of Radiology, Massachusetts General Hospital and Harvard Medical School, 75 Blossom Court, Suite 220, Boston, MA 02114, USA

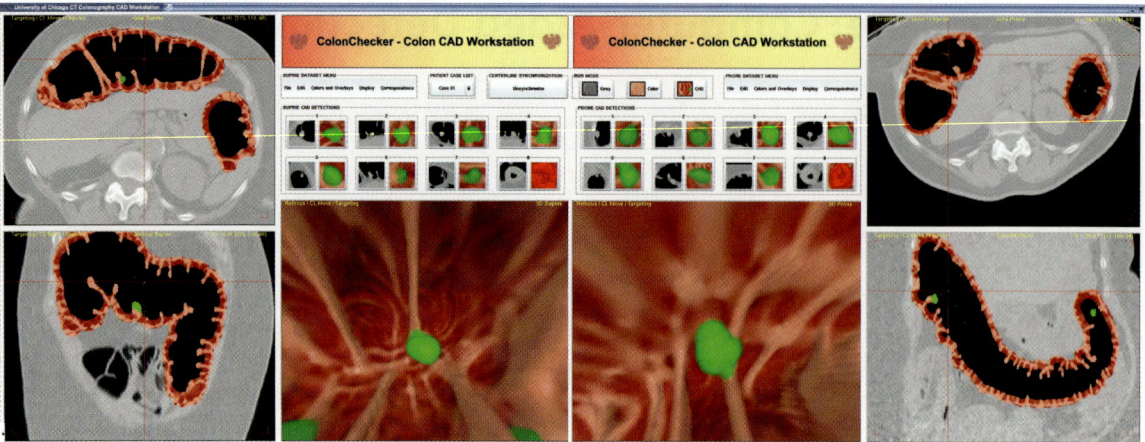

Fig. 11.1. Prototype colon CAD workstation

multiplanar reconstruction (MPR) views of the supine and prone scans of a patient, respectively, with the computer-extracted colonic wall superimposed. The bottom middle two images show the corresponding 3D endoluminal views of the colon. Polyps detected by CAD are shown as a list of icons on the middle row of the screen. By clicking on one of the icons, one can jump to the corresponding polyp on a 3D endoluminal view and/or an MPR view. The polyp (green) is displayed in both supine and prone views if it is found in the corresponding regions in these two views (see Sect. 11.5.2). CAD output is integrated into the 2D MPR and 3D endoluminal views by use of the coloring scheme that delineates the detected polyps and the normal structures in the colonic lumen (see Sect. 11.2).

The latest prototype CAD systems yield a clinically acceptable high sensitivity and a low false-positive rate (see Sect. 11.4), and they are becoming integrated into the 3D workstation for CTC examinations and thus into clinical workflow. However, some technical and clinical challenges still remain as open problems for CAD to become a clinical reality.

The remainder of this chapter describes the benefits of CAD, the fundamental CAD scheme, detection performance of CAD, pitfalls in CAD, and the current and future challenges in CAD.

11.2
Why CAD?

Although CTC is a promising alternative screening tool for colon cancer (DACHMAN and YOSHIDA 2003; PICKHARDT 2005; VAN GELDER et al. 2005), currently three key obstacles have held the clinical practicality of CTC at bay: (1) the variable diagnostic performance of CTC across studies (DACHMAN 2002; MULHALL et al. 2005), (2) the need for a full colon cleansing preparation, which is one of the major sources of poor patient compliance in colon cancer screening (GLUECKER et al. 2003; RISTVEDT et al. 2003), and (3) expertise required of the readers for interpreting the examination (BODILY et al. 2005; FLETCHER et al. 2005).

The first problem was partly addressed by PICKHARDT et al. (PICKHARDT et al. 2003), who showed that, based on 1233 asymptomatic patients, CTC could have a high by-polyp sensitivity of 93.9% for polyps >8 mm. This was superior even to that of optical colonoscopy. However, other large trials showed much lower sensitivity: a prospective trial on 703 asymptomatic patients reported by Johnson. et al. (JOHNSON et al. 2003a), a multicenter trial at 8 hospitals on 314 patients, also reported by Johnson et al. (JOHNSON et al. 2003b), a prospective multicenter trial at 9 hospitals on 615 patients by Cotton et al. (COTTON et al. 2004), and the most recent prospective multicenter trial at 15 hospitals on 617 patients by ROCKEY et al. (ROCKEY et al. 2005). Therefore, a larger clinical trial with the state-of-the art CT scanner and interpretation method needs to be conducted to address the first concern.

The second problem was partly addressed by LEFERE et al. (LEFERE et al. 2002, 2004a, b), who showed that dietary fecal-tagging CTC could be a viable alternative to full colon cleansing. However, the third obstacle remains problematic. In particular, the detection performance among readers can be quite variable, which may be one of the factors for the large variation in the results of reported large-scale clinical trials (FLETCHER et al. 2005).

CAD for CTC is attractive because it has the potential to overcome the third obstacle, i.e., polyps and masses detected by CAD have the potential to increase radiologists' detection performance and to reduce variability of the detection accuracy among readers.

An improvement in the detection performance can be achieved because CAD can reduce radiologists' perceptual errors during the detection of polyps. These perceptual errors may be caused by the presence of normal structures that mimic polyps or by variable conspicuity of polyps, depending on the display method (BEAULIEU et al. 1999; FLETCHER et al. 1999; JOHNSON and DACHMAN 2000; KARADI et al. 1999; MCFARLAND 2002). The absence of visual cues that normally exist with colonoscopy, such as mucosal color changes and a large number of images for each patient, also makes image interpretation tedious and susceptible to perceptual error.

A reduction of variability can be achieved because CAD can provide objective and consistent results. The performance of a radiologist may be influenced by his or her skill and experience. Moreover, a variety of circumstances, including distraction, fatigue, as well as time constraints in a busy clinical practice, influence the diagnostic performance. Although radiologists may detect a type of polyp in the majority of cases, the same persons may miss the same type of polyp under different circumstances. Use of CAD can potentially overcome this lack of consistency of radiologists, and thus it can be useful for reducing variability among readers in identifying polyps in CTC, as demonstrated by CAD for mammography and chest radiography (JIANG et al. 2001; KOBAYASHI et al. 1996) as well as the studies described in Sect. 11.4.2.

11.3
CAD Techniques for Detection of Polyps

To date, most of the CAD schemes developed in academia and in industry comprise of the following four fundamental steps: (1) extraction of the colonic wall from the CTC images, (2) detection of polyp candidates in the extracted colon, (3) characterization of false positives, and (4) discrimination between false positives and polyps. A brief description of each of these steps is provided below. More technical details on the fundamental CAD scheme can be found in recent review articles (YOSHIDA and DACHMAN 2004, 2005).

In the first step of the extraction of the colonic wall, either fully automated (MASUTANI et al. 2001; NÄPPI et al. 2002a, 2004b; WYATT et al. 2000) or semi-automated (CHEN et al. 2000; IORDANESCU et al. 2005; SUMMERS et al. 2000) methods are used. Most of these methods use the thresholding of the CTC data based on the CT values characteristic of the colonic wall and the contrast between the colonic wall and the air in the colonic lumen as a means of extracting the colon.

In the second step, polyp candidates are detected by use of morphologic features that characterize the shape differences among polyps, folds, and the colonic wall. Figure 11.2a shows an example colonoscopy image of a 6-mm polyp in the sigmoid colon. As schematically shown in the middle column, polyps tend to appear as bulbous, cap-like structures adhering to the extracted colonic wall, whereas folds appear as elongated, ridge-like structures, and the colonic wall itself appears as a large, nearly flat, cup-like structure. To characterize these morphologic differences, various methods have been developed, including use of a volumetric shape index and curvedness (YOSHIDA et al. 2002a; YOSHIDA and NÄPPI 2001), surface curvature with a rule-based filter (SUMMERS et al. 2000), sphere fitting (KISS et al. 2002), and overlapping surface normal method (PAIK et al. 2004). Figure 11.2b shows pseudo-coloring of the colonic lumen that visualizes the result of the shape analysis based on the volumetric shape index. The shape index determines to which of the following five topologic classes a voxel belongs: cup, rut, saddle, ridge, or cap. Color coding of the anatomic structures in the colonic lumen based on these classes can thus differentiate among polyps (green), folds (pink), and colonic walls (brown) effectively (NÄPPI et al. 2005b).

Typically, the polyp candidates thus detected include a large number of false positives, many of which are caused by prominent folds and by feces (YOSHIDA et al. 2002a, 2002b). Various methods characterizing false positives based on geometric and texture features have been developed for reduction of their number, include volumetric texture analysis (NÄPPI and YOSHIDA 2002), CT attenuation (SUMMERS et al. 2001), random orthogonal shape section (GOKTURK et al. 2001), and optical flow (ACAR et al. 2002).

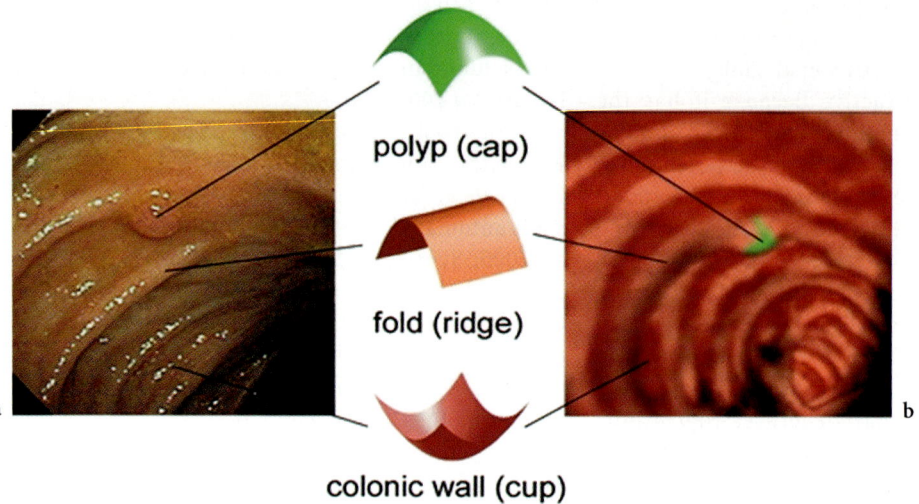

Fig. 11.2a,b. Schematic illustration of the geometric modeling of the structures in the colonic lumen. (Reprint, with permission, from YOSHIDA and DACHMAN 2004)

The final detected polyps are obtained by application of a statistical classifier based on the image features to the differentiation of polyps from false positives. Investigators use parametric classifiers such as quadratic discriminant analysis (YOSHIDA and NÄPPI 2001), non-parametric classifiers such as artificial neural networks (JEREBKO et al. 2003b; KISS et al. 2002; NÄPPI et al. 2004b), a committee of neural networks (JEREBKO et al. 2003a), and a support vector machine (GOKTURK et al. 2001). In principle, any combination of features and a classifier that provides a high classification performance should be sufficient for the differentiation task.

The CAD output is displayed, in a 3D workstation, as a list of detected polyps (YOSHIDA et al. 2004b) (Fig. 11.1) or integrated in 2D MPR and 3D endoluminal views of the colon by use of, for example, the coloring scheme that delineates the detected polyps and the normal structures in the colonic lumen (NÄPPI et al. 2005b) as shown in Fig. 11.3. For each pair in this figure, the left image shows an axial CT image containing a polyp (arrow), and the right image shows its 3D endoscopic view by perspective volume rendering. The color coding is based on the above shape index analysis (Fig. 11.2). Figure 11.3a shows a 6-mm sessile polyp in cecum and Fig. 11.3b shows a 5.3-mm polyp in cecum, both of which were missed by a radiologist at first reading. Figure 11.3c shows a 7-mm polyp in the transverse colon, and Fig. 11.3d shows an 11-mm sessile polyp in the hepatic flexure. All of these polyps are clearly segmented from folds and the colonic wall by use of CAD.

11.4 Performance in the Detection of Polyps

11.4.1 Performance of CAD

Several academic institutions have conducted clinical trials to demonstrate the performance of their CAD systems (KISS et al. 2002; NÄPPI et al. 2004b; NÄPPI and YOSHIDA 2003; PAIK et al. 2004; SUMMERS et al. 2001; YOSHIDA et al. 2002a, b; YOSHIDA and NÄPPI 2001) that implement the full CAD scheme in the previous section or a part of it. In these studies, optical colonoscopy was used as the gold standard, i.e., the locations of the polyps detected by CAD were compared with the "true" locations of polyps that were determined visually in CTC data sets based on colonoscopy reports. In most of theses studies, the performance of CAD was evaluated on CTC cases that were collected retrospectively at a single institution, and that were acquired with a protocol that is currently widely used for CTC, i.e., standard precolonoscopy cathartic bowel cleansing, insufflation of the colon with room air or carbon dioxide, and standard-dose CT scanning with CT parameter settings such as the following: a collimation of 2.5–5.0 mm, pitch of 1–2, a tube current of 50–200 mA, and a reconstruction interval of 1.25–3.0 mm.

Among the studies published in peer-reviewed journals that describe a full CAD scheme, the CAD scheme developed at the University of Chicago yielded a 95% by-polyp sensitivity, with an average of 1.5 false positives per patient (0.7 false positives per

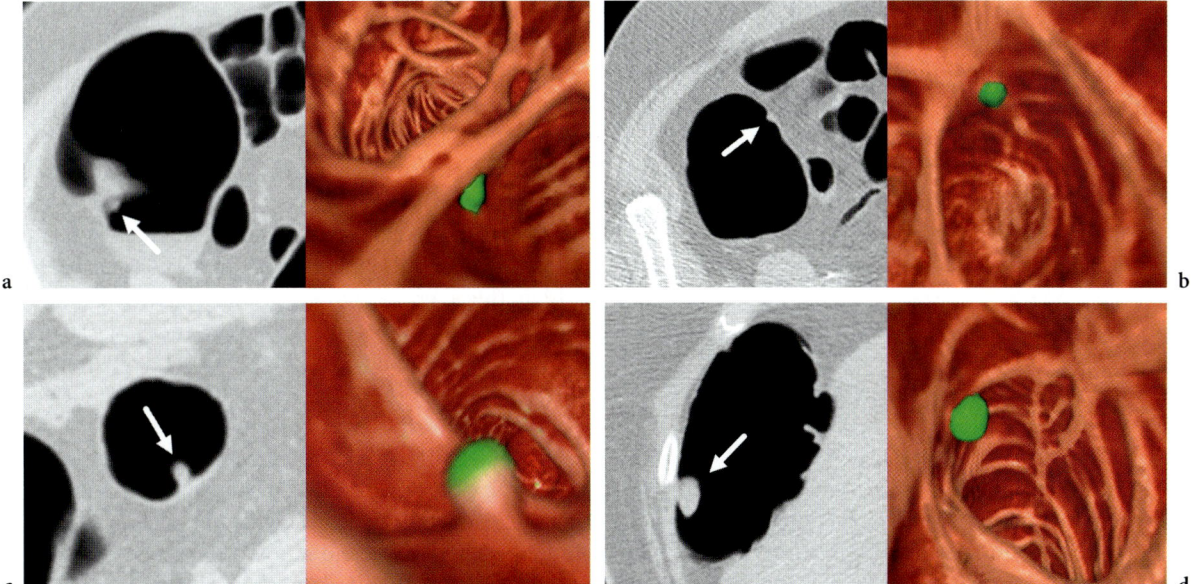

Fig. 11.3a–d. Example of polyps detected by CAD. (Reprint, with permission, from YOSHIDA and DACHMAN 2005)

data set), based on 72 patients (144 data sets), including a total of 21 polyps ≥5 mm in 14 patients. In a by-patient analysis, the sensitivity was 100%, with 1.3 false positives per patient (NÄPPI and YOSHIDA 2003). The same group reported, in a follow-up study that was published in a conference proceedings paper, a 93% by-polyp sensitivity with 4.0 false positives per patient (2.0 false positives per data set) based on 121 patients (242 data sets), including a total of 42 polyps ≥5 mm in 28 patients (NÄPPI et al. 2004b). Figure 11.4 shows a free-response receiver-operating characteristic (FROC) curve that shows the sensitivity of this CAD scheme as a function of the average number of false positives per data set. Generally, sensitivity of CAD increases as the number of false positives increases.

The CAD system at the University Hospital Gasthuisberg achieved an 80% by-polyp sensitivity, with 8.2 false positives per patient (4.1 false positives per data set), based on 18 patients, with 15 polyps ≥5 mm in 9 patients (KISS et al. 2002). In this study, fecal tagging was used for most of the cases. A group at Stanford reported a 100% sensitivity with 7.0 false positives per data set (only the supine data set of each patient was used) based on 8 patients that included a total of 7 polyps >10 mm in 4 patients (PAIK et al. 2004). The sensitivity was less than 50% at the same false positive rate for 11 polyps between 5 and 9 mm that were found in 3 of the above 8 patients. A group at the NIH reported a 90% sensitivity with 15.7 false positives per data set, based on 40 patients (80 data sets) that included a total of 39 polyps ≥3 mm in 20 patients (JEREBKO et al. 2003b). In a separate study, they reported that multiple artificial neural networks could potentially be employed to increase the sensitivity by an average of 6.9% and to reduce the false-positive rate by 30–36% (JEREBKO et al. 2003a, YAO et al. 2004).

These studies indicate that CAD is promising in detecting polyps with high sensitivity and a low false-positive rate. It appears that the detection performance can reach up to 100% by-patient sensitivity with 1.3 false positives per patient for polyps ≥5 mm (NÄPPI and YOSHIDA 2003). Generally, however, the performance of CAD systems appears to range between 70 and 100% by-patient sensitivity for

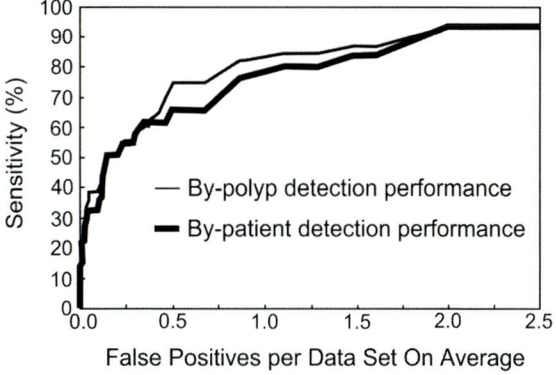

Fig. 11.4. Free-response receiver-operating characteristic curve showing the performance of CAD in the detection of polyps

polyps ≥6 mm, with 2–8 false positives per patient. A meta-analysis of the reported performance of CTC showed that, for human readers, the pooled by-patient sensitivity for polyps ≥10 mm and for those 6–9 mm was 85 and 70%, respectively (MULHALL et al. 2005). Comparing this performance with that of CAD, it appears that the performance, especially the sensitivity, of CAD is approaching that of an average human reader.

11.4.2
Improvement of Radiologists' Detection Performance

The ultimate goal of CAD is to improve the performance of radiologists in the detection of polyps and masses. Thus, establishing the sensitivity and specificity of CAD is only the first step in the evaluation of the benefit of CAD; CAD must be shown to improve the performance of radiologists.

It should be noted that CAD does not have to be as accurate as are expert radiologists to improve the detection performance of human readers. Computers make detection errors, as do human beings. However, together they can improve the diagnostic performance. Such a tendency can be found in an early clinical study by Summers et al. (SUMMERS et al. 2002), who examined the complementary role of CAD in radiologists' detection performance based on 25 polyps >10 mm in 40 asymptomatic high-risk patients. Two radiologists participated in the study. The sensitivity of both the two radiologists and that of CAD was only 48%; however, CAD showed that 4 of 13 polyps were missed by radiologists, thus increasing the potential sensitivity to 64%.

A recent observer performance study, which evaluated the effect of CAD on radiologists in an environment that closely resembles a clinical interpretation environment of CTC, showed that CAD could substantially improve radiologists' detection performance (DACHMAN et al. 2004; OKAMURA et al. 2004). Four observers with different levels of reading skill (two experienced radiologists, a gastroenterologist, and a radiology resident) participated in the study, in which an observer read 20 CTC data sets (including 11 polyps 5–12 mm in size), first without and then with CAD. The observer rated the confidence level regarding the presence of at least one polyp ≥5 mm in the colon. As shown in Fig. 11.5, the detection performance, measured by the area under the receiver-operating characteristic curve (A_z) (METZ 2000), increased for all of the observers when they used CAD, regardless of the different levels of their reading skill. The average A_z values without and with CAD were 0.70 and 0.85, respectively, and the difference was statistically significant ($p=0.025$). The increase in the A_z value was the largest for the gastroenterologist (0.21) among the four observers.

Another observer study was conducted by Mani et al. (MANI et al. 2004) based on 41 CTC cases, in which the average by-polyp and by-patient detection performance for 3 observers increased from 63 to 74% and from 73 to 90%, respectively, for 12 polyps ≥10 mm in 10 subjects, although the differences were not statistically significant.

These small-scale studies show the potential of CAD in increasing radiologists' detection performance, especially for those with less experience as indicated by the second study. A larger scale study needs to be conducted to show convincingly the benefits of CAD in improving the detection performance, in reducing the variability of the detection accuracy among readers, and in bringing the detection accuracy of inexperienced readers up to that of experienced readers.

11.5
CAD Pitfalls

11.5.1
CAD False Negatives

Knowing the pattern of the false negatives in CAD is important for improved sensitivity when the output of CAD is used as a detection aid. The types of false negatives included in CAD results are similar to

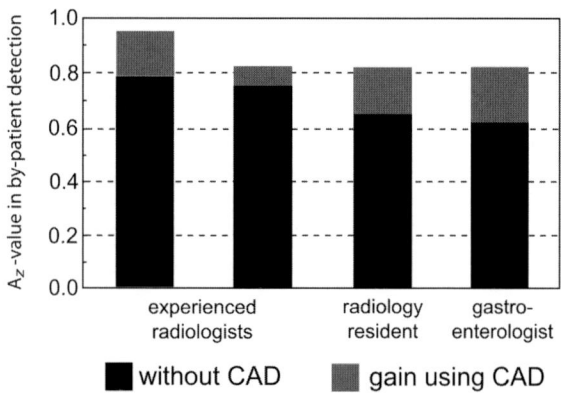

Fig. 11.5. Improvement of detection performance of human reader by use of CAD in the detection of polyps

those encountered by radiologists (YOSHIDA et al. 2002a,b). Most of the CAD techniques depend on a shape analysis that assumes that polyps appear to have a cap-like shape, i.e., they appear as polypoid lesions. Therefore, polyps that do not protrude sufficiently into the lumen (e.g., diminutive polyps and flat lesions), whose shape deviates significantly from polypoid (e.g., infiltrating carcinoma), those that lose a portion due to the partial volume effect, those that are located in a collapsed region of the colon, or those that are submerged in fluid, may be missed by CAD. Improvement of the CAD techniques for reliable detection of these types of polyps remains for future investigation.

Representative examples of CAD false negatives are shown in Figure 11.6. Figure 11.6a shows a magnified view of a 6-mm polyp at the proximal transverse colon (white arrow), and Fig. 11.6b shows its 3D endoscopic view (white arrow). This polyp was located in a narrow valley where two folds merge, and thus the shape of the polyp was distorted. Moreover, a motion artifact made the polyp appear blurred, and thus it was a false-negative polyp. The neighboring polyp (black arrow), located below the convergence of the two folds, was detected by CAD because it was less distorted than the above polyp. Figure 11.6c shows a 7-mm polyp in the sigmoid colon, and Fig. 11.6d shows an 8-mm polyp in the sigmoid colon. These polyps appear smaller than expected from their size, mainly because they lost a portion due to the partial volume effect, and thus these polyps were false-negative polyps in CAD.

11.5.2
CAD False Positives

False positives may lead to unnecessary further workups such as polypectomy by colonoscopy; therefore, knowledge about the pattern of CAD false positives is important for dismissing them. Studies showed that most of the false positives detected by CAD tend to exhibit polyp-like shapes, and the major causes of CAD false positives are the following (YOSHIDA et al. 2002a,b). Approximately half (45%) of the false positives are caused by folds or flexural pseudotumors. They consist of sharp folds at the sigmoid colon, folds prominent on the colonic wall,

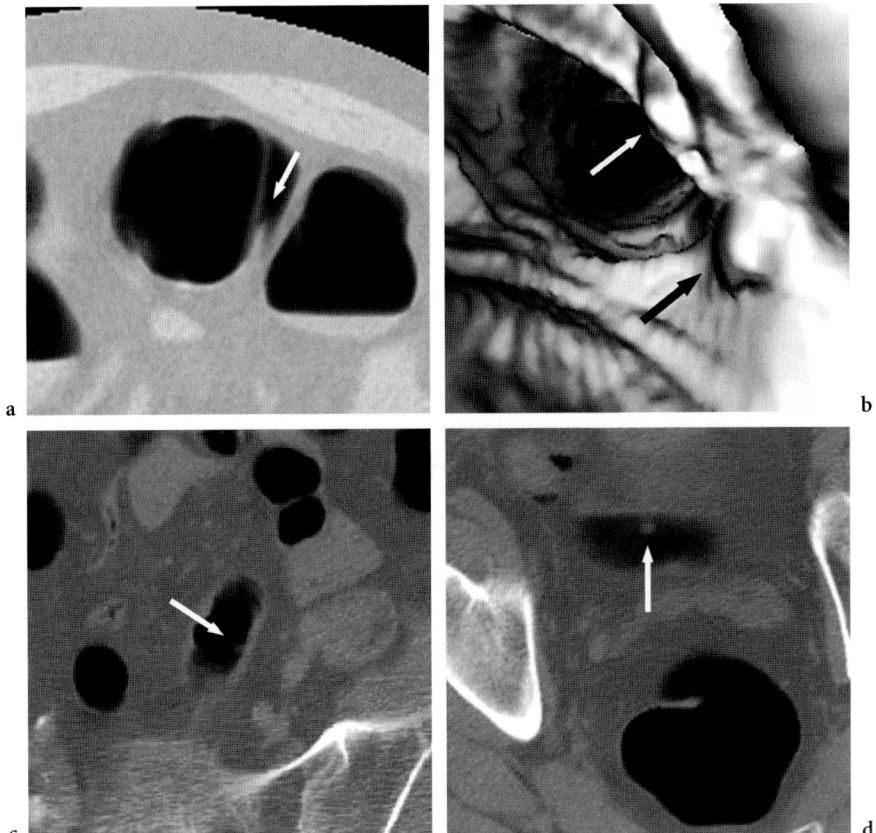

Fig. 11.6a–d. Example of CAD false negatives. (Reprint, with permission, from YOSHIDA and DACHMAN 2005)

two converging folds, ends of folds in the tortuous colon, and folds in the not-well-distended colon. One-fifth (20%) are caused by solid stool, which is often a major source of error for radiologists as well. Approximately 15% are caused by residual materials inside the small bowel and stomach, and 10% are caused by the ileocecal valve. Among other causes of false positives are rectal tubes, elevation of the anorectal junction by the rectal tube, and motion artifacts, each amounting to less than 3%.

Representative examples of CAD false positives are shown in Figure 11.7. Figure 11.7a shows a prominent fold (*arrow*). The tip of the fold appeared to be a cap-like structure, and thus it was incorrectly identified by CAD as a polyp. Figure 11.7b shows a piece of solid stool (*arrow*). This polyp-mimicking stool has a cap-like appearance and a solid internal texture pattern, and thus it was detected incorrectly as a polyp. Figure 11.7c shows an ileocecal valve (*arrow*). The tip of the ileocecal valve often has the cap-like appearance of a polyp and thus can be a cause of false positives in CAD. Figure 11.7d shows the residual materials (*arrow*) inside the small bowel and stomach. Although a majority of the small bowel and stomach is removed in the colon extraction step, a small piece of them may be extracted along with the colon, and thus residual materials in the small bowel and stomach can cause false-positive detections.

Studies show that radiologists can dismiss the majority of these false positives relatively easily based on their characteristic locations and appearance (DACHMAN et al. 2002). For example, false positives due to ileocecal valves and the rectal tube can easily be dismissed based on their anatomic location and shape; a semi-automated recognition of ileocecal valves may make this already easy task even easier (SUMMERS et al. 2004). Solid stool can be distinguished from polyps by visual correspondence analysis between prone and supine views; this relatively elaborate process can be facilitated by a computer aid (see Sect. 11.5.2).

However, there are types of false positives, such as solid stool that mimics the shape of polyps and adheres to the colonic wall, which are difficult to differentiate from polyps even for an experienced

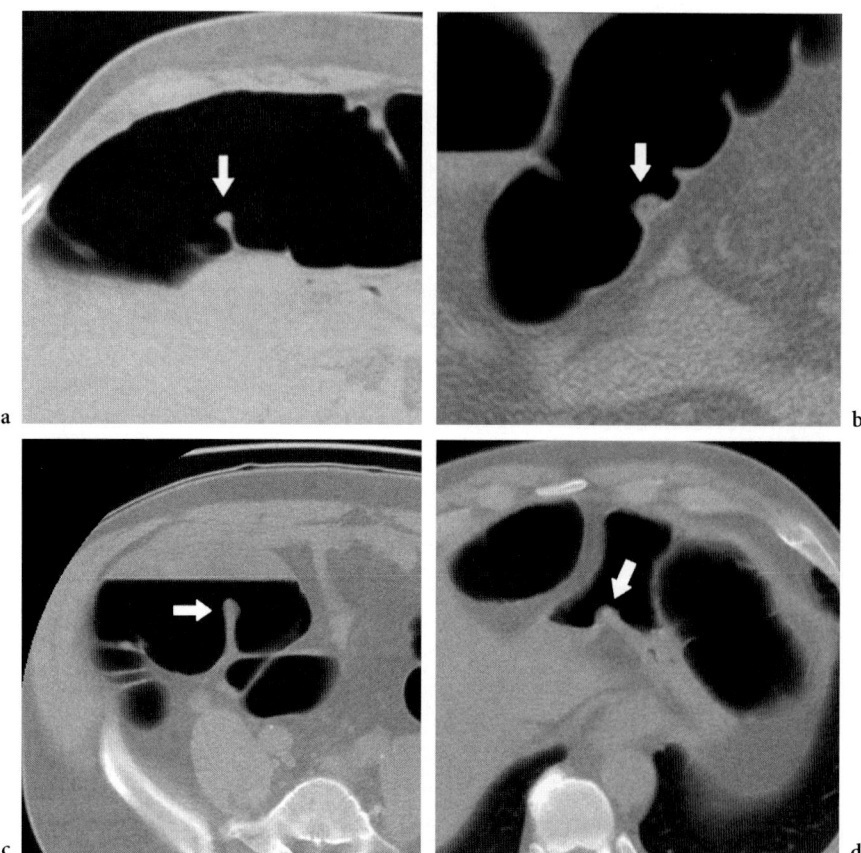

Fig. 11.7a–d. Example of CAD false positives. (Reprint, with permission, from YOSHIDA and DACHMAN 2005)

radiologist. Moreover, the pattern of the false positives may differ as new CAD techniques are developed. More research is required for establishing how radiologists can remove these false positives to make a correct final diagnosis reliably.

11.6
Current and Future Challenges

During the past several years, many of the challenges that were facing CAD in its early stage of development (SUMMERS and YOSHIDA 2003; SUMMERS 2002) have been extensively investigated and partially solved. However, some challenges remain as open problems. Also, new challenges are facing CAD as the methods for acquisition and interpretation of CTC images evolve. Some of the current and future challenges of CAD are described in the following sections.

11.6.1
Detection and Extraction of Colorectal Masses

Despite the importance of the detection of cancers, only a very small number of CAD schemes have been developed for detection of colorectal masses that are likely to be cancers. This is probably because colorectal masses are generally considered to be easily seen by radiologists due to their size and invasiveness. On the contrary, it is not easy for CAD to detect and accurately delineate entire mass regions; instead, CAD tends erroneously to report local surface bumps of a mass as several polyps.

The detection of both polyps and masses by CAD would be a more efficient computer aid in the interpretation of CTC examinations than is the detection of polyps alone. If masses are not detected by CAD, radiologists need to perform a careful and complete review of all CTC cases for the presence of masses, which may increase the reading time. Moreover, accurate detection of masses may depend on radiologists' experience and on how rapidly they read the cases (MORRIN et al. 2003). Therefore, the application of CAD to the detection of masses could improve the diagnostic accuracy of CTC by reducing potential reading errors due to reader fatigue, inexperience, or a too rapid reading. Furthermore, without explicit mass detection, CAD could also confuse radiologists by presenting portions of masses as several polyps.

Automated detection of masses poses challenges for CAD because they may appear as intraluminal types (lobulated, polypoid, or circumferential) or nonintraluminal types (mucosal wall-thickening type of growth pattern or masses that block the colon), both of which have a wide variation in shape characteristics. Only a few CAD schemes for the detection of colorectal cancers have addressed this challenge (NÄPPI et al. 2002b, 2004a). One of these studies (NÄPPI et al. 2004a) used a fuzzy merging method and wall-thickening analysis for delineation of intraluminal and non-intraluminal masses, respectively. The CAD scheme detected 93% of masses (13 of the 14 masses) in 82 patients and extracted their regions, with 0.21 false positives per patient on average. Figure 11.8a shows a 50-mm intraluminal circumferential mass with apple-core morphology, and Figure 11.8b shows its endoscopic view. The entire mass region was extracted by the mass detection method, as indicated by the white regions in Figure 11.8c,d.

Preliminary results indicate that CAD has the potential to detect colorectal masses in CTC with high accuracy. However, further research and a large-scale evaluation are needed for development of a CAD scheme that detect and delineate various types of masses reliably.

11.6.2
Use of Correspondence Between Supine and Prone Views

Use of both supine and prone data sets of a patient is important for improving the specificity in the detection of polyps, because the mobility of a suspicious lesion between supine and prone views can differentiate polyps from stool (CHEN et al. 1999; MORRIN et al. 2002). A real polyp tends to stay at the same location in the supine and prone views of the colon, whereas a piece of stool tends to move around in the colon, and thus, the stool can be found in different locations when supine and prone views are compared.

However, in order for CAD to find such movement, it is necessary to establish a location correspondence between the supine and prone views. This is often a challenging task because the colon can be substantially deformed when the patient's position is changed from supine to prone. Moreover, some parts of the colon can be displaced and collapsed at this positional change.

Most of the previous studies on correspondence between the supine and prone views were aimed

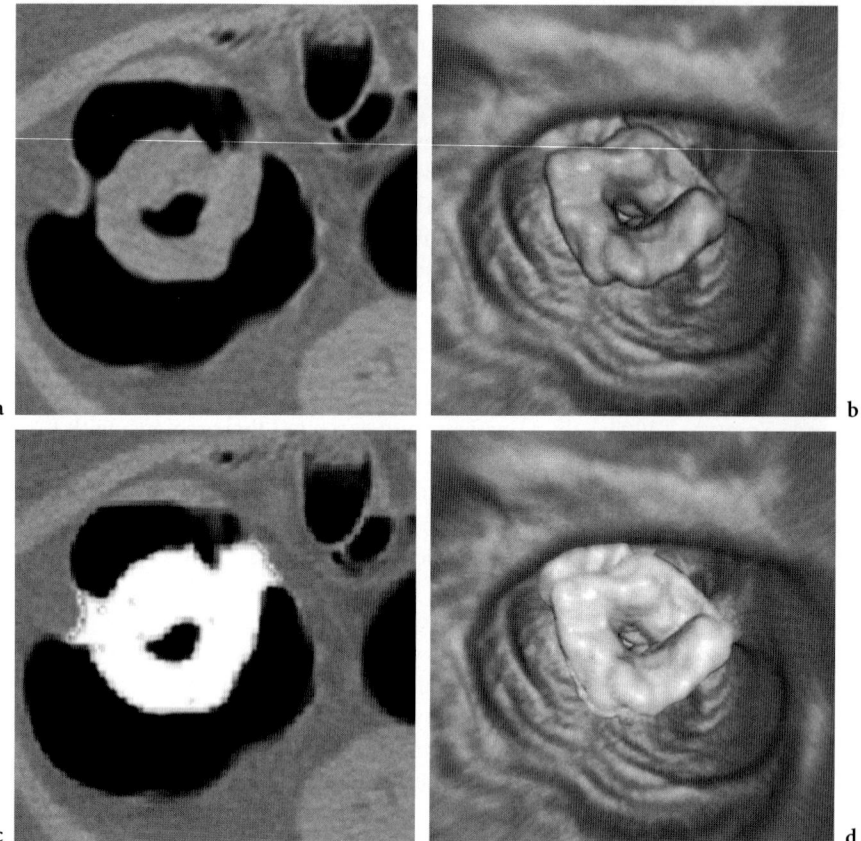

Fig. 11.8a–d. Detection of masses

at matching the polyp pairs after they are detected (IORDANESCU and SUMMERS 2003; LI et al. 2004; NAIN et al. 2002). Such a method would permit radiologists easily to identify the matched polyps in both views for subsequent detailed examination. For example, the CAD user interface in Figure 11.1 provides such a polyp matching function as shown in the middle two windows on the screen.

Only a few studies have addressed the challenge of using the supine-prone correspondence for improving the detection performance of CAD. One of these established a regional correspondence between supine and prone data sets of a patient by dividing of the colon into overlapped regions (NÄPPI et al. 2005a). Figure 11.9 shows an example of the overlapped regions, in which a narrow region (light gray) indicates the overlap between the two neighboring regions (dark gray and black). In this study, a polyp candidate was kept as a detected polyp if both of the corresponding regions in the supine and prone views contain the polyp candidate (gray circle). On the other hand, if only one of the corresponding regions contains a polyp candidate, it was removed as a false-positive detection (white circle). Use of this region-based correspondence method in CAD reduced the number of false-positive detections by 20% while maintaining a 90% by-patient detection sensitivity (NÄPPI et al. 2005a).

The preliminary result is encouraging; however, further investigations need to be conducted for demonstrating that the use of both the prone and supine views is truly useful for CAD to achieve a high specificity.

11.6.3
Effect of Fecal Tagging and Digital Bowel Cleansing

Tagging of feces, especially fluid, by an oral contrast agent such as a barium suspension or water-soluble iodinated contrast material, is a promising method for differentiating residual feces from polyps and thus improving the accuracy in the detection of polyps (BIELEN et al. 2003; LEFERE et al. 2002, 2004a, b, ; PICKHARDT et al. 2003; THOMEER et al. 2003).

The Future: Computer-Aided Detection

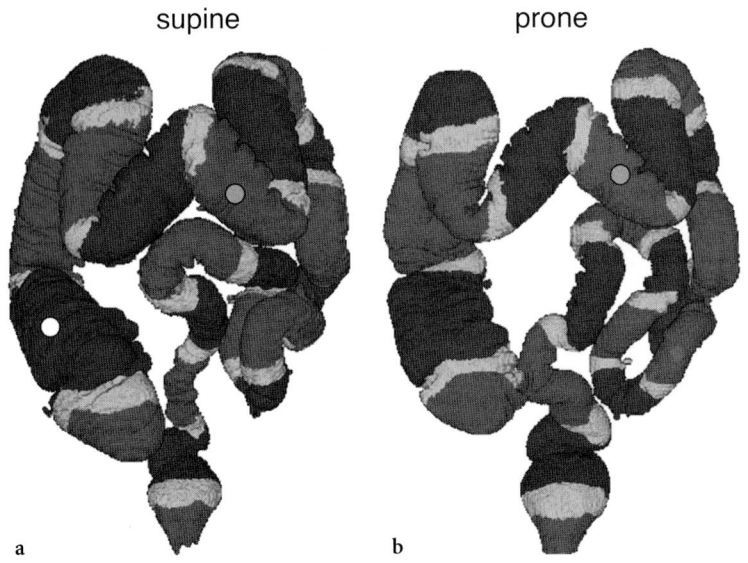

Fig. 11.9a,b. Region-based supine-prone correspondence method for reduction of false-positive detections. (Reprint, with permission, from YOSHIDA and DACHMAN 2005)

Digital bowel cleansing is an emerging technology for removing the tagged stool and fluid, and thus it is useful for reducing bowel cleansing while maintaining the accuracy of human readers in detecting polyps (PICKHARDT and CHOI 2003; ZALIS and HAHN 2001; ZALIS et al. 2003, 2004b).

Tagging of feces introduces an additional challenge to CAD because reduced bowel cleansing tends to introduce a large amount of fecal residue, some of which may be tagged well, whereas some may not be tagged completely. Such a mixture of tagged and untagged stool can be a cause of false positives in CAD (YOSHIDA et al. 2004a). Figure 11.10 shows examples of stool (arrows) adhering to the colonic wall that were not tagged by the barium-based tagging regimen and thus were erroneously detected as polyps by CAD.

Moreover, digital cleansing may introduce artifacts because of the partial volume effect and a suboptimal mucosal reconstruction method, especially at the interface of air and tagged fluid along the colonic wall or at the interface of air, fluid, and a fold (ZALIS et al. 2004a). Digital cleansing may also create 3D artifacts that simulate polyps because incomplete cleansing due to suboptimal opacification of luminal fluid can result in artifacts that may have the appearance of polyposis (PICKHARDT and CHOI 2003), which can be a cause of false positives in CAD. Current investigations of CAD for fecal-tagging cases with cathartic preparation (SUMMERS et al. 2005) and with reduced or minimum preparation (YOSHIDA et al. 2004a; ZALIS et al. 2004a) are encouraging in that CAD showed the potential to detect polyps not only in the dry region of the colon, but also submerged in the tagged fluid. The left image in Figure 11.11 shows an example of a polyp (black arrow) that was submerged in the tagged fluid; this polyp was correctly detected and segmented by CAD, as indicated by the black region in the right image.

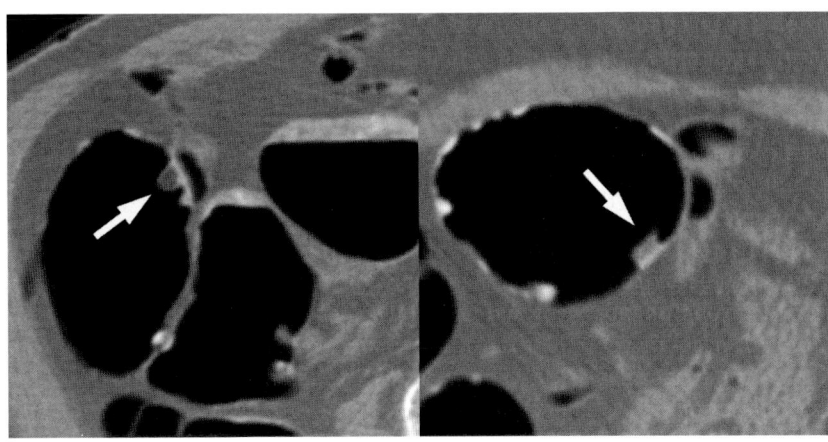

Fig. 11.10. Example of false positives in CAD for fecal-tagging CTC. (Courtesy of P. Lefere, M.D., Stedelijk Ziekenhuis, Roeselare, Belgium)

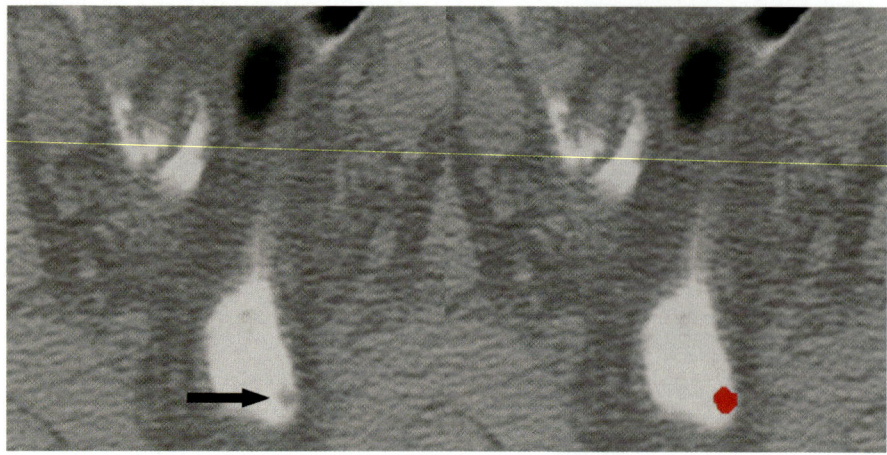

Fig. 11.11. Example of a true positive in CAD for fecal-tagging CTC. (Courtesy of Michael Zalis, M.D., Massachusetts General Hospital, Boston, MA)

Although encouraging, the results of these studies are limited and are not conclusive; therefore, CAD for fecal-tagging CTC remains a subject for future research.

11.6.4
CAD for Rapid Interpretation: First Reader Paradigm

Some researchers proposed that CAD can reduce the interpretation time if radiologists focus on a small number of regions indicated by a CAD scheme. A reduction in time is most likely to occur when CAD is used as a first reader. Such a paradigm, often called "CAD as a first reader" (EVANCHO 2002; MANI et al. 2004), can possibly be used for separating out negative CTC cases even before radiologists read the cases. However, such a separation is likely to come with an increased number of missed abnormalities, because there is always a trade-off between sensitivity and specificity in CAD due to the fact that the diagnostic performance of a CAD scheme is represented by a receiver-operating characteristic curve (METZ 2000). In other words, when a CAD scheme is set to yield a high true-negative rate (i.e., a high specificity), the price we need to pay is a high false-negative rate (i.e., a low sensitivity).

Thus far, no study has shown convincingly that CAD can shorten the interpretation time of CTC examinations, although some commercial CAD systems are advertised to be used in a similar manner to a first reader, and thus they imply that their CAD systems would reduce radiologists' interpretation time. In fact, conventional use of CAD as a second reader may increase the interpretation time, because additional time is needed for examining the possible lesions found by CAD but not by a human reader. However, such an increase in time is expected to be small, as demonstrated in CAD for mammography (JIANG et al. 1999), or the total reading time may be unchanged, as demonstrated by a recent observer study (MANI et al. 2004). Further studies need to be conducted for evaluation of the effect of CAD for rapid interpretation of CTC examinations as well as the efficacy of the use of CAD as a first reader.

11.7
Conclusion

CAD techniques for CTC have advanced substantially during the last several years. As a result, a fundamental CAD scheme for the detection of polyps has been established, and commercial products are now appearing. Thus far, CAD shows the potential for detecting polyps and cancers with high sensitivity and with a clinically acceptable low false-positive rate. However, CAD for CTC needs to be improved further for more accurate and reliable detection of polyps and cancers. There are a number of technical challenges that CAD must overcome, and the resulting CAD systems should be evaluated based on large-scale, multi-center, prospective clinical trials. If the assistance in interpretation offered by CAD is shown to improve the diagnostic performance substantially, CAD is likely to make CTC a cost-effective clinical procedure, especially in the screening setting.

In the future, no matter what types of visualization method (endoscopic, virtual dissection view, etc.) and reading method (2D primary or 3D primary reading) are widely used, it is expected that the detection of polyps by CTC will make use of some form of CAD. As the benefits of CAD are established, it will become more difficult to justify not using it, just as it would be difficult for a radiologist to justify not using a magnifying glass for reading mammographic films. CAD will be a powerful diagnostic tool that will provide radiologists with an opportunity to expand their sphere of influence by placing these CAD systems under their control, rather than losing procedures irretrievably to other specialists.

References

Acar B, Beaulieu CF, Gokturk SB et al. (2002) Edge displacement field-based classification for improved detection of polyps in CT colonography. IEEE Trans Med Imaging 21:1461–1467

Astley SM, Gilbert FJ (2004) Computer-aided detection in mammography. Clin Radiol 59:390–399

Beaulieu CF, Jeffrey RB Jr, Karadi C et al. (1999) Display modes for CT colonography. Part II. Blinded comparison of axial CT and virtual endoscopic and panoramic endoscopic volume-rendered studies. Radiology 212:203–212

Bielen D, Thomeer M, Vanbeckevoort D et al. (2003) Dry preparation for virtual CT colonography with fecal tagging using water-soluble contrast medium: initial results. Eur Radiol 13:453–458

Bodily KD, Fletcher JG, Engelby T et al. (2005) Nonradiologists as second readers for intraluminal findings at CT colonography. Acad Radiol 12:67–73

Chen D, Liang Z, Wax MR et al. (2000) A novel approach to extract colon lumen from CT images for virtual colonoscopy. IEEE Trans Med Imaging 19:1220–1226

Chen SC, Lu DS, Hecht JR et al. (1999) CT colonography: value of scanning in both the supine and prone positions. Am J Roentgenol 172:595–599

Cotton PB, Durkalski VL, Pineau BC et al. (2004) Computed tomographic colonography (virtual colonoscopy): a multicenter comparison with standard colonoscopy for detection of colorectal neoplasia. JAMA 291:1713–1719

Dachman AH (2002) Diagnostic performance of virtual colonoscopy. Abdominal Imaging 27:260–267

Dachman AH, Yoshida H (2003) Virtual colonoscopy: past, present, and future. Radiol Clin North Am 41:377–393

Dachman AH, Näppi J, Frimmel H et al. (2002) Sources of false positives in computerized detection of polyps in CT colonography. Radiology 225(P):303

Dachman AH, Yoshida H, Parsad N et al. (2004) Observer performance study for evaluation of the effect of computer-aided detection of polyps in CT colonography. Am J Roentgenol 182:76

Doi K (2004) Overview on research and development of computer-aided diagnostic schemes. Semin Ultrasound CT MR 25:404–410

Evancho AM (2002) Computer-aided diagnosis: blessing or curse? Radiology 225:606; author reply 606–607

Fletcher JG, Johnson CD, MacCarty RL et al. (1999) CT colonography: potential pitfalls and problem-solving techniques. Am J Roentgenol 172:1271–1278

Fletcher JG, Booya F, Johnson CD et al. (2005) CT colonography: unraveling the twists and turns. Curr Opin Gastroenterol 21:90–98

Gluecker TM, Johnson CD, Harmsen WS et al. (2003) Colorectal cancer screening with CT colonography, colonoscopy, and double-contrast barium enema examination: prospective assessment of patient perceptions and preferences. Radiology 227:378–384

Gokturk SB, Tomasi C, Acar B et al. (2001) A statistical 3-D pattern processing method for computer-aided detection of polyps in CT colonography. IEEE Trans Med Imaging 20:1251–1260

Iordanescu G, Summers RM (2003) Automated centerline for computed tomography colonography. Acad Radiol 10:1291–1301

Iordanescu G, Pickhardt PJ, Choi JR et al. (2005) Automated seed placement for colon segmentation in computed tomography colonography. Acad Radiol 12:182–190

Jerebko AK, Malley JD, Franaszek M et al. (2003a) Multiple neural network classification scheme for detection of colonic polyps in CT colonography data sets. Acad Radiol 10:154–160

Jerebko AK, Summers RM, Malley JD et al. (2003b) Computer-assisted detection of colonic polyps with CT colonography using neural networks and binary classification trees. Med Phys 30:52–60

Jiang Y, Nishikawa RM, Schmidt RA et al. (1999) Improving breast cancer diagnosis with computer-aided diagnosis. Acad Radiol 6:22–33

Jiang Y, Nishikawa RM, Schmidt RA et al. (2001) Potential of computer-aided diagnosis to reduce variability in radiologists' interpretations of mammograms depicting microcalcifications. Radiology 220:787–794

Johnson CD, Dachman AH (2000) CT colonography: the next colon screening examination? Radiology 216:331–341

Johnson CD, Harmsen WS, Wilson LA et al. (2003a) Prospective blinded evaluation of computed tomographic colonography for screen detection of colorectal polyps. Gastroenterology 125:311–319

Johnson CD, Toledano AY, Herman BA et al. (2003b) Computerized tomographic colonography: performance evaluation in a retrospective multicenter setting. Gastroenterology 125:688–695

Karadi C, Beaulieu CF, Jeffrey RB Jr et al. (1999) Display modes for CT colonography. Part I. Synthesis and insertion of polyps into patient CT data. Radiology 212:195–201

Kiss G, Van Cleynenbreugel J, Thomeer M et al. (2002) Computer-aided diagnosis in virtual colonography via combination of surface normal and sphere fitting methods. Eur Radiol 12:77–81

Kobayashi T, Xu XW, MacMahon H et al. (1996) Effect of a computer-aided diagnosis scheme on radiologists' performance in detection of lung nodules on radiographs. Radiology 199:843–848

Lefere PA, Gryspeerdt SS, Dewyspelaere J et al. (2002) Dietary fecal tagging as a cleansing method before CT colonography: initial results – polyp detection and patient acceptance. Radiology 224:393–403

Lefere PA, Gryspeerdt SS, Baekelandt M et al. (2004a) Laxative-free CT colonography. Am J Roentgenol 183:945–948

Lefere PA, Gryspeerdt SS, Baekelandt M et al. (2004b) CT

colonography after fecal tagging with a reduced cathartic cleansing and a small volume of barium. Am J Roentgenol 182:75–76

Li P, Napel S, Acar B et al. (2004) Registration of central paths and colonic polyps between supine and prone scans in computed tomography colonography: pilot study. Med Phys 31:2912–2923

Mani A, Napel S, Paik DS et al. (2004) Computed tomography colonography: feasibility of computer-aided polyp detection in a "first reader" paradigm. J Comput Assist Tomogr 28:318–326

Masutani Y, Yoshida H, MacEneaney PM et al. (2001) Automated segmentation of colonic walls for computerized detection of polyps in CT colonography. J Comput Assist Tomogr 25:629–638

McFarland EG (2002) Reader strategies for CT colonography. Abdom Imaging 27:275–283

Metz CE (2000) Fundamental ROC analysis. In: Beutel J, Kundel HL, Metter RLV (eds) Handbook of medical imaging. SPIE Press, Bellingham, WA, USA, pp 751–770

Morrin M, Sosna J, Kruskal J et al. (2003) Diagnostic performance of radiologists with differing levels of expertise in the evaluation of CT colonography. Radiology 226(P):365

Morrin MM, Farrell RJ, Keogan MT et al. (2002) CT colonography: colonic distention improved by dual positioning but not intravenous glucagon. Eur Radiol 12:525–530

Mulhall BP, Veerappan GR, Jackson JL (2005) Meta-analysis: computed tomographic colonography. Ann Intern Med 142:635–650

Nain D, Haker S, Eric W et al. (2002) Intra-patient prone to supine colon registration for synchronized virtual colonoscopy. In: Dohi T, Kikins R (eds) Lecture notes in computer science. Springer, Berlin Heidelberg New York, pp 573–580

Näppi J, Yoshida H (2002) Automated detection of polyps with CT colonography: evaluation of volumetric features for reduction of false-positive findings. Acad Radiol 9:386–397

Näppi J, Yoshida H (2003) Feature-guided analysis for reduction of false positives in CAD of polyps for computed tomographic colonography. Med Phys 30:1592–1601

Näppi J, Dachman AH, MacEneaney P et al. (2002a) Automated knowledge-guided segmentation of colonic walls for computerized detection of polyps in CT colonography. J Comput Assist Tomogr 26:493–504

Näppi J, Frimmel H, Dachman AH et al. (2002b) Computer aided detection of masses in CT colonography: techniques and evaluation. Radiology 225(P):406

Näppi J, Frimmel H, Dachman AH et al. (2004a) Computerized detection of colorectal masses in CT colonography based on fuzzy merging and wall-thickening analysis. Med Phys 31:860–872

Näppi J, Frimmel H, Dachman AH et al. (2004b) A new high-performance CAD scheme for the detection of polyps in CT colonography. In: Sonka M, Fitzpatrick JM (eds) Medical imaging 2004: image processing. SPIE, pp 839–848

Näppi J, Okamura A, Frimmel H et al. (2005a) Region-based supine-prone correspondence for reduction of false positive CAD polyp candidates in CT colonography. Acad Radiol 12(6):695–707

Näppi J, Frimmel H, Yoshida H (2005b) Virtual endoscopic visualization of the colon by shape-scale signatures. IEEE Trans Inf Technol Biomed 9:120–131

Okamura A, Dachman AH, Parsad N et al. (2004). Evaluation of the effect of CAD on observers' performance in detection of polyps in CT colonography. In: Lemke HU, Vannier MW, Inamura K, Farman AG, Doi K, Reiber JHC (eds) CARS–Computer Assisted Radiology and Surgery. Elsevier, Chicago, IL, USA, pp989–992

Paik DS, Beaulieu CF, Rubin GD et al. (2004) Surface normal overlap: a computer-aided detection algorithm with application to colonic polyps and lung nodules in helical CT. IEEE Trans Med Imaging 23:661–675

Pickhardt PJ (2005) CT colonography (virtual colonoscopy) for primary colorectal screening: challenges facing clinical implementation. Abdom Imaging 30:1–4

Pickhardt PJ, Choi JH (2003) Electronic cleansing and stool tagging in CT colonography: advantages and pitfalls with primary three-dimensional evaluation. Am J Roentgenol 181:799–805

Pickhardt PJ, Choi JR, Hwang I et al. (2003) Computed tomographic virtual colonoscopy to screen for colorectal neoplasia in asymptomatic adults. N Engl J Med 349:2191–2200

Ristvedt SL, McFarland EG, Weinstock LB et al. (2003) Patient preferences for CT colonography, conventional colonoscopy, and bowel preparation. Am J Gastroenterol 98:578–585

Rockey DC, Paulson E, Niedzwiecki D et al. (2005) Analysis of air contrast barium enema, computed tomographic colonography, and colonoscopy: prospective comparison. Lancet 365:305–311

Summers R, Yoshida H (2003) Future directions of CT colonography: computer-aided diagnosis. In: Dachman AH (ed) Atlas of virtual colonoscopy. Springer, berlin Heidelberg New York, pp 55–62

Summers RM (2002) Challenges for computer-aided diagnosis for CT colonography. Abdom Imaging 27:268–274

Summers RM, Beaulieu CF, Pusanik LM et al. (2000) Automated polyp detector for CT colonography: feasibility study. Radiology 216:284–290

Summers RM, Johnson CD, Pusanik LM et al. (2001) Automated polyp detection at CT colonography: feasibility assessment in a human population. Radiology 219:51–59

Summers RM, Jerebko AK, Franaszek M et al. (2002) Colonic polyps: complementary role of computer-aided detection in CT colonography. Radiology 225:391–399

Summers RM, Yao J, Johnson CD (2004) CT colonography with computer-aided detection: automated recognition of ileocecal valve to reduce number of false-positive detections. Radiology 233:266–272

Summers RM, Franaszek M, Miller MT et al. (2005) Computer-aided detection of polyps on oral contrast-enhanced CT colonography. Am J Roentgenol 184:105–108

Thomeer M, Carbone I, Bosmans H et al. (2003) Stool tagging applied in thin-slice multidetector computed tomography colonography. J Comput Assist Tomogr 27:132–139

van Gelder RE, Florie J, Stoker J (2005) Colorectal cancer screening and surveillance with CT colonography: current controversies and obstacles. Abdom Imaging 30:5–12

Wyatt CL, Ge Y, Vining DJ (2000) Automatic segmentation of the colon for virtual colonoscopy. Comput Med Imaging Graph 24:1–9

Yao J, Miller M, Franaszek M et al. (2004) Colonic polyp segmentation in CT colonography based on fuzzy clustering and deformable models. IEEE Trans Med Imaging 23:1344–1352

Yoshida H, Dachman AH (2004) Computer-aided diagnosis for CT colonography. Semin Ultrasound CT MR 25:419–431

Yoshida H, Dachman AH (2005) CAD techniques, challenges, and controversies in computed tomographic colonography. Abdom Imaging 30:26–41

Yoshida H, Näppi J (2001) Three-dimensional computer-aided diagnosis scheme for detection of colonic polyps. IEEE Trans Med Imaging 20:1261–1274

Yoshida H, Masutani Y, MacEneaney P et al. (2002a) Computerized detection of colonic polyps at CT colonography on the basis of volumetric features: pilot study. Radiology 222:327–336

Yoshida H, Näppi J, MacEneaney P et al. (2002b) Computer-aided diagnosis scheme for detection of polyps at CT colonography. Radiographics 22:963–979

Yoshida H, Lefere P, Näppi J et al. (2004a) Computer-aided detection of polyp in CT colonography with dietary fecal tagging: pilot assessment of performance. Radiology 227(P):577

Yoshida H, Näppi J, Parsad N et al. (2004b) ColonChecker: a state-of-the-art CAD workstation for detection of polyps in CT colonography. Radiology 227(P):809

Zalis M, Yoshida H, Näppi J et al. (2004a) Evaluation of false positive detections in combined computer-aided polyp detection and minimal preparation/digital subtraction CT colonography (CTC). Radiology 227(P):578

Zalis ME, Hahn PF (2001) Digital subtraction bowel cleansing in CT colonography. Am J Roentgenol 176:646–648

Zalis ME, Perumpillichira J, Del Frate C et al. (2003) CT colonography: digital subtraction bowel cleansing with mucosal reconstruction: initial observations. Radiology 226:911–917

Zalis ME, Perumpillichira J, Hahn PF (2004b) Digital subtraction bowel cleansing for CT colonography using morphological and linear filtration methods. IEEE Trans Med Imaging 23:1335–1343

12 Quality and Consistency in Reporting CT Colonography

Abraham H. Dachman and Michael Zalis

CONTENTS

12.1 Introduction 153
12.2 Screening vs Non-Screening Cohorts 153
12.3 Defining the Patient Preparation and CT Technique 153
12.4 Interpretation Method 154
12.5 Lesion Size and Colonic Segment Location 155
12.6 Lesion Morphology 157
12.7 Definition of the "Gold Standard" 157
12.8 By-Patient Data 158
12.9 Synchronous Lesions; Reporting of Data By-Polyp 158
12.10 Future Considerations 158
12.11 Conclusion 158
References 158

12.1 Introduction

The assessment of new technology such as CT colonography (CTC) is usually based on the evidence presented in the peer reviewed literature (Bruzzi et al. 2001; Sosna et al. 2003; Dachman 2002). A summary or combined metric of performance is often based on a meta-analysis of multiple reports. A typical meta-analysis, as often seen for clinical drug trials, requires a reasonable uniformity in methodology. The difficulties in conducting a statistically valid meta-analysis in virtual colonoscopy have been summarized previously (Dachman 2002). Sosna et al. performed a meta-analysis of CTC data (Sosna et al. 2003) and found only 14 papers in the peer reviewed literature meeting their criteria for inclusion. However these data assume a fundamental homogeneity of technique of exam performance, interpretation and reporting. Recent articles have emphasized the need for uniformity in presenting and reporting CTC data (Dachman and Zalis 2004; Zalis et al. 2005). In this chapter we review the factors that should be considered when the researcher reports results. Also, the informed reader should seek this information when reading reports of CTC trials. Even in a non-research setting, an internal audit of the success of a new CTC screening program is often desired. This chapter will guide radiologists and administrators as to the data that should be recorded and reported.

12.2 Screening vs Non-Screening Cohorts

The diagnostic performance in a screening cohort might be poorer than in a cohort with a high prevalence of disease. It is useful to know what percentage of cases are truly screening, meaning average risk for colorectal cancer (CRC), the risk factor being age 50 years or older, vs above average risk patients. Above average risk patients are those with a family history of CRC (particularly in a first degree relative), a personal history of CRC or colonic adenomas, or signs or symptoms suggestive of a colonic abnormality (e.g. blood in the stool, weight loss, anemia, etc.).

12.3 Defining the Patient Preparation and CT Technique

The effect of preparation is important, not only in terms of cleansing of the colon of residual stool, but also of residual fluid. Most CTC reports have been done on consenting research patients who are already scheduled to undergo a non-research conventional colonoscopy. The preparation is often chosen by the gastroenterologist. A colonic lavage

---

A. H. Dachman, MD, FACR
The University of Chicago, Department of Radiology, MC 2026, 5841 S. Maryland Ave., Chicago, IL 60645, USA
M. E. Zalis, MD
Massachusetts General Hospital, Dept of Radiology (White 270), 55 Fruit St., Boston, MA 02114, USA

with 4 L of polyethylene glycol is know to leave significant residual fluid which can hide polyps unless a unique strategy is used to reveal polyps submerged in fluid. Granted, in a well-distended colon, the use of both supine and prone views will theoretically move the fluid and reveal the polyp on at least one view, reader confidence is affected by not seeing the lesion on both views and sometimes the segment is collapsed on one view, thus precluding the possibility of correct diagnosis. Therefore in CTC screening, when the preparation is chosen by the radiologist a relatively "dry" preparation is preferred, using phosphosoda or magnesium citrate. Bisacodyl tablets can also be used to reduce residual rectal fluid. Polyps submerged in fluid can be revealed by use of additional decubitus views, use of intravenous contrast or use of fluid tagging with barium and/or water soluble orally administered contrast. Thus differences in these techniques can affect the diagnostic quality of the CTC and affect the validity of combining data from different investigators.

Recent evidence points to the efficacy of stool and residual fluid tagging, independent of the use of electronic subtraction (or "cleansing") by specialized software programs (IANNACONNE et al. 2004; McFARLAND and ZALIS 2004). Data should be analyzed separately for patients undergoing tagging regimens and those that do not. Details of tagging options are discussed elsewhere in this book.

Controversy also remains regarding the use of spasmolytics: glucagon (primarily used in the United States) and Buscopan (used in Europe, but not approved for use in the United States). These drugs may affect patient comfort (and thus the reporting of patient satisfaction) and colonic distention. Spasmolytics may theoretically improve or hinder colonic distention. On the one hand, colonic spasm is minimized. However the ileocecal valve may become incompetent allowing reflux of gas into the small bowel. The effect of ileocecal valve reflux will depend on the method of distension. If a mechanical pump is used which keeps the colon distended at a set pressure, then the reflux may not hinder colonic distension. If manual distension is used, additional gas insufflation just prior to scanning will be needed to compensate for the gas refluxed into the small bowel. For these reasons, reporting of medication used, its route and dosage and timing of administration, is also important.

The CT parameters will also impact the quality of the 2D, multiplanar and 3D reconstructed images. The details of scanner type, collimation, pitch, detector array for volume scanner, gantry rotation time, kVp, mA, mAs, radiation dose modulation, reconstruction kernel, reconstruction slice thickness and interval, pixel size, will all be important. Because of the complexity of these parameters, often data combined from different institutions is combined based on broad groups focusing on only key parameters such as: single vs multidetector scan; collimation over 3 mm vs 3 mm and less; high dose vs low radiation dose (a very subjective term since a wide range of dosages have been used). Other seemingly less important factors, many nevertheless, are significant, such as the method of breath hold. Older papers used multiple breath holds or a breath hold followed by quiet breathing. Volume CT scanners such as 16, 32, 40 and 64 slice scanners are capable of shorter breath holds (depending on the detector array and collimation used) thus minimizing artifacts due to respiratory motion.

12.4
Interpretation Method

The method of interpretation will undoubtedly affect reading time and probably diagnostic exam performance. Over the history of CTC, a wide range of software packages with varying capabilities have been used. In fact, software for CTC is still advancing rapidly and it is not uncommon to find that by time a peer-reviewed manuscript is in press, the software version used has been updated or is even no longer available. For this reason software platforms should be specified by vendor, version and other factors that can affect evaluation, such as: single vs dual monitor reading, mouse vs button control of navigation, automated vs manual fly-though. In the case of volume rendering, display parameters such as opacity and threshold should be reported in addition to standard window and grayscale level. For surface rendering displays, parameters such as threshold, contrast, lighting default settings should be reported. For both methods, it is important for investigators to report the field-of-view employed for scanning, and what if any zooming was employed during the interpretation of studies. Little head-to-head comparison has been made of these different viewing factors and the reporting of this data could assist in retrospective analysis of their affects (McFARLAND 2002).

Because it may affect reading time, the hardware platform upon which images are evaluated should also be specified. In particular, authors should report both the number of processors utilized in the display system and their clock speed. As cost analysis of CTC will be an important aspect of its evaluation, it is useful to separate interpretation time from the time needed to fill out research case report forms.

Many authors have used confidence scales to help in interpreting data (PICKHARDT et al. 2004b). This is another source of variation between authors in how confidence scales and ROC curves are generated. We suggest that rating scales for any issues such as: a) quality of distension, b) residual fluid, c) residual solid stool, d) confidence that a polyp is present at particular size criteria, uses a four- or five-point scale with discrete verbal descriptors of each of the points.

When more than one reader's results are reported, clarify if the interpretations are independent or represent a consensus. Independent, multiple-observer studies are preferred. If reading time is reported, specify if this includes the time required to document the findings.

There should always be a retrospective analysis of the cause of false positive and false negative interpretations of CTC and CC, when those data are available.

12.5
Lesion Size and Colonic Segment Location

The Boston Working Group previously published guidelines on the reporting of colonic lesion features (Table 12.1) and the classification of colonic findings for the purposes of suggested follow up (Table 12.2). Some of those parameters will be explained here as they impact the reporting of CTC data.

The matching of conventional colonoscopy (CC) and CTC for size and location is required in order to understand the diagnostic accuracy of the technique. Every effort should be made to measure accurately the size of each lesion detected. Ideally, during endoscopy use of a caliper tool is ideal. Normally only an estimate is made by comparing the polyp to the size of the open forceps. Measurement of polyps by comparison to open forceps requires that the forceps be held as closely as possible to the lesion, a point that should be emphasized as a quality control measure. Thus polyp size as reported by CC is usually at best an estimate. Lesion localization to a colonic segment is also a rough estimate by CC, because the endoscopist has little direct extraluminal reference by which to correlate the position of the endoscope within the colon. Even with new methods, such as a magnetic device attached to the endoscope that indicates endoscope location on the patient's skin, CC may be subject to overestimation of distance of the lesion from the rectum due to stretching of the colon by the endoscope. Thus comparison for lesion location is best done by review of a recorded video of the endoscopy when available. The matching of lesions between CC and CTC should include lesion relationship to folds (on-a-fold vs in between folds) and lesion morphology (sessile, pedunculated, and flat). When multiple lesions are present, sequence of lesions can be helpful as well. Because video recording the entirety of each colonoscopy exam is not always feasible, an alternative is for the endoscopist to acquire still snapshots of pertinent views of colon anatomy. These images can demonstrate colon pathology in relation to local normal anatomy and can be readily compared with the rendered endoluminal reconstructions that are available on all commercial CTC display stations. These matching techniques should substitute for a simple "segment" analysis of lesion location, and reporting investigators should clearly state what method they employed to compare size and position of polyps. Caution should be used before concluding that a lesion found by CTC – but not CC – is a false positive, even if video endoscopy is available for review. Pickhardt et al. have shown that some of these represent false negative exams by OC due to a polyp being hidden behind a fold (PICKHARDT et al. 2004a).

Table 12.1. Feature descriptors of colonic lesions

Lesion size (mm)	For lesions 6 mm or greater, single largest dimension of polyp head (excluding stalk if present) in either, MPR, or 3D views. The type of view employed for measurement should be stated
Morphology	Sessile–broad based lesion the width of which is greater than the vertical height
	Pedunculated–polyp with stalk
	Flat–vertical height less than 3 mm above the surrounding normal colonic mucosa
Location	Refer to named standardized colonic segmental divisions: rectum, sigmoid, descending, transverse, ascending, and cecum
Attenuation	Soft tissue density
	Fat

Table 12.2. Classification of colonic findings and suggested follow-up

C0. Inadequate study/awaiting prior comparisons	Inadequate prep: cannot exclude lesions >10 mm due to fluid/feces
	Inadequate insufflation: one or more colonic segments collapsed on both views
	Awaiting prior colon studies for comparison
C1. Normal colon or benign lesion; continue routine screening[a]	No visible abnormalities of the colon
	No polyp ≥6 mm
	Lipoma or inverted diverticulum
	Non-neoplastic findings, e.g. colonic diverticula
C2. Indeterminate lesion; surveillance recommended, or endoscopy[b]	Polyp 6–9 mm, <3 in number
	Findings indeterminate; cannot exclude polyps ≥6 mm
C3. Polyp, possibly advanced adenoma; follow-up colonoscopy recommended	Polyp ≥10 mm
	Three or more polyps, each 6–9 mm
C4. Colonic mass, likely malignant; surgical consultation recommended[c]	Lesion compromises bowel lumen; demonstrates extra colonic invasion

[a] Every 5–10 years
[b] Evidence suggests surveillance can be delayed at least three years, subject to individual patient circumstance
[c] Communicate to referring physician as per accepted guidelines for communication, such as ACR Practice Guideline for Communication: Diagnostic Radiology. Subject to local practice, endoscopic biopsy may be indicated

We favor the use of a six segment scheme when reporting the colonic segment location of a polyp. We suggest avoiding "hepatic flexure" and "splenic flexure" as separate segments. While the point of the flexure however is usually well-defined as the radiologic splenic and hepatic flexure – the first sharp curve in the colon at its most cephalad point – there is no defining transition between the flexure and the adjacent ascending, transverse or descending colon for the endoscopist. We suggest use of rectum, sigmoid, descending, transverse, ascending and cecum to report lesion location. We recognize that the defining points of the sigmoid are a matter of judgment of the radiology investigator and can vary according to the anatomy of each patient.

There remain differing opinions as to the best way to measure lesions. In most cases, lesion size can be measured accurately on magnified 2D multiplanar images. A notable exception is lesions that are oval which may be more accurately measured on 3D endoluminal views. We propose that for standardization, the largest single dimension be reported for a given lesion (analogous to RISC criteria for solid tumors), on 2D for round lesions and on 2D or 3D for oval lesions. Placing electronic cursors on the edge of a polyp on the 3D view is subject to error in that placement just beyond the edge of the polyp may markedly overestimate polyp size if the cursor is really placed on a nearby or distant colonic surface. As a result, we urge caution when making size measurements primarily on 3D endoluminal reconstructions. Investigators may wish to confirm correct placement of 3D cursors in another view before recording a measurement. While ideally, the average of several lesion measurements should be reported, but we recognize that this may not be feasible in all cases due to time constraints. Lesion shape should be given, e.g. round or oval, although the largest dimension should be used for reporting size. For pedunculated lesions the stalk diameter and length should be estimated. The selection of a particular window and level will also affect the apparent size of a lesion. We prefer lung window settings. In any event, the setting used should be specified.

To promote further standardization of reporting, we suggest that investigators should report polyps based on the following standard size categories: under 5 mm, ≥5 to <10 mm and ≥10 mm. Since large masses have a different conspicuity and clinical significance compared to polyps, they should be reported separately. More detailed data by exact size threshold (e.g. 6 mm, 7 mm, 8 mm and 9 mm sizes) is desirable. There is mounting evidence that a 6 or 7 mm size cut off is optimal and that reporting smaller lesions will adversely impact exam specificity. Annular cancers and masses 4.0 cm or larger be reported and analyzed separately from polyps. The size distributions of reported polyps has been a particularly frustrating issue in attempting to summarize reports, as some have used 7 mm or 8 mm size groupings. In some publications it is unclear how diminutive polyps (less than 5 mm) have been categorized. The data are overwhelming that specificity of CTC drops to unacceptable levels if lesions <5 mm are reported. In addition, there is growing consensus that the clinical significance of these diminutive polyps is quite small. The conclusion concerning clinical significance is based on the extremely low prevalence of carcinoma to be found in resected specimens of this size, and the fact that a large percentage of these lesions are hyperplastic in histology, hence carrying no malignant potential. In non-research situations, the lesions size can be first estimated by comparison to a scale on the 2D images. If the lesions is clearly <5 mm, time can be saved by not trying to measure or problem-solve these potential polyps.

When comparing lesion size to biopsy or pathology specimens, the report should indicate if the specimen was fresh or fixed. In either case, the lesion size as reported by the pathologist is likely to be smaller than that observed by either radiologist or endoscopist due to the combination of lack of blood flow and consequence of the fixation process.

The histology of the polyp should be categorized as adenoma (tubular, villous or mixed), adenocarcinoma, hyperplastic or normal mucosa. Hyperplastic polyps (and mucosal tags) are not pre-malignant, and several authors have suggested that hyperplastic polyps may flatten and be less conspicuous in well-distended or over-distended colons. In the case of diminutive lesions or difficult resections, the endoscopist is not always able to retrieve sufficient material to provide pathologic diagnosis. However, when available, this data aids in our understanding the prevalence and clinical significance of lesions. In addition, the ability to correlate of diagnostic performance to histology will be an important aspect of the validation of CTC since only the adenomatous lesions are pre-malignant. Therefore we recommend reporting sensitivity data for adenomatous lesions separately and for all lesions separately.

12.6
Lesion Morphology

Polyps should be reported with morphologic data in addition to size, as lesions with sessile or flat morphology are thought to confer a different risk of harboring carcinoma. Another important area of interest is the diagnostic performance of CTC for detecting flat lesions-polyps that primarily infiltrate along the colon mucosa and hence do not markedly impinge into the colon lumen (FIDLER et al. 2002). A recent review of the National Polyp Study showed that flat lesions, as defined by pathologists, do not have an increased risk of dysplasia or carcinoma, independent of the lesion size (O'BRIAN et al. 2004). Fidler et al. (FIDLER et al. 2002) have shown that flat lesions are less common than previously reported and that these lesions were also often hyperplastic. We propose that for reporting purposes, a flat lesion should be a one whose height is no more that 3 mm above the surrounding normal mucosa. (Avoid defining flat lesions as those whose height is 50% of the lesion diameter.) Accordingly, when a flat lesion is suspected, we recommend that authors report the additional dimension of lesion height. While lesion height may be easily measured from the CTC images, we recognize that lesion height from endoscopy may only be an estimate and is not normally reported unless prospectively requested. We propose that flat lesions should be further subdivided in those that are infiltrative with no perceptible raised component, and those that are raised and project into the lumen. The justification is that the latter may be more conspicuous to the CTC reader and may be more amenable to detection by shaped-based computer-aided diagnosis programs. Reporting the morphology of lesions more comprehensively will assist in fully evaluating the performance of CTC, since there may be differences in sensitivity related to morphology, particularly for flat lesions. In addition, to maximize our ability to retrospectively analyze the performance of CTC, we recommend that authors specify if flat or infiltrative lesions are visible only on one particular window/level setting. Analysis of this visualization data may permit future refinement of recommended reading protocols.

12.7
Definition of the "Gold Standard"

The often reported miss rate for CC of 6% for polyps 1 cm or larger, is based on a single small study of back-to-back CCs (REX et al. 1997). CTC studies suggest the CC miss rate may be 12% (PICKHARDT et al. 2004a). Several strategies are being employed by some multicenter trials to address this issue, including the segmental unblinding of the colonoscopist during the removal of the endoscope (PICKHARDT et al. 2003). In this method, CTC results are reported segment by segment, after the endoscopist has made his/her own independent evaluation of a segment of colon. If there is a discrepancy between the reported CTC finding and CC, the endoscopist is able to re-advance the scope in attempt to find and confirm the presence or absence of a polyp. This comparison is particularly important to reduce the false positive rate for CTC that may be due to true lesions that are not initially detected by endoscopy. Clearly, CC is our best arbitrary "standard", but it is important that we recognize its limitations. When possible, all follow up data should be used for comparison of lesion matching, including surgical findings and follow up endoscopy.

When a follow up exam such as a second colonoscopy, flexible sigmoidoscopy, barium enema or surgical resection of colon changes the "truth", the by-patient data should be presented both with and without this follow up data.

12.8
By-Patient Data

Using size and histologic criteria outlined above, the by-patient sensitivity, specificity, positive and negative predictive values of CTC should be reported with their confidence intervals and p values. Inclusion criteria often mix ACS average risk and above average risk patients. The data should be reported both combined and separated by risk stratification for colorectal cancer. Newly recognized risk factors such as association with ovarian carcinoma in women should be sought.

12.9
Synchronous Lesions; Reporting of Data By-Polyp

The presence of synchronous polyps in the same patient could be handled in a variety of ways that could bias reported results. For example, in clinical practice, one might argue that the observation of even a single significant sized lesion on CTC will result in a colonoscopy follow-up examination. Hence, one could argue that, in order to decrease reading time and reader fatigue, a detailed search for synchronous lesion is unnecessary if a significant lesion has already been detected. However, CC may be incomplete in 2–10% of patients and since the actual miss-rate for CC is estimated at 6–12% for 10 mm lesions, we suggest that both clinical and research based CTC interpretation involve a complete evaluation of the entire colon. Alternately, synchronous lesions could artificially increase by-polyp sensitivity by increasing dwell-time in evaluating one segment of colon; if one spends more time evaluating a polyp candidate; there is a greater likelihood in detecting a second adjacent lesion when one is present). Because of these complex biases that could affect sensitivity, the number of patients with synchronous lesions, the lesion sizes and histologies in those patients should be specified.

12.10
Future Considerations

The impact of current research on stool opacification, electronic subtraction of fluid and stool and integration of computer aided diagnosis is uncertain but likely to improve patient acceptance and ease of interpretation (DACHMAN and YOSHIDA 2003). In evaluating stool opacification the dosing regimen should be detailed. In comparing CAD to observer studies we suggest that CAD be evaluated as a "second opinion" similar to its use in mammography.

12.11
Conclusion

The uniform terminology and reporting of CTC data will lead to a better understanding of true exam performance and better patient management recommendations (Table 12.2). This quality and consistency is beneficial to both academic and non-academic settings. We hope that an understanding of the complex interaction of the parameters discussed above will facilitate a better analysis and reporting of clinical trials and even review of exam performance within individual clinical practices where CTC is introduced as a new screening too.

References

Bruzzi JF, Moss AC, Fenlon HM (2001) Clinical results of CT colonoscopy. Eur Radiol 11(11):2188–2194

Dachman AH (2002) Diagnostic performance of virtual colonoscopy. Abdom Imaging 27:260–267

Dachman AH, Yoshida H (2003) Virtual colonography: past, present, and future. Radiol Clin North Am 41:377–393

Dachman AH, Zalis ME (2004) Quality and consistency in CT colonography and research reporting. Radiology 230:319–323

Fidler JL, Johnson CD, MacCary RL, Welch TJ, Hara AK, Harmsen WS (2002) Detection of flat lesions in the colon with CT colonography. Abdom Imaging 27:292–300

Iannacone R, Laghi A, Catalano C, Mangiapane F, Lamazza A, Schillaci A et al. (2004) Computed tomographic colonography without cathartic preparation for the detection of colorectal polyps. Gastroenterology 127;1300–1311

McFarland EG (2002) Reader strategies for CT colonography. Abdom Imaging 27:275

McFarland EG, Zalis ME (2004) CT colonography: progress toward colorectal evaluation without catharsis. Gastroenterology 127(5):1623–1626

O'Brien MJ, Winawer SJ, Zauber AG, Bushey MT, Sternberg SS, Gottlieb LS, Bond JH, Waye JD, Schapiro M (2004) Flat adenomas in the National Polyp Study (NPS) are not associated with an increased risk of high grade dysplasia initially nor during surveillance. [Work carried out for the National Polyp Study Workgroup]. Clin Gastro Hepatol 2:905–911

Pickhardt PJ, Choi JR, Hwang I, Butler JA, Puckett ML, Hildebrandt HA, Wong RK, Nugent PA, Mysliwiec PA, Schindler WR (2003) Computed tomographic virtual colonoscopy to screen for colorectal neoplasia in asymptomatic adults. N Engl J Med 4 349(23):2191–2200

Pickhardt PJ, Nugent PA, Mysliwiec PA, Choi JR, Schindler WR (2004a) Location of adenomas missed by optical colonoscopy. Ann Intern Med 7 141(5):352–359

Pickhardt PJ, Choi JR, Nugent PA, Schindler WR (2004b) The effect of diagnostic confidence on the probability of optical colonoscopic confirmation of potential polyps detected on CT colonography: prospective assessment in 1,339 asymptomatic adults. Am J Roentgenol 183(6):1661–1665

Rex DK, Cutler CS, Lemmel GT et al. (1997) Colonoscopic miss rates of adenomas determined by back-to-back colonoscopies. Gastroenterology 112:24–28

Sosna J, Morrin MM, Kruskal JB, Lavin PT, Raptopoulous V (2003) CT colonography for detecting colorectal polyps: a meta-analysis. Am J Roentgenol 181:1593–1598

Zalis ME, Barrish M, Choi RJ, Dachman A, Fenlon J, Ferrucci J, Glick S, Laghi A, Macari M, McFarland E, Morrin M, Pickhardt P, Soto J, Yee J (2005) C-RADS. CT Colonography Reporting and Data System (C-RADS): a Consensus Statement. Radiology. [Work carried out for the Working Group on Virtual Colonoscopy l.]. Radiology 236: 3–9

13 Virtual Colonoscopy Beyond Polyp Detection?

Thomas Mang, Wolfgang Schima, Andrea Maier, and Peter Pokieser

CONTENTS

13.1 Introduction 161
13.2 Diverticular Disease 161
13.3 Inflammatory Bowel Disease 164
13.3.1 Ulcerative Colitis 164
13.3.2 Crohn's Disease 165
13.4 Colorectal Carcinoma 167
13.5 Colorectal Lymphoma 170
13.6 Surveillance Post-Surgery or Post-Intervention 171
References 172

13.1 Introduction

Currently, there are two main indications for CT colonography (CTC). First, polyp detection, in patients with an increased risk for colorectal cancer, or in asymptomatic patients, with an average risk, for screening purposes. The second common indication is incomplete or failed colonoscopy, where CT colonography is useful for complete colon visualization; for example, to detect additional lesions proximal to a stenotic cancer (Morrin et al. 1999; Macari et al. 1999). In addition to these main indications, there are several other conditions where the role of CT colonography is not yet clearly defined. Some of these conditions may lead to colon obstruction, in which case CTC is performed after incomplete colonoscopy. However, CTC may also be used for surveillance of these conditions, per se, as an alternative to colonoscopy or barium enemas. Diverticular disease is the most common colonic disease in the Western world and often leads to diverticulitis. CTC is helpful in the assessment of not only the lumen, but also any extramural changes (Table 13.1). At chronic stages of inflammatory bowel diseases, CT colonography can provide information about the extent of the disease and about stenosis and prestenotic regions, as well as the extracolonic extent and complications of the diseases. There is little experience about the feasibility of CT colonography in the evaluation of colonic lymphoma or for post-surgical or post-interventional surveillance.

Although the primary target lesion for CT colonography is defined as the adenomatous polyp, CT colonography has the ability to provide unique information about many other pathologic conditions.

13.2 Diverticular Disease

Diverticular disease is the most common colonic disease in the Western world, affecting 10–30% of people at age 50 years and 30–60% at age 80 years. However, the disease is asymptomatic in the majority of patients. Together with aging, longstanding low dietary fiber is the main predisposing factor for diverticular disease. Other etiological factors have been suggested, including increased consumption of red meat, fat, and salt.

An early stage of the disease is the so-called prediverticulosis, which is characterized by thickening

Table 13.1. CTC features of diverticular disease

Diverticula
Gas filled outpouching of colon wall in 2D
Complete dark ring in 3D
Cave: *polypoid pseudolesion* in VE "en face"
Impacted diverticula
Polypoid pseudolesion in 3D
Incomplete ring shadowing in 3D
2D Pathognomonic: filled with air, stool, retained barium, CM wall enhancement
Diverticulitis
Wall thickening with CM enhancement
Stenosis and pericolic fat stranding
VE: Nonspecific

T. Mang, MD; W. Schima, MD; A. Maier, MD; P. Pokieser, MD
Department of Radiology, Medical University of Vienna, Waehringer Gürtel 18–20, 1090 Vienna, Austria

of the muscular layer, shortening of the taeniae, and luminal narrowing. With advancing disease, caliber and haustral abnormalities appear. This results in a global and regular wall thickening of >4 mm of long colonic segments with prominent semicircular folds, shortened interhaustral segments (concertina appearance), and a reduced colonic distensibility (LEFERE et al. 2003) (Fig. 13.1a–c).

Most of the diverticula are pseudodiverticula, which are herniations of the mucosa, muscularis mucosae, and submucosa through the circular muscularis propria layer at weak points in the colonic wall where nutrient arteries penetrate the muscularis propria. Rarely, true diverticula (most often at the proximal colon) are found, which are characterized by an outpouching of mucosa, submucosa, and the muscularis propria. The radiological features of the two types of diverticula are not distinguishable. The CTC appearance of diverticula is easily recognized as air-filled outpouchings of the colonic wall on 2D images. On the virtual endoscopic (VE) images, the diverticular orificium can be recognized as a complete dark circumferential ring when seen en face. Because of the complete dark ring, diverticula may simulate polyps when seen en face on VE images (FENLON et al. 1998) (Fig. 13.2a–c).

Differential diagnostic problems can occur if a diverticula inverts into the colonic lumen or is impacted with stool. A diverticulum may occasionally invert into the colonic lumen and produce a pseudopolypoid lesion on 2D and 3D images. The corresponding VE image is nonspecific and shows a polypoid lesion (Fig. 13.3a,b). The 2D images are essential to arrive at the correct diagnosis: inverted diverticula with pseudopolypoid shape sometimes contain some air, residual stool, or fat attenuation because of a central umbilication in the inverted part of the diverticulum, or due to an inclusion of perisigmoidal fat (FENLON 2002).

A more common finding than inverted diverticula, diverticula impacted with fecal material may appear as a raised lesion and mimic polyps on VE images. On the 2D images, a hyperdense ring with a hypodense center containing air or stool, or even retained barium from prior examinations, can be found in such a lesion (HARA et al. 1997) (Fig. 13.4a,b).

Inflammation of the diverticula leads to symptomatic diverticulitis, which occurs in two-thirds of cases in the sigmoid colon. Complications that may develop are pericolic abscess, perforation, hemorrhage, fistula formation, and post-inflammatory stenosis. For diagnosis of acute diverticulitis, CT without colon distension is the primary imaging modality. Significant findings for diverticulitis are cone-shaped mild wall thickening with involvement of a long segment (>10 cm) with increased contrast enhancement, pericolic fat stranding, and fluid at the root of the mesentery (Fig. 13.5). The most important differential diagnosis for diverticulitis is colon cancer. In contrast, extensive wall thickening with short extension (<5 cm), especially with shoulder formation and pericolonic lymph nodes, is suspicious for neoplasms (CHINTAPALLI et al. 1999).

Presently, CT colonography has no role in the diagnosis of acute diverticulitis, and, in addition, the distension of the colon may lead to perforation. In selected cases, CTC may help in the differential diagnosis between diverticulitis and cancer after the acute inflammatory episode has subsided.

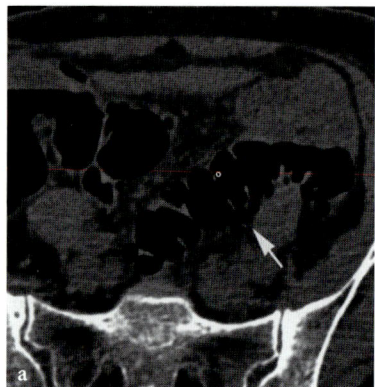 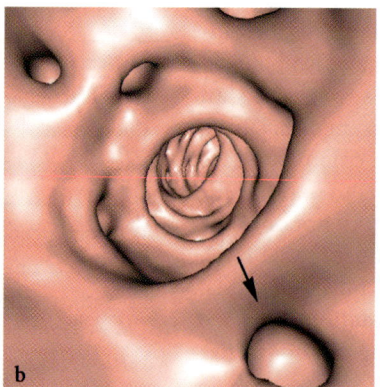 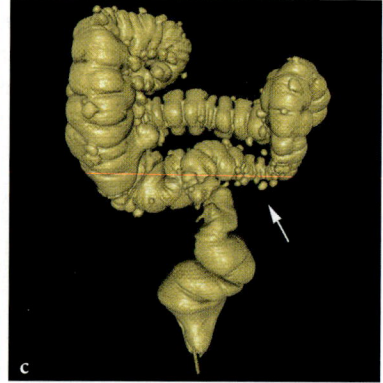

Fig. 13.1a–c. Diverticulosis: **a** axial planes show multiple gas-filled outpouchings of colon wall in nearly all parts of the colon (*arrow*); **b** VE shows complete dark rings (*arrow*); **c** global volume rendering views show the extent of the disease with reduced colonic distension (concertina appearance), especially in the sigmoid colon (*arrow*)

Fig. 13.2a,b. Polyp vs diverticula: **a** VE shows complete dark ring at the diverticulum (*arrow*); **b** incomplete ring shadowing at the polyp (*arrow*)

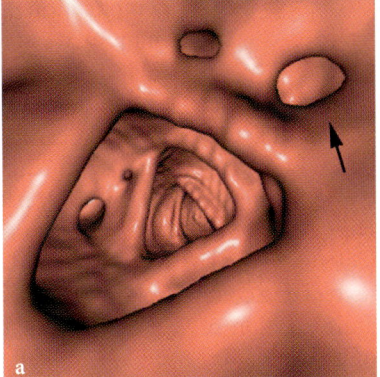 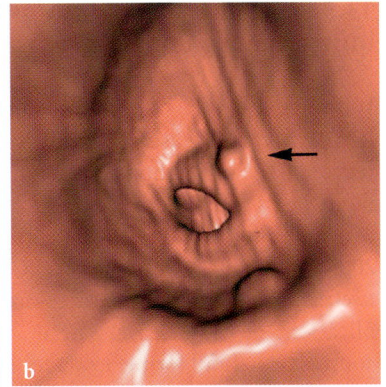

Fig. 13.3a,b. Inverted diverticulum: pseudopolypoid shape on virtual endoscopic images. On 2D images, these lesions contain some air, residual stool, or fat attenuation because of a central umbilication in the inverted part of the diverticulum or due to an inclusion of perisigmoidal fat. (Used with permission of LEFERE et al. 2003)

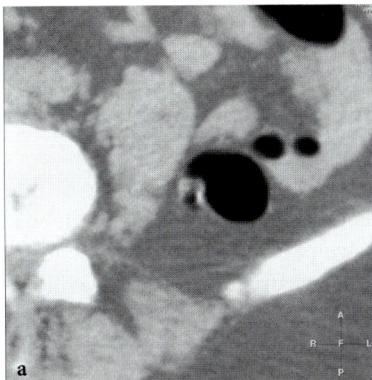 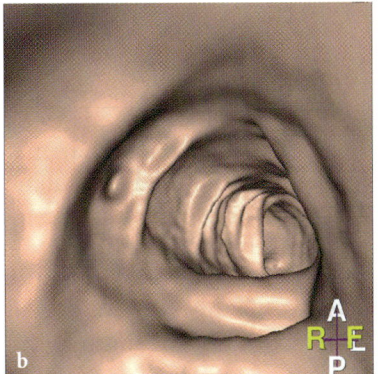

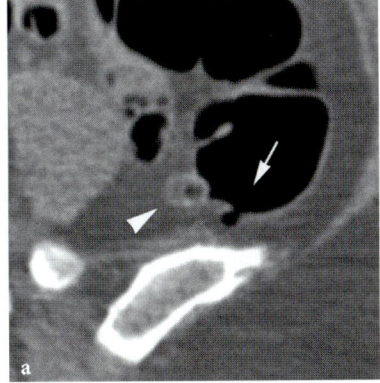 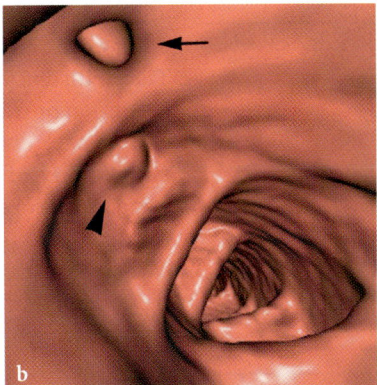

Fig. 13.4a,b. Normal (*arrow*) and stool-impacted diverticulum (*arrowhead*). VE shows complete dark ring at the normal diverticulum and incomplete ring shadowing at the impacted diverticulum simulating a polypoid lesion. On 2D images in the impacted diverticulum, a hyperdense ring with a hypodense center can be found

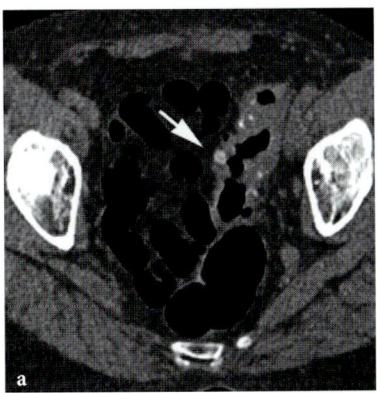 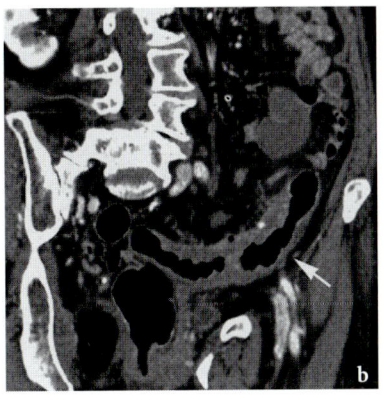

Fig. 13.5a,b. Diverticulitis axial unenhanced (a) and curved multiplanar view with IV contrast (b): Wall thickening of a long segment (*arrow*) with CM enhancement, diverticula, stenosis, and fat stranding

13.3
Inflammatory Bowel Disease

Within the group of inflammatory bowel diseases (IBD), Crohn's disease (CD) and ulcerative colitis (UC) represent the most important conditions. CT colonography helps to assess the colon proximal to a stenosis, which cannot be passed with endoscopy (OTA et al. 2003) (Table 13.2). Furthermore, CT colonography is useful for evaluating the extracolonic extent and complications of the disease. The i.v. administration of contrast is helpful for the evaluation of inflammatory wall changes (HARVEY et al. 2001).

13.3.1
Ulcerative Colitis

Ulcerative colitis is an inflammatory bowel disease limited to the mucosa and submucosa of the colon. The disease typically begins in the rectum and continuously extends proximally to involve part of the colon or the entire colon (pancolitis). In 10–40% of cases, the distal ileum is also inflamed, which is referred to as backwash ileitis. The most severe

Table 13.2. CTC features of inflammatory bowel disease

Discrete irregular wall thickening (continuous vs. discontinuous)
Flattening or disappearance of haustra
Increased CM enhancement of wall
Stenosis
Pseudopolyps
Cobblestone pattern (Crohn)
Fibrofatty proliferation around colon (Crohn > UC)
Lymph nodes (Crohn > UC)
Abscess, fistula, pseudotumor (Crohn)
Cancer (UC >> Crohn)

complication is the toxic megacolon, which appears in up to 5% of cases and carries the risk of perforation and peritonitis (Fig. 13.6a,b).

Although there is little experience in the evaluation of ulcerative colitis with CT colonography, the early subtle inflammatory mucosal changes, such as the granular pattern of the mucosa or tiny punctuate ulcers known from double contrast barium enema, may be beyond current spatial resolution of CT colonography.

Progression of the disease leads to hyperemia and submucosal edema, which then results in thickening and stratification of the wall, and is accompanied by increased paracolic vascularity. Increased ulceration and pseudopolyps appear and the mucosa becomes friable. Lymph node enlargement is only slight. The appearance of abscess or fistula formation is uncommon. In these acute stages, the benefit of CT colonography, in contrast to conventional colonoscopy, seems to be questionable. In case of toxic megacolon, there is an absolute contraindication to insufflation of air due to the extreme risk of perforation. In case of acute colitis without signs of toxic megacolon, CTC should be performed with caution. There are only a few reports about colonic perforations due to CTC (SOSNA et al. 2005). However, in most cases, stenotic or otherwise diseased colons were affected and ulcerative colitis has been reported as one of these predisposing conditions (COADY-FARIBORZIAN et al. 2004). The air distension of the colon may lead to intramural laceration or frank perforation (Fig. 13.7a–c.)

Subacute and chronic forms lead to thickening and rigidity of the wall. Narrowing of the colonic lumen and foreshortening of the colon may occur (MACARI and BALTHAZAR 2001). The bowel loses its haustral pattern, which can result in a tubular "lead pipe" appearance. Post-inflammatory polyps may be present. As a result of inflammation, there may be proliferation of the pericolic fat (Fig. 13.8a–c.).

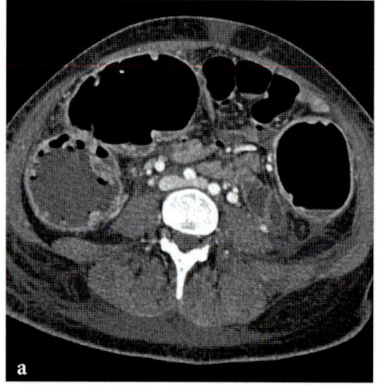 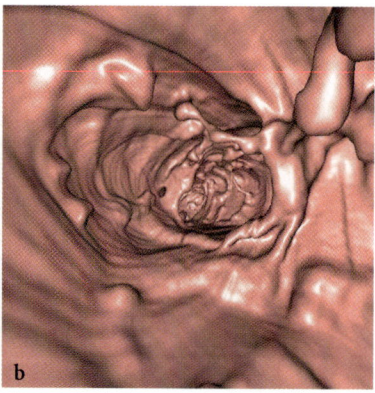

Fig. 13.6a,b. Toxic megacolon (no colonic insufflation was performed): colonic dilatation with intraluminal air and fluid (**a**). The luminal contour is distorted and anhaustral. Diffuse slight wall thickening with increased CM enhancement of the whole colon and ill-defined nodular/pseudopolypoid surface (**a,b**). There is an absolute contraindication for insufflation of air due to the extreme risk of perforation!

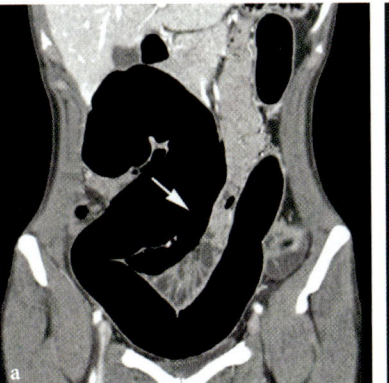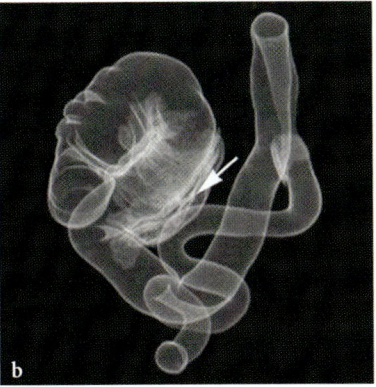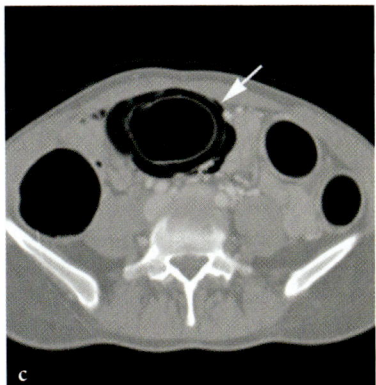

Fig. 13.7a–c. Acute ulcerative colitis with perforation due to air insufflation: discrete diffuse wall thickening with increased CM enhancement of the whole colon (**a**). Total flattening and disappearance of the haustra with a tubular appearance of the colon (**a,b**). Focal paracolic air formations around the transverse colon are a sign of perforation (*arrow*) (**a–c**)

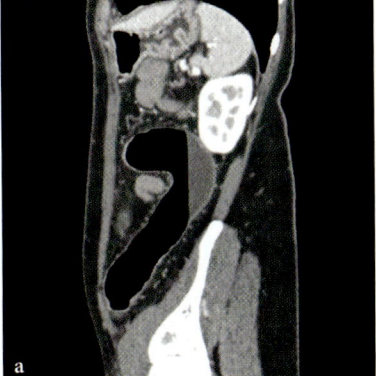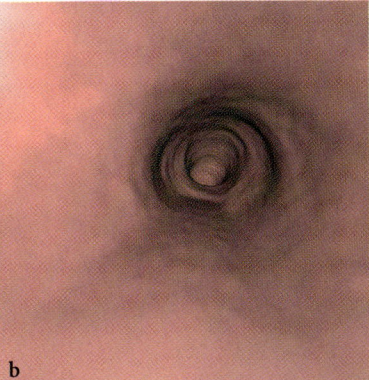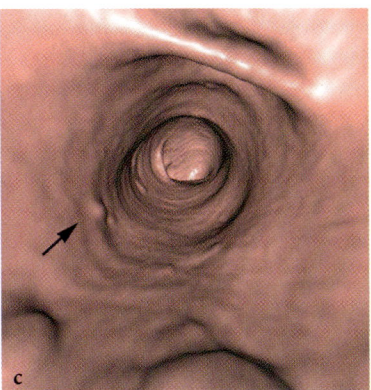

Fig. 13.8a–c. Chronic ulcerative colitis: **a,b** narrowing of the colonic lumen and foreshortening of the colon with total flattening and disappearance of the haustra, leading to tubular appearance ("lead pipe") of the colon; **c** pseudopolyps (*arrow*)

The risk of development of colorectal cancer increases with the extent and the duration of the disease. Focal wall thickening, shoulder formation, or large polypoid lesions are suspicious for the development of colorectal cancer (Fig. 13.9. a–c). Differentiation between an inflammatory stenosis in ulcerative colitis and cancer is the domain of endoscopy with biopsy, but CTC may be used as an adjunct in patients with an endoscopically non-assessable colon.

13.3.2
Crohn's Disease

Crohn's disease may involve segments of the whole GI tract. However, Crohn's disease most often affects the terminal ileum and the proximal colon. Unlike ulcerative colitis, Crohn's disease typically affects the GI tract in a discontinuous way (so-called skip lesions) and the inflammatory process is transmural in nature.

CT usually misses the early stages of Crohn's disease (BIANCONE et al. 2003). With progression of the disease, mural thickening and luminal narrowing occur. The outer contour of the colon wall is irregular. The degree of contrast enhancement of the bowel wall correlates with the severity of the disease (GORE et al. 1996). As a result of the hyperemia from the inflammatory process, the local mesenteric vessels are dilated and widely spaced, which has been described as the "comb sign." A progressive increase in higher-density pericolic fat is called fibrofatty proliferation and is an attempt by the body to contain the inflammatory process, resulting in separation of the bowel loops. Usually, multiple mesenteric lymph nodes, measuring <10 mm in the short axis diameter, are present. Extensive, intersecting linear transverse and longitudinal ulcerations can result

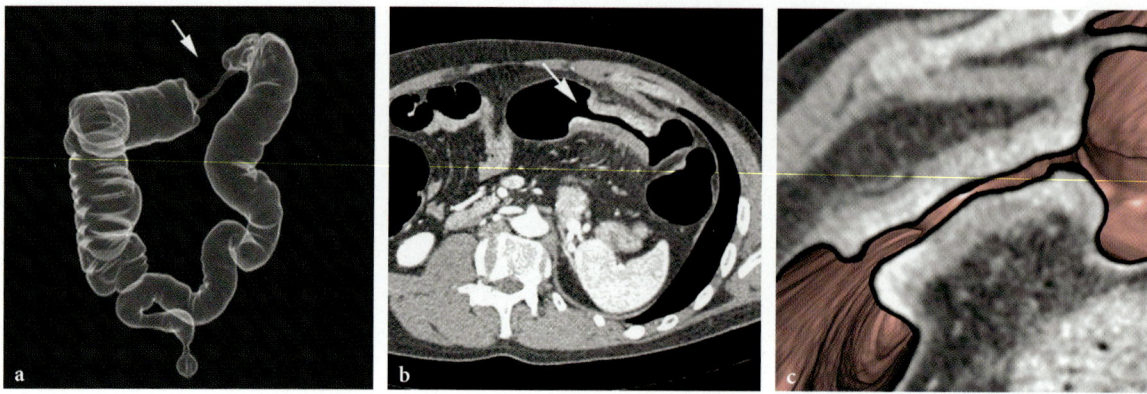

Fig. 13.9a–c. Ulcerative colitis with stenotic cancer in the transverse colon (*arrow*): local flattening and disappearance of the haustra in the sigmoid and descending colon (**a**). Focal, stenotic, circular wall thickening with shoulder formation in the transverse colon, with soft tissue attenuation and CM enhancement (**b,c**). Combined 2D+3D view of the stenotic cancer (**c**)

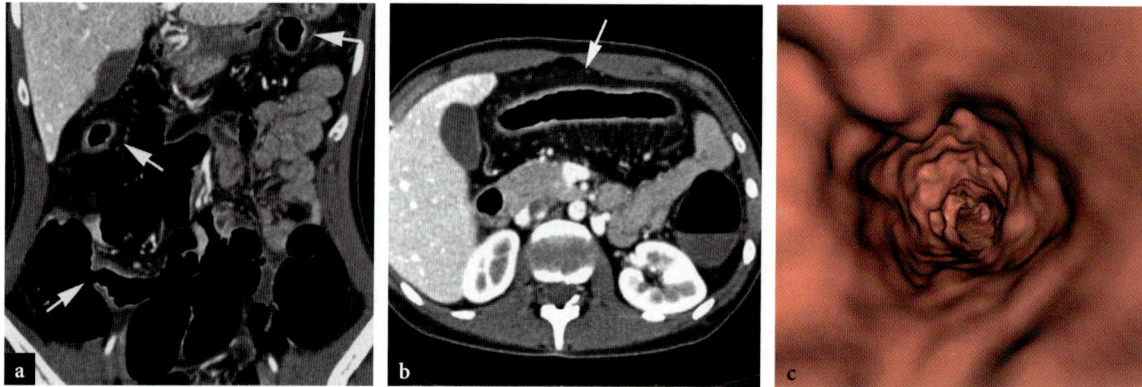

Fig. 13.10a–c. Crohn's disease: Skip lesions (*arrow*) in the terminal ileum and the transverse colon (**a,b**). Irregular wall thickening and stenosis of the transverse colon with pericolic fat stranding and flattening and disappearance of the haustra (*arrow*) (**b**). Virtual colonoscopy shows luminal narrowing and cobblestone pattern

in the so called "cobblestone pattern," which can be evaluated with virtual endoscopic images (Tarjan et al. 2000). With progression of the disease, the transmural inflammation is accompanied by irreversible fibrosis. (Fig. 13.10a–c)

Frequent complications are fistula, abscesses, adhesions, and stenosis, leading to bowel obstruction. Fistula can appear as ill-defined soft tissue bands extending into the paraintestinal fat. After colonic air insufflation, small amounts of air can sometimes be present in the fistulas, resulting in a better delineation (Tarjan et al. 2000). On endoluminal views, the fistula opening is sometimes depicted (Fig. 13.11b). A Fistula opening may be seen at the top of a pseudopolypoid lesion of granulation tissue formation. In these cases, the combination of 3D and 2D images may provide sufficient information for complex disease. Abscesses are most frequently associated with small bowel disease or ileocolitis and may extend into adjacent tissues, bowel loops, or organs. Stenosis in Crohn's disease shows, in many cases, circular cone-shaped wall thickening with increased CM enhancement and involvement of a longer segment. In other cases, short stenoses with wall thickening and abrupt shoulders at the proximal and distal end occur, which makes differentiation from malignant stenosis impossible (Figs. 13.11a and 13.12a–c). Perforations are uncommon and usually contained. Conglomerate masses are present if there is an involvement of multiple bowel segments or a large bowel segment with fistulation and abscess formation (Fig. 13.11c).

There is a slightly increased risk of developing colorectal cancer and lymphoma as a complication of the disease. These neoplasms mostly affect the small bowel. The presence of lymph node enlargement >10 mm in the short axis diameter should raise suspicion for malignancy.

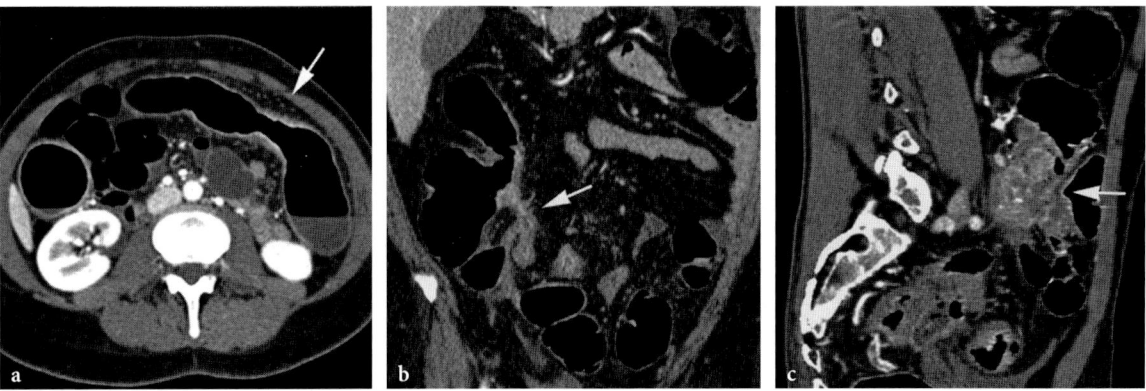

Fig. 13.11. a Crohn's disease: stenosis in the transverse colon (*arrow*). b Ileo-cecal fistula (*arrow*) and stenosis in the ascending colon. c Conglomerate mass between cecum and small bowel loops (*arrow*)

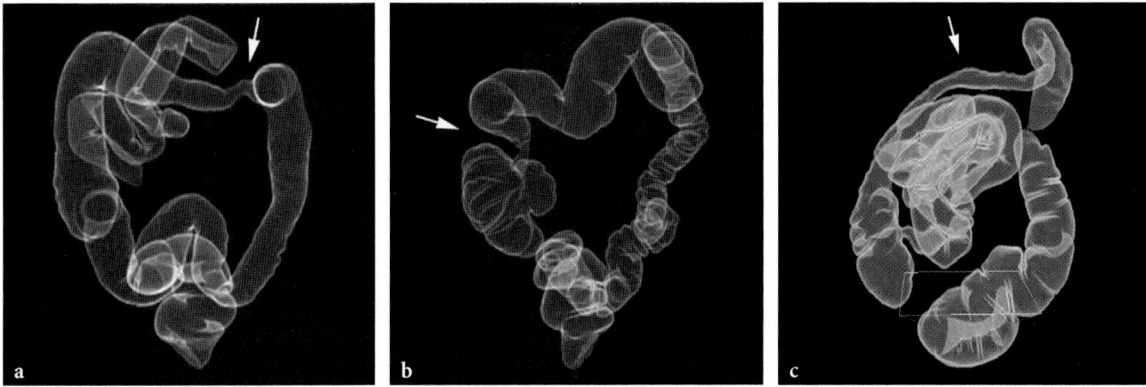

Fig. 13.12a–c. Crohn's disease: various forms of stenoses (*arrow*) and disappearance of the haustra in three different patients

For evaluation of the small bowel involvement, CT enteroclysis is the preferred technique. There is little experience about the feasibility of CT colonography in Crohn's disease. Published results indicate that CT colonography can be helpful in the evaluation of colonic involvement, especially if conventional colonoscopy is incomplete (BIANCONE et al. 2003). In addition, the extracolonic extent and complications of the disease can be evaluated.

13.4
Colorectal Carcinoma

Adenocarcinomas are the most common colonic primary tumors. The peak incidence is between 50 and 70 years of age. Approximately 90% arise from benign adenomatous polyps. Most carcinomas show an exophytic, polypous type of growth with frequent central degeneration. Adenocarcinomas tend to infiltrate the bowel wall circumferentially and 50% are found in the rectum, and 25% in the sigmoid. In up to 5% of cases, a synchronous carcinoma is present (Fig. 13.18a,b).

The main indication for CT colonography in colorectal cancer is the evaluation of the pre-stenotic colon to detect additional tumors or polyps (GENLON et al. 1999; MORIN et al. 2000a; NERI et al. 2002) (Table 13.3). CT colonography also offers information about local tumor invasion, lymph nodes, and distant metastases (FILIPPONE et al. 2004; CHUNG et al. 2005; IANNACCONE et al. 2005). For this purpose, the i.v. administration of contrast media is indicated (MORRIN et al. 2000b). The role of CT colonography for T staging of known colorectal cancer is still a matter of discussion because primary tumors are resected, even if metastases are present, to prevent bowel obstruction. Less invasive surgical approaches, such as local tumor resection (mucosal

Table 13.3. CTC features of colorectal carcinoma

Focal, asymmetric or circular wall thickening
Annular stricture
Wall irregularity
CM enhancement
Pericolic invasion (pericolic soft tissue stranding)
Local lymphadenopathy
Metastases
T Staging
T1: Invasion of the mucosa and submucosa
T2: Infiltration of the muscularis propria
T3: Infiltration of pericolic fat
T4: Invasion of adjacent organs

Reliable differentiation between mucosal /submucosal invasion (T1) and infiltration of the muscularis propria (T2) with CT is still not possible

resection) in stages below T3, may indicate the need for a re-evaluation of the role of CT colonography in T staging.

Unlike polypoid lesions, which are more easily detected on 3D endoluminal views, invasive mass lesions are better depicted on 2D images, which allow mural and extramural evaluation (PICKHARDT 2004).

Colorectal cancer typically shows extensive focal polypoid, asymmetric, or circular wall thickening with short extension (<5 cm), especially with shoulder formation (FENLON et al. 1998; TAYLOR et al. 2003a). Colorectal carcinomas show moderate enhancement with intravenous contrast (OTO et al. 2003; SOSNA et al. 2003) (Fig. 13.13a,b). CT differentiation between stage T1 (invasion of mucosa and/or submucosa) and T2 (invasion of the muscularis propria) is not feasible, but tumor extension beyond the colon wall (T3), characterized by stranding, an indistinct boundary, and nodular protrusions into pericolic fat tissue, is readily appreciated by CT (Fig. 13.14a,b). Tumor infiltration to adjacent organs (T4) is most likely if the carcinoma shows a broad-based contact, no intervening fat planes, and indistinct boundaries

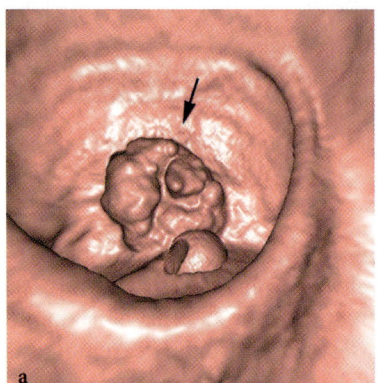
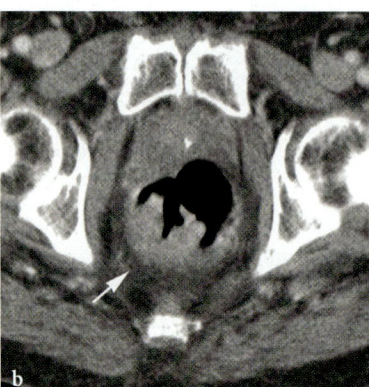

Fig. 13.13a,b. Polypoid rectal cancer (*arrow*): large polypoid, lobulated mass in the rectum (**a,b**). The lesion shows soft tissue attenuation and CM enhancement (**b**)

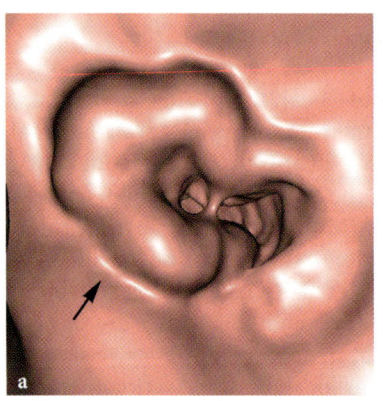
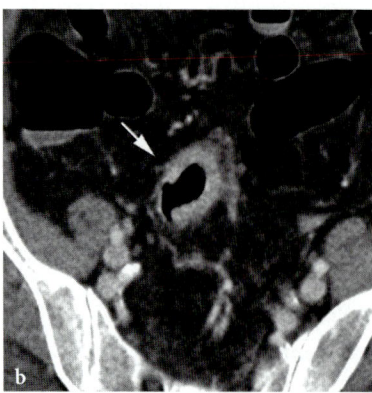

Fig. 13.14a,b. Semicircular sigmoid carcinoma (*arrow*): focal, asymmetric, semicircular wall thickening with shoulder formation in the sigmoid colon (**a,b**). The lesion shows CM enhancement and pericolic soft tissue stranding (**b**)

to other organs (Fig. 13.15a,b). Pericolonic lymph nodes and distant metastasis are signs of progression of the disease and can be evaluated with 2D planes.

The most common pitfalls are inflammatory stenosis and the segmental colonic spasm. Inflammatory and post-inflammatory stenosis more often show cone-shaped mild wall thickening with involvement of a long segment (>10 cm) and pericolonic fat stranding. Sometimes fluid is present at the root of the mesentery (CHINTAPALLI et al. 1999) (compare Figs. 13.10b and 13.11a, vs Fig. 13.14 and 13.15).

Segmental colonic spasm is a physiological luminal narrowing due to peristaltic muscular contraction of the colon. The administration of antispasmotic drugs, such as butylscopolamine (Buscopan) and glucagon may reduce the appearance of spasms and improve colonic distension (TAYLOR et al. 2003b). Often, these pseudostenoses disappear during the examination when changing the position from prone to supine or vice versa. In such cases, the evaluation of the second series can be diagnostic to see whether the pseudostenosis disappears when the spasm relaxes (Fig. 13.16a–d).

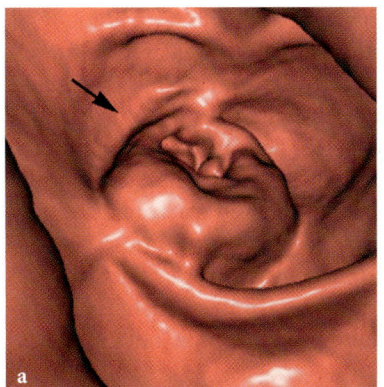
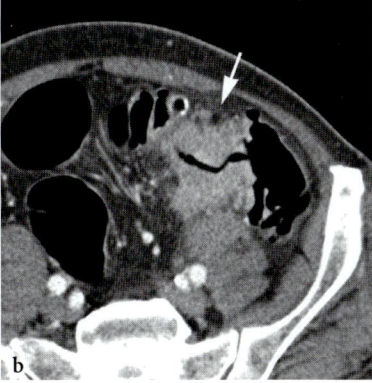

Fig. 13.15a,b. Circular sigmoid carcinoma T4 (*arrow*): focal, symmetric, circular wall thickening with shoulder formation and pericolic soft tissue stranding in the sigmoid colon (a,b). The lesion shows a broad-based contact, no intervening fat planes and indistinct boundaries to the psoas muscle, indicative of infiltration (b)

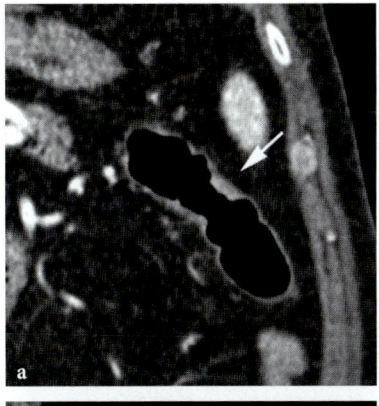
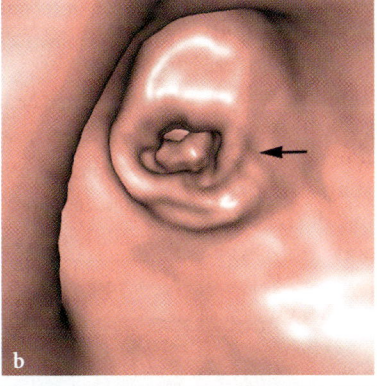
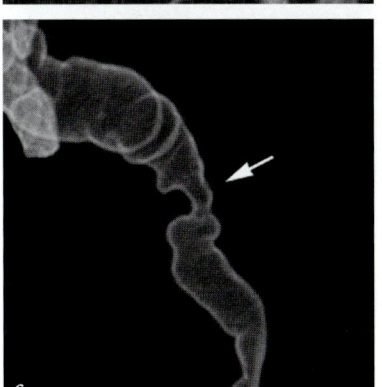
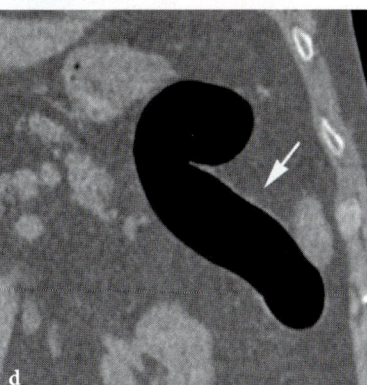

Fig. 13.16a–d. Segmental colonic spasm in the descending colon (*arrow*): focal, irregular circular wall thickening with shoulder formation in the supine position (a–c). The lesion shows soft tissue attenuation and CM enhancement (a). Normal colon wall without wall thickening or stenosis in the prone position (d). It is important to identify the same segment as in the supine position

13.5 Colorectal Lymphoma

Lymphoma involves the colon either as a primary neoplasm or as a part of a disseminated disease. In contrast to the small bowel, where lymphomas are the most frequent primary, lymphomas in the colon are rare. In secondary colonic lymphoma, the involvement of the gastrointestinal tract follows a previously diagnosed extraabdominal lymphoma (O'CONNELL and THOMPSON 1978; MEGIBOW et al. 1983).

The primary colonic lymphoma is usually found in middle-aged or elderly people. Males are twice as often affected as females. Common symptoms include abdominal pain, weight loss, and changing bowel habits with an average duration of about 4–6 months. Primary colonic lymphomas occur more frequently in the setting of inflammatory bowel disease and immunosuppression and are found most commonly in the cecum or the rectum (BRENETON et al. 1983) (Fig. 13.17a–c).

The radiological appearance can be classified as focal or diffuse. The most common focal type is the intraluminal mass (O'CONNELL and THOMPSON 1978). These polypoid lesions are lobulated, broad-based, and sessile with or without central ulcerations with only slight CM enhancement. They are often morphologically indistinguishable from adenomatous polyps.

The focal appearance can also consist of an infiltration that results in pronounced eccentric or circumferential bowel wall thickening. As a consequence, the intestinal lumen may be narrowed. However, unlike colon cancer, lymphoma can also show a dilated caliber in the form of an "aneurysmal" dilatation due to infiltration and destruction of the myenteric plexus (MONTGOMERY and CHEW 1997). Ulcerations, necrosis, and fistulae between adjacent bowel loops may appear. Regional, mesenteric, and retroperitoneal lymphadenopathy may be present. Another focal form of lymphoma is the endo-eccentric mass with large ulcerations involving adjacent bowel loops where fistulae can appear (O'CONNELL and THOMPSON 1978).

The diffuse form presents with multiple polypoid lesions and is called diffuse mucosal nodularity or malignant lymphomatous polyposis (O'CONNELL and THOMPSON 1978; CALLAWAY et al. 1997). The polyps appear smooth and sessile but can also be irregular or pedunculated. Often, the entire colon or a long segment is involved.

The radiologic patterns of primary colonic lymphoma, such as intraluminal masses, polyps, stenosis, and polyposis, are often quite similar to those of carcinomatous stenosis, adenomatous polyps, and familial polyposis, and can also be evaluated by CT colonography (Table 13.4). The possibility of lymphoma should be considered when cecal tumors involve the terminal ileum, when tumors do not invade the pericolonic fat or adjacent structures and when there are secondary findings such as splenomegaly or bulky abdominal lymph node enlarge-

Table 13.4. CTC features of colorectal lymphoma

Common in cecum and rectum (primary / secondary)
Focal, asymmetric or circular wall thickening, lymphomatid polyposis
Lumen dilated or stenotic
Slight CM enhancement
Ulceration, necrosis, fistula
Pericolic invasion (pericolic soft tissue stranding)
Pericolic lymphadenopathy

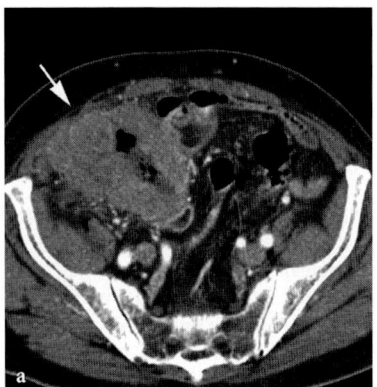 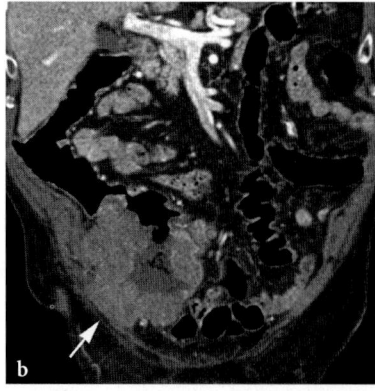 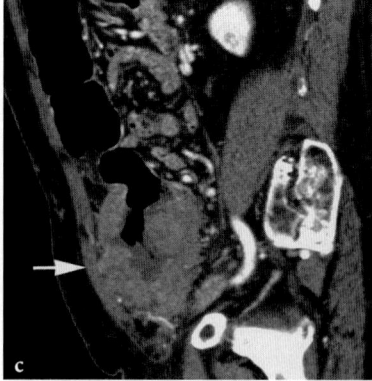

Fig. 13.17a–c. Colorectal lymphoma, axial, coronal, and sagittal view: Circumferential bowel wall thickening of the cecum with moderate CM enhancement (*arrow*). Consequently, the intestinal lumen is narrowed. Focal wall defects as a sign of an early fistula

ment (WYATT et al. 1994). However, in most cases, a reliable radiological differentiation is not possible and the specific diagnosis is only possible with histology. In cases of stenosis or incomplete colonoscopy, CTC could be helpful in the evaluation of the pre-stenotic colon. Extracolonic involvement, fistulae and lymphadenopathy can easily be evaluated with planar images.

13.6
Surveillance Post-Surgery or Post-Intervention

With regard to post-surgical conditions in the colon, there is no general agreement about the use of CT colonography. Contrast-enhanced CT colonography has the potential to detect local recurrence, metachronous disease, and distant metastases in patients with a history of invasive colorectal cancer (FLETCHER et al. 2002; LAGHI et al. 2003; NERI et al. 2005).

Currently, endoscopy or barium enemas are performed in many cases after colonic surgery for routine surveillance, to detect tumor recurrence, or to discover a metachronous cancer. After partial colonic resection, particularly, some of these control examinations could be replaced by contrast-enhanced CT colonography. In most cases, CT colonography allows visualization of the entire colon, which is important for demonstrating the post-surgical anatomic conditions. Two-dimensional views offer information about the wall morphology of the anastomosis. This is important because the majority of local recurrences are extraluminal and therefore endoscopically occult. Only one third to one half of local recurrences have an intraluminal component (BARKIN et al. 1988; WANEBO et al. 1989). Most colonic anastomoses at CT colonography will not demonstrate excess of soft tissue. However, benign findings like polypoid granulation tissue or benign nodularity can be seen frequently endoscopically and at CT colonography.

Neoplasms or inflammatory conditions on the anastomosis can lead to focal or circular wall thickening, increased CM enhancement, and pericolic fat stranding (Figs. 13.18a,b and 13.19a,b).

Polypoid filling defects and enhancing mucosal soft tissue at colonic anastomosis are nonspecific findings on CT colonography in patients with a history of colorectal cancer and can represent granulation tissue, inflammation or recurrent or metachronous disease.

Therefore differentiation between granulation tissue, inflammatory stenosis and cancer recurrence is the domain of endoscopy with biopsy, if possible. Pericolonic lymph nodes and distant metastasis can be evaluated with 2D planes.

Treatment of large bowel obstruction using self-expanding metal stents is now well-established and widely disseminated. Stenting is used in patients with incurable disease for definitive palliation, or preoperatively for patients where curative resection is possible (CAMUNEZ et al. 2000).

Follow-up of the location and the lumen of a stent may be feasible with CT colonography. Particularly if endoscopy is incomplete or if stents could not be passed by conventional colonoscopy, CT colonography could be an alternative for contrast enema. CT colonography provides additional information about the location and the lumen of the stent and the proximal colon (Fig. 13.20a–c). In case of re-obstruction because of tumor recurrence, the additional 2D displays demonstrate the morphology of the stent-stenosis, which might be helpful for further treatment. During the same procedure, the extracolonic conditions of the disease (metastases, lymph nodes) can be evaluated.

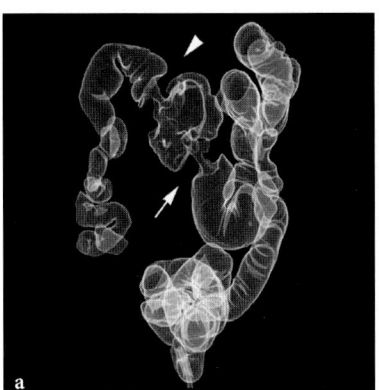 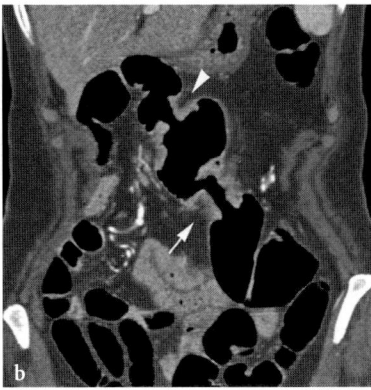

Fig. 13.18a,b. Right hemicolectomy: CT colonography reveals a second cancer in the transverse colon (*arrow*) and a cancer recurrence at the entero-colic anastomosis (*arrowhead*), which was not diagnosed by endoscopy

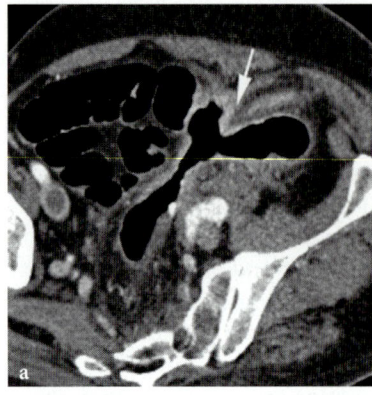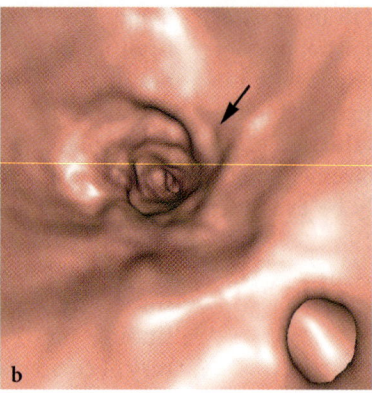

Fig. 13.19a,b. Inflammatory stenosis at the anastomosis after colonic resection: Mild wall thickening with stenosis and pericolic fat stranding (*arrow*). Virtual colonoscopy shows luminal narrowing (*arrow*) and a diverticula

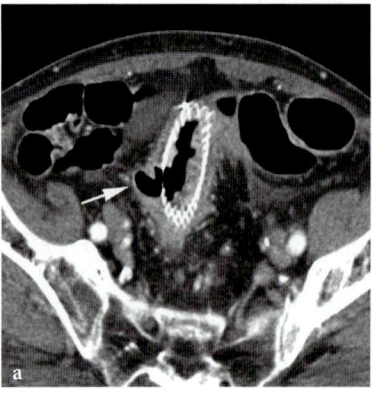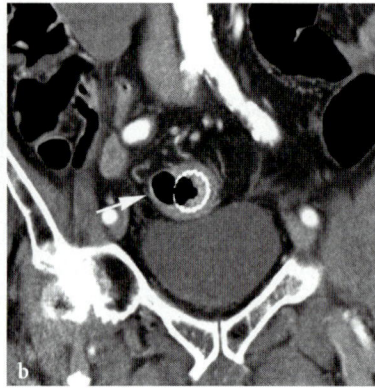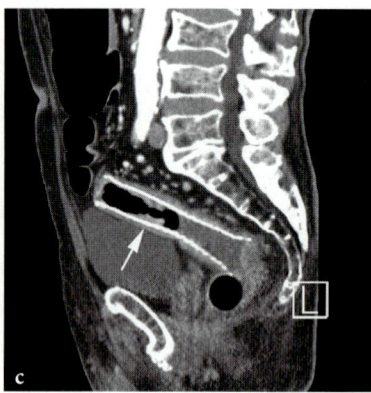

Fig. 13.20a–c. Rectal carcinoma with rectal stent for palliation, axial, coronal, and sagittal view: Stent fracture (*arrow*) with air leakage (**a,b**). Beginning tumor invasion (*arrow*) in the stent graft (**c**)

References

Barkin JS, Cohen ME, Flaxman M, Lindblad AS, Mayer RJ, Kalser MH, Steinberg SM (1988) Value of a routine follow-up endoscopy program for the detection of recurrent colorectal carcinoma. Am J Gastroenterol 83(12):1355–1360

Biancone L, Fiori R, Tosti C, Marinetti A, Catarinacci M, De Nigris F, Simonetti G, Pallone F (2003) Virtual colonoscopy compared with conventional colonoscopy for stricturing postoperative recurrence in Crohn's disease. Inflamm Bowel Dis 9(6):343–350

Bruneton JN, Thyss A, Bourry J, Bidoli R, Schneider M (1983) Colonic and rectal lymphomas. A report of six cases and review of the literature. Rofo 138(3):283–287

Callaway MP, O'Donovan DG, Lee SH (1997) Case report: malignant lymphomatous polyposis of the colon. Clin Radiol 52(10):797–798

Camunez F, Echenagusia A, Simo G, Turegano F, Vazquez J, Barreiro-Meiro I (2000) Malignant colorectal obstruction treated by means of self-expanding metallic stents: effectiveness before surgery and in palliation. Radiology 216(2):492–497

Chintapalli KN, Chopra S, Ghiatas AA, Esola CC, Fields SF, Dodd GD III (1999) Diverticulitis versus colon cancer: differentiation with helical CT findings. Radiology 210(2):429–435

Chung DJ, Huh KC, Choi WJ, Kim JK (2005) CT colonography using 16-MDCT in the evaluation of colorectal cancer. Am J Roentgenol 184(1):98–103

Coady-Fariborzian L, Angel LP, Procaccino JA (2004) Perforated colon secondary to virtual colonoscopy: report of a case. Dis Colon Rectum 47(7):1247–1249

Fenlon HM (2002) CT colonography: pitfalls and interpretation. Abdom Imaging 27(3):284–291

Fenlon HM, Clarke PD, Ferrucci JT (1998) Virtual colonoscopy: imaging features with colonoscopic correlation. Am J Roentgenol 170(5):1303–1309

Fenlon HM, McAneny DB, Nunes DP, Clarke PD, Ferrucci JT (1999) Occlusive colon carcinoma: virtual colonoscopy in the preoperative evaluation of the proximal colon. Radiology 210(2):423–428

Filippone A, Ambrosini R, Fuschi M, Marinelli T, Genovesi D, Bonomo L (2004) Preoperative T and N staging of colorectal cancer: accuracy of contrast-enhanced multi-detector row CT colonography–initial experience. Radiology 231(1):83–90

Fletcher JG, Johnson CD, Krueger WR, Ahlquist DA, Nelson H, Ilstrup D, Harmsen WS, Corcoran KE (2002) Contrast-enhanced CT colonography in recurrent colorectal carcinoma: feasibility of simultaneous evaluation for metastatic disease, local recurrence, and metachronous neoplasia in colorectal carcinoma. Am J Roentgenol 178(2):283–290

Gore RM, Balthazar EJ, Ghahremani GG, Miller FH (1996) CT features of ulcerative colitis and Crohn's disease. Am J Roentgenol 167(1):3–15

Hara AK, Johnson CD, Reed JE (1997) Colorectal lesions: evaluation with CT colonography. Radiographics 17(5):1157–1167

Harvey CJ, Renfrew I, Taylor S, Gillams AR, Lees WR (2001) Spiral CT pneumocolon: applications, status and limitations. Eur Radiol 11(9):1612–1625

Iannaccone R, Laghi A, Passariello R (2005) Colorectal carcinoma: detection and staging with multislice CT (MSCT) colonography. Abdom Imaging 30(1):13–19

Laghi A, Iannaccone R, Bria E, Carbone I, Trasatti L, Piacentini F, Lauro S, Vecchione A, Passariello R (2003) Contrast-enhanced computed tomographic colonography in the follow-up of colorectal cancer patients: a feasibility study. Eur Radiol 13(4):883–889

Lefere P, Gryspeerdt S, Baekelandt M, Dewyspelaere J, van Holsbeeck B (2003) Diverticular disease in CT colonography. Eur Radiol 13 Suppl 4:L62–L74

Macari M, Balthazar EJ (2001) CT of bowel wall thickening: significance and pitfalls of interpretation. Am J Roentgenol 176(5):1105–1116

Macari M, Berman P, Dicker M, Milano A, Megibow AJ (1999) Usefulness of CT colonography in patients with incomplete colonoscopy. Am J Roentgenol 173(3):561–564

Megibow AJ, Balthazar EJ, Naidich DP, Bosniak MA (1983) Computed tomography of gastrointestinal lymphoma. Am J Roentgenol 141(3):541–547

Montgomery M, Chew FS (1997) Primary lymphoma of the colon. Am J Roentgenol 168(3):688

Morrin MM, Kruskal JB, Farrell RJ, Goldberg SN, McGee JB, Raptopoulos V (1999) Endoluminal CT colonography after an incomplete endoscopic colonoscopy. Am J Roentgenol 172(4):913–918

Morrin MM, Farrell RJ, Raptopoulos V, McGee JB, Bleday R, Kruskal JB (2000a) Role of virtual computed tomographic colonography in patients with colorectal cancers and obstructing colorectal lesions. Dis Colon Rectum 43(3):303–311

Morrin MM, Farrell RJ, Kruskal JB, Reynolds K, McGee JB, Raptopoulos V (2000b) Utility of intravenously administered contrast material at CT colonography. Radiology 217(3):765–771

Neri E, Giusti P, Battolla L, Vagli P, Boraschi P, Lencioni R, Caramella D, Bartolozzi C (2002) Colorectal cancer: role of CT colonography in preoperative evaluation after incomplete colonoscopy. Radiology 223(3):615–619

Neri E, Vagli P, Picchietti S, Vannoci F, Bardine A, Bartolozzi C (2005) CT Colonography in the follow up of patients with partial colectomy. Eur Radiol 15(3):164

O'Connell DJ, Thompson AJ (1978) Lymphoma of the colon: the spectrum of radiologic changes. Gastrointest Radiol 2(4):377–385

Ota Y, Matsui T, Ono H, Uno H, Matake H, Tsuda S, Sakurai T, Yao T (2003) Value of virtual computed tomographic colonography for Crohn's colitis: comparison with endoscopy and barium enema. Abdom Imaging 28(6):778–783

Oto A, Gelebek V, Oguz BS, Sivri B, Deger A, Akhan O, Besim A (2003) CT attenuation of colorectal polypoid lesions: evaluation of contrast enhancement in CT colonography. Eur Radiol 13(7):1657–1663

Pickhardt PJ (2004) Differential diagnosis of polypoid lesions seen at CT colonography (virtual colonoscopy). Radiographics 24(6):1535–1556

Sosna J, Morrin MM, Kruskal JB, Farrell RJ, Nasser I, Raptopoulos V (2003) Colorectal neoplasms: role of intravenous contrast-enhanced CT colonography. Radiology 228(1):152–156

Sosna J, Blachar A, Amitai, M, Bar-Ziv J (2005) Assessment of the risk of colonic perforation at CT colonography. Eur Radiol 15(3):16

Tarjan Z, Zagoni T, Gyorke T, Mester A, Karlinger K, Mako EK (2000) Spiral CT colonography in inflammatory bowel disease. Eur J Radiol 35(3):193–198

Taylor SA, Halligan S, Bartram CI (2003a) CT colonography: methods, pathology and pitfalls. Clin Radiol 58(3):179–190

Taylor SA, Halligan S, Goh V, Morley S, Bassett P, Atkin W, Bartram CI (2003b) Optimizing colonic distention for multi-detector row CT colonography: effect of hyoscine butylbromide and rectal balloon catheter. Radiology 229(1):99–108

Wanebo HJ, Llaneras M, Martin T, Kaiser D (1989) Prospective monitoring trial for carcinoma of colon and rectum after surgical resection. Surg Gynecol Obstet 169(6):479–487

Wyatt SH, Fishman EK, Hruban RH, Siegelman SS (1994) CT of primary colonic lymphoma. Clin Imaging 18(2):131–141

14 Pictorial Overview of Normal Anatomy, Mimics of Disease, and Neoplasia at CT Colonography

Joel G. Fletcher and Fargol Booya

CONTENTS

14.1 Introduction 175
14.2 Intrinsic Features of the Normal Colon 176
14.2.1 Hemorrhoids 176
14.2.2 Diverticulosis 176
14.2.3 Folds 178
14.2.4 Collapse and Contraction 178
14.2.5 Ileo-cecal Valve 181
14.2.6 Inverted Appendiceal Stump and Appendiceal Intussusception 181
14.3 Benign Findings 183
14.3.1 Lipomas 183
14.3.2 Diverticulitis 183
14.4 Intracolonic and Extracolonic Processes Mimicking Disease 183
14.4.1 Stool 183
14.4.2 Fluid 185
14.4.3 Extrinsic Compression 185
14.4.4 Technical Artifacts 185
14.5 Colonic Neoplasia at CT Colonography 185
14.5.1 Polyps 185
14.5.2 Carcinomas 190
14.6 Conclusion 190
References 192

14.1 Introduction

Interpretation of CT colonography data requires a radiologist to interrogate interactively a high spatial resolution, three-dimensional dataset of the air-filled human colon. Optimal scanning and interpretive techniques can yield diagnostic results on a par with optical colonoscopy (Yee et al. 2001; Pickhardt 2003; Macari et al. 2004). While colonic neoplasia can have a variety of appearances at CT colonography, the spectrum of neoplastic disease within the colorectum, and the methods used to examine the CT dataset, are well-defined. The purpose of this chapter is to review pictorially the spectrum of normal and pathological findings within the human colon at CT colonography.

Examination of CT colonography datasets generally involves two steps: (1) screening the colorectum for suspicious abnormalities, (2) problem-solving to determine if suspicious abnormalities represent neoplasia or benign or normal findings. Preliminary screening of the colorectum for suspicious lesions may be performed using either 2D axial and 2D multiplanar reformatted images (Dachman et al. 1998; Macari et al. 2000), or reviewing the 3D endoluminal surface of the colon (Pickhardt et al. 2003). Two-dimensional screening involves panning through enlarged 2D images from anus to cecum using lung window settings to detect intraluminal filling defects, usually followed by reverse screening of the colon with narrower window settings (e.g., bone window settings), in order to detect focal regions of colonic wall thickening. Three-dimensional screening typically involves viewing forward and reverse endoluminal fly-throughs (i.e., perspective, volume renderings) of the colorectum from anus to cecum, but can also rely upon other three-dimensional endoluminal renderings of the human colon (Fletcher et al. 2001). The aim of both screening techniques is to quickly identify all potential lesions, which can then be interrogated electronically using the computer workstation.

Standard problem-solving techniques are employed once suspicious filling defects are identified using 2D or 3D screening methods. First, the morphology of filling defects are examined using 2D multiplanar and 3D endoluminal images. Most polyps possess a typical polypoid morphology on both 2D and 3D images. If a filling defect remains suspicious, the internal attenuation and textural features are subsequently displayed by changing the CT window settings. Stool will often contain internal locules of air, while lipomas possess internal fat attenuation. Neoplasms possess soft tissue attenuation, in the absence of partial volume effects. Finally, the appearance of suspicious lesions is compared between supine and prone datasets (Fletcher et al.

J. G. Fletcher, MD; F. Booya, MD
Department of Radiology, Mayo Clinic Rochester, 200 First Street, SW, Rochester, MN 55905, USA

2000). While stool will generally change positions with gravity, most lesions retain a fixed geometry with respect to the colon between the supine and prone positions. Rarely, additional scanning with intravenous contrast or repositioning with re-inflation of the colon is used (MORRIN et al. 2000). By investigating the colon systematically using these problem-solving techniques, questionable filling defects can be confidently diagnosed as intraluminal neoplasms or benign findings.

The purpose of this chapter is to elucidate the spectrum of findings that radiologists may encounter within the colon at CT colonography. Illustrations are generously employed to expand the visual understanding of the spectrum of normality (FLETCHER et al. 1999; MACARI and MEGIBOW 2001; MACARI et al. 2003), with only a brief review of the appearances of neoplasia (HARA et al. 1997), which are highlighted elsewhere in the text. We first examine intrinsic features of the normal colon, followed by common benign findings encountered at CT colonography. Intraluminal and extracolonic processes that may simulate disease will be juxtaposed to the common appearance of colonic neoplasia found at CT colonography. The spectrum of findings associated with neoplasia will be reviewed.

14.2
Intrinsic Features of the Normal Colon

Unlike endoscopists, most radiologists examine the colon from the rectum to the cecum. The spectrum of normal findings within the colon are therefore discussed in this order.

14.2.1
Hemorrhoids

Internal hemorrhoids can be seen as smoothly marginated and curved filling defects that project into the rectal vault, lying adjacent to the rectal tube tip (Fig. 14.1). In contradistinction, low rectal cancers will normally have shouldering, and arise some distance from the anus itself. Physical examination usually confirms the presence of internal hemorrhoids. If the remainder of the colorectum has been cleared of significant lesions, a limited proctoscopic or sigmoidoscopic examination can be performed, if digital examination is nondiagnostic.

14.2.2
Diverticulosis

Diverticular disease is exceedingly common, and is seen as focal outpouchings of the colonic lumen projecting beyond the colonic wall on 2D axial and 2D MPR images. Three-dimensional endoluminal images demonstrate the internal orifices projecting from the colonic lumen (Fig. 14.2 and Fig. 14.3). Occasionally, muscular hypertrophy of diverticulosis can cause colonic wall thickening, but in these segments, we usually observe diverticula interposed throughout the regions of colonic wall thickening. Filling defects can be associated with diverticular disease. The most

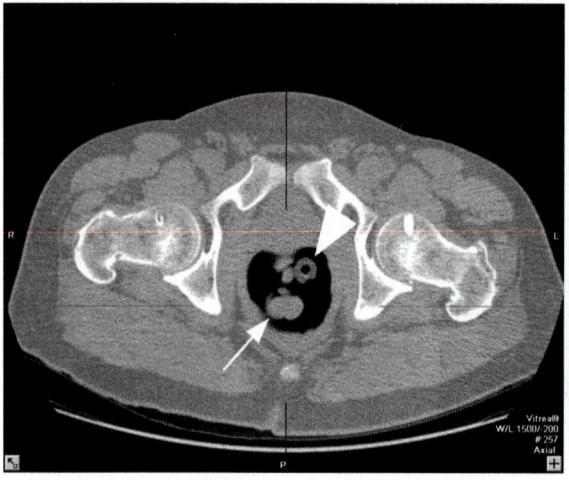 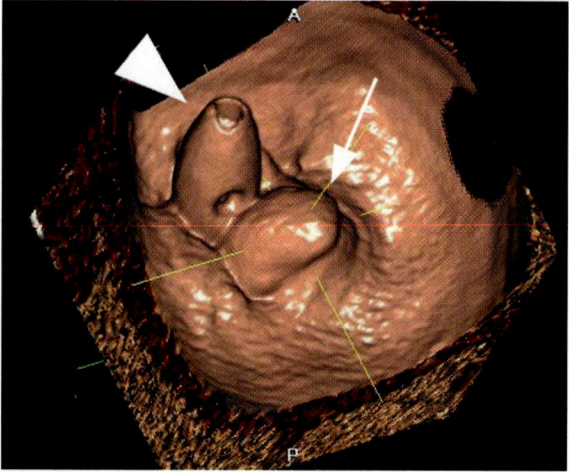

Fig. 14.1a,b. Sixty-eight-year-old male with large internal hemorrhoids at endoscopy. **a)** axial CT image, **b)** 3D endoluminal image at CT colonography. Note the smoothly marginated and curved filling defects (*arrow*) that project into the rectal vault, lying adjacent to the rectal tube tip (*arrowhead*)

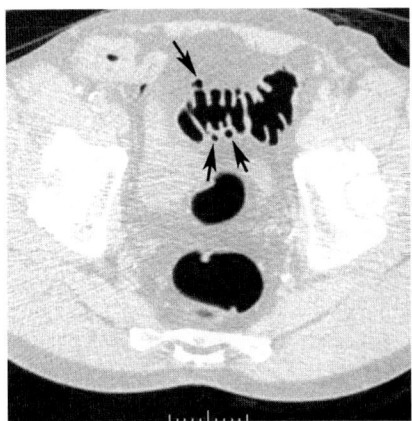
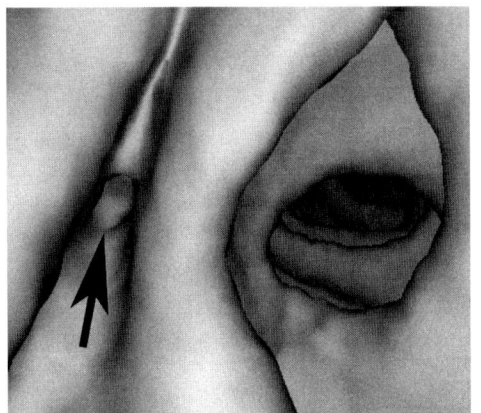
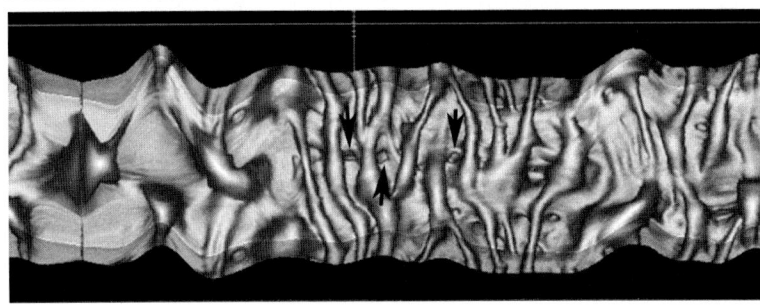

Fig. 14.2.a Diverticulosis in a patient with normal CT Colonography. Note the focal outpouchings of the colonic lumen on 2D axial image. **b,c** 3D endoluminal images showing diverticular (*arrows*) orifices projecting from the colonic lumen on 3D endoluminal images

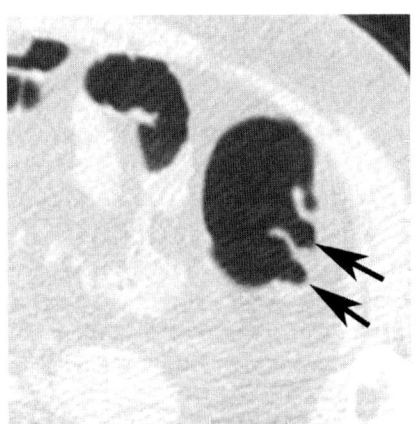
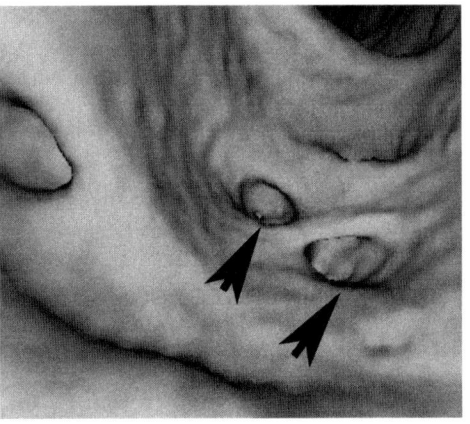
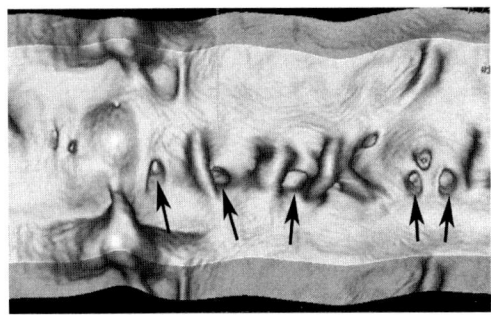

Fig. 14.3a–c. Diverticulosis in a normal patient: **a** note the focal outpouchings of the colonic diverticula on 2D MPR images (*arrows*); **b,c** diverticular orifices projecting from the colonic lumen on 3D endoluminal images (*arrows*)

common of these is the stool-containing diverticulum (Fig. 14.4). Stool can be recognized by its heterogeneous internal attenuation characteristics, the presence of intra-lesional air, and pointed edges on 3D endoluminal views. The fact that a filling defect also projects beyond the colonic wall also indicates the presence of the diverticulum or intramural lesion (as opposed to the neoplastic mucosal lesions). Frequently divertic-

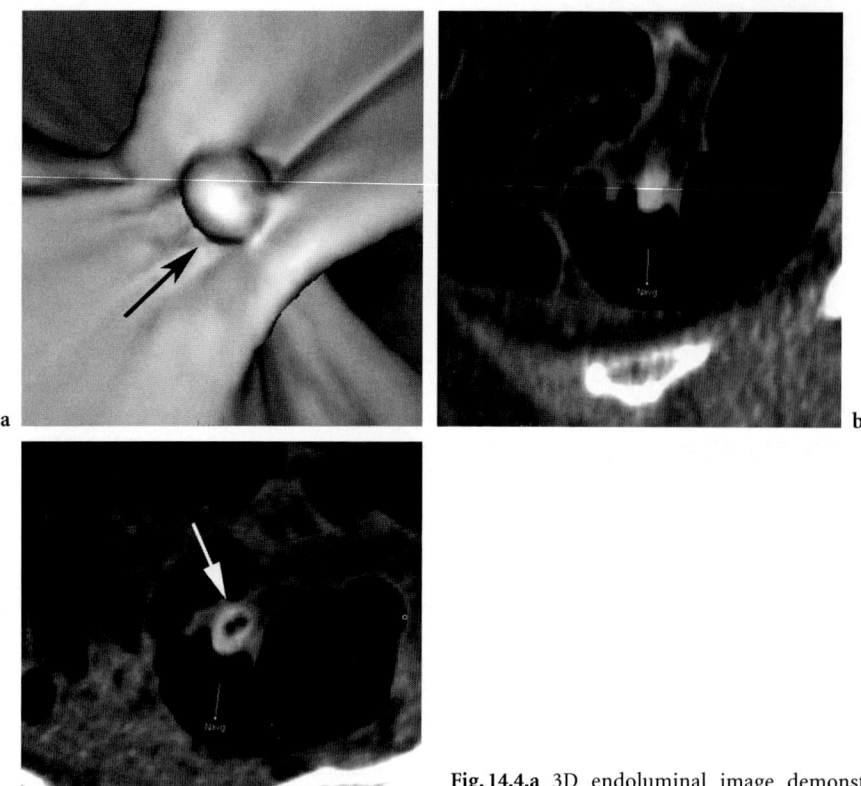

Fig. 14.4.a 3D endoluminal image demonstrates a polypoid filling defect. **b,c** 2D images with soft tissue windows show the filling defect to project beyond the colonic wall into the pericolonic fat (**b**) and contain barium and air (**b,c**), indicating the defect is retained stool and barium within a diverticulum

ula will have residual barium from prior radiographic examination. An inverted diverticulum occurs when the diverticular outpouching intussuscepts into the colonic lumen. In such cases, the perienteric fat can be seen within the filling defect.

14.2.3
Folds

Colonic folds can be particularly complex, particularly in the flexures and rectum. Fused folds are common in these locations (Fig. 14.5). Fused folds are simply recognized by their three-dimensional shape. Occasionally one may visualize focal thickening within a fold. Folds can be distinguished from polyps due to the obtuse margins, internal attenuation (which will often contain some fat) and the nonfocality of the lesion. Thickened folds are usually seen in regions of suboptimal colonic distension, so comparison with the complementary dataset in a different position with improved distention will frequently assist in the identification of thickened folds (Fig. 14.6).

14.2.4
Collapse and Contraction

Luminal collapse can be confused with malignant scirrhous tumors by radiologists learning CT colonography (FIDLER et al. 2004). Imaging patients in two positions has been shown by multiple observers to result in complementary distension and can be employed to distend collapsed bowel (CHEN et al. 1999; FLETCHER et al. 2000; YEE et al. 2003). In general, the patient should be rolled such that the collapsed bowel loop is in the most nondependent location (Fig. 14.7). Contraction can appear as a focal area of wall thickening, which can mimic an annular-constricting lesion. Delayed imaging in another position usually will allow for the colonic bowel segment to relax (Fig. 14.8). Alternatively glucagon can be given when this is suspected. In our experience annular constricting neoplasms, which do not have well-defined soft tissue shoulders, can be mistaken for collapse by inexperienced readers (Fig. 14.9). These lesions will retain the marked colonic wall thickening and irregularity to the intraluminal margins of the mass, potentially

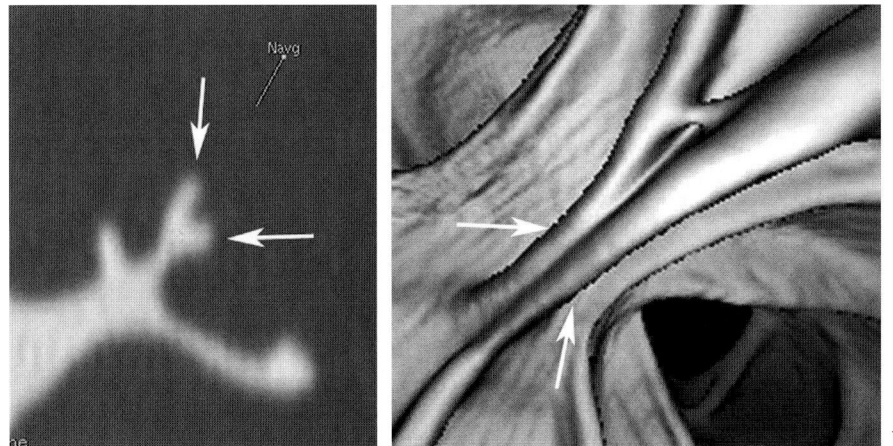

Fig. 14.5a,b. Complex colonic folds can mimic polyps on 2D images. These folds are particularly common in the colonic flexures They can easily be recognized by comparing: **a** 2D image (*arrows*); **b** 3D endoluminal image (*arrows*)

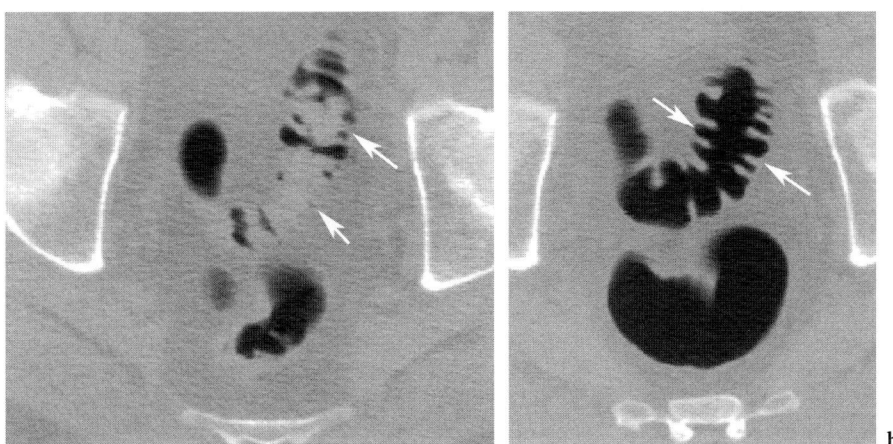

Fig. 14.6.a Thickened folds in a suboptimally distended sigmoid colon (*arrows*). **b** Repositioning distends the sigmoid colon to allow easily for the recognition of colonic folds (*arrows*)

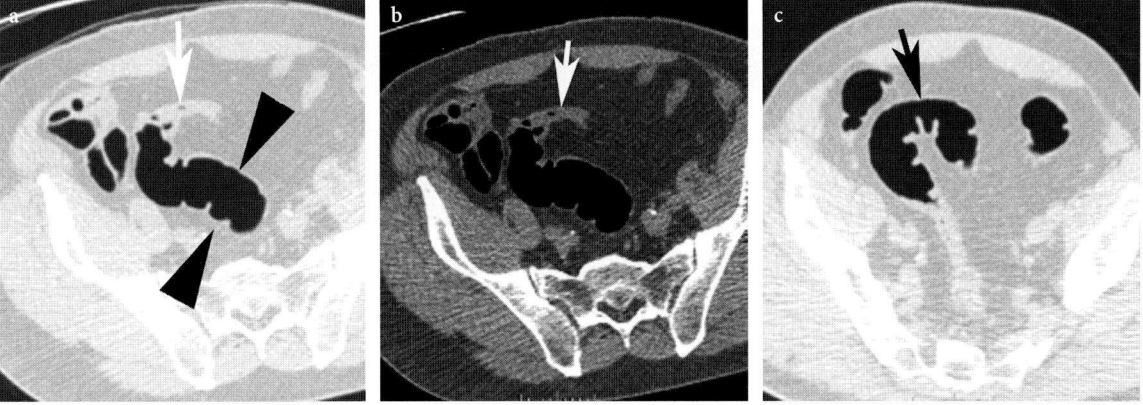

Fig. 14.7.a,b A collapsed sigmoid loop (*white arrow*) demonstrates a smooth transition to distal distention (*black arrowheads*). **c** Inflation in the complimentary position (*black arrow*)

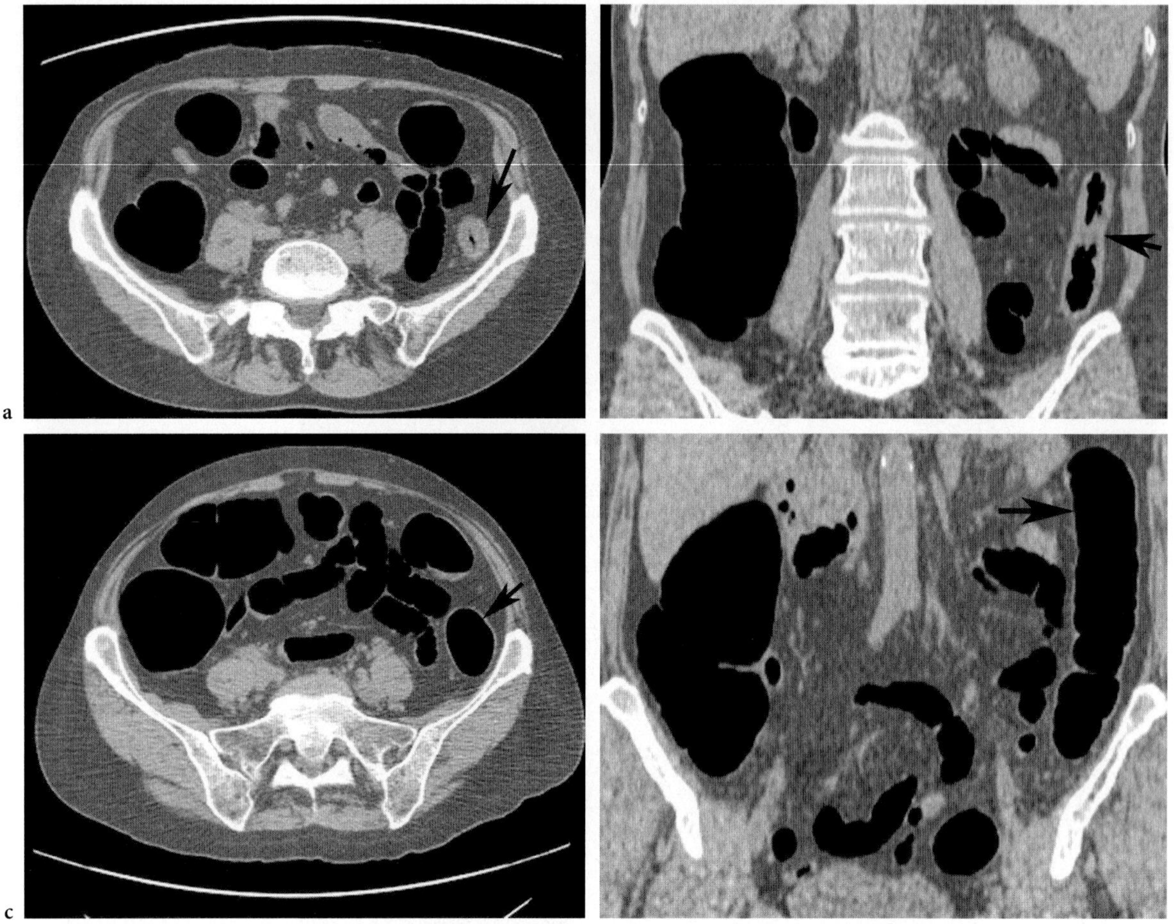

Fig. 14.8.a,b Colonic contraction in the descending colon (*arrow*) causes focal wall thickening. **c,d** Delayed imaging in a complimentary position shows inflation of previously contracted descending colon (*arrows*)

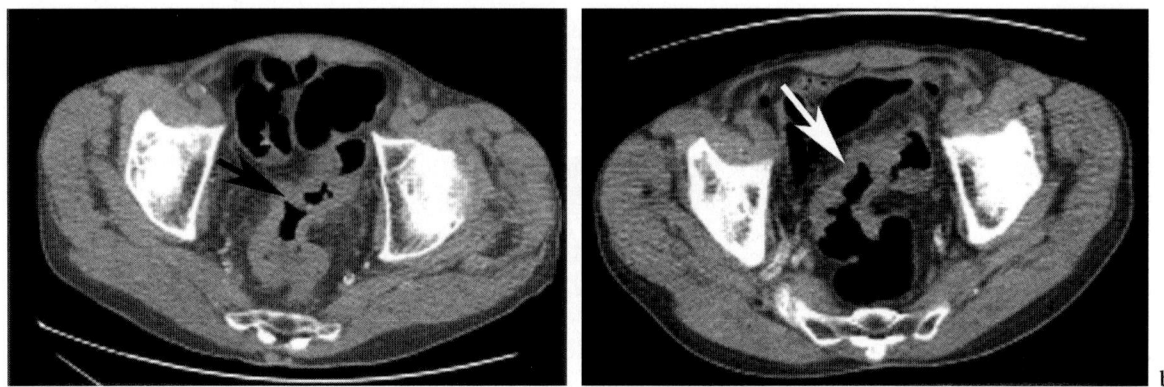

Fig. 14.9a,b. Annular constricting cancers should not be confused with collapse. Colonic wall thickening and intraluminal irregularity observed in these types of lesion are persistent in complimentary positions. Note the persistent non-distension that is present in both supine (**a**) and prone (**b**) images

extending into the pericolonic tissues (if invasive), as other large carcinomas.

14.2.5
Ileo-cecal Valve

The ileo-cecal valve is the entry point for small bowel enteric contents as they dump into the cecum. It is important to understand that the ileo-cecal valve is located within a fold within the cecum. The valve should be symmetric with respect to the valve orifice on 2D and 3D views. By narrowing the window and level settings to soft tissue settings, one can visualize the internal fatty attenuation of the valve and its associated fold, and distinguish this from suspicious filling defects (Figs. 14.10 and 14.11). Several normal variants of ileo-cecal valve morphology have been described (MACARI and MEGIBOW 2001), but an assessment of the 2D and 3D morphology and internal attenuation is usually sufficient. Lipomatous ileo-cecal valves retain benign features we have previously described, only appearing larger and more bulbous, with a homogenous fatty internal attenuation (Fig. 14.12).

14.2.6
Inverted Appendiceal Stump and Appendiceal Intussusception

An inverted appendiceal stump can appear identical to a polyp (Fig. 14.13), and is located at the site of prior appendectomy. Both the appendiceal stump and intraluminal neoplasm will enhance with intravenous contrast. Close correlation with the clinical history of incidental inversion-ligation appendectomy may be revealing, but in cases where clinical history is incomplete, endoscopic correlation may be required. Appendiceal intussusception can also occur. Barium enema has the advantage of being able to attempt reduction of the intussusception manually, so that the filling defect disappears during reduction. In CT colonography, this is usu-

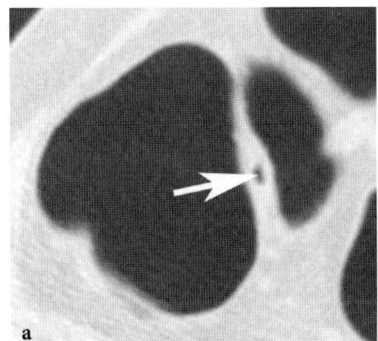 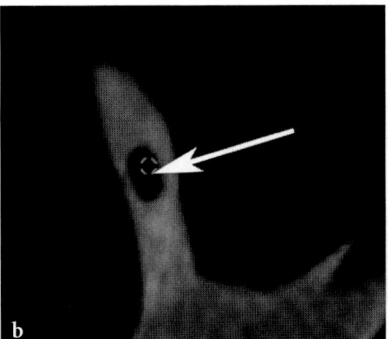 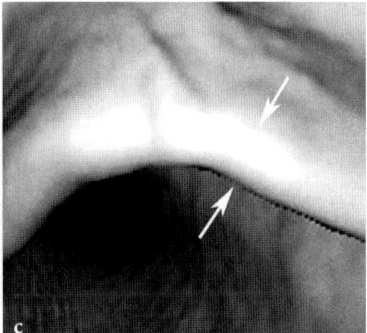

Fig. 14.10a–c. Normal ileo-cecal valve. The valve should be symmetric with respect to the valve orifice on: **a** 2D view; **c** 3D view; **b** by narrowing the window and level settings to soft tissue settings, one can visualize the internal fatty attenuation of the valve and its associated fold (*arrow*)

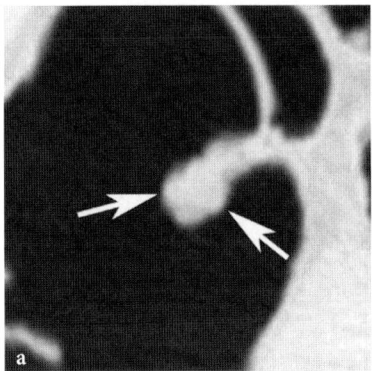 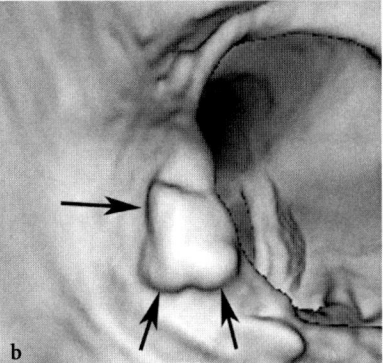 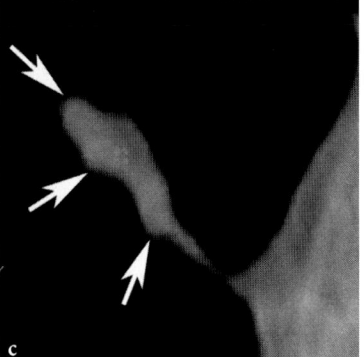

Fig. 14.11a–c. Ileo-cecal valve with lobulated polypoid filling defects on: **a** 2D view; **b** 3D views (*arrows*) without symmetry; **c** soft tissue windows revealed internal soft tissue attenuation (*arrow*). Endoscopy demonstrated an adenoma of ileo-cecal valve

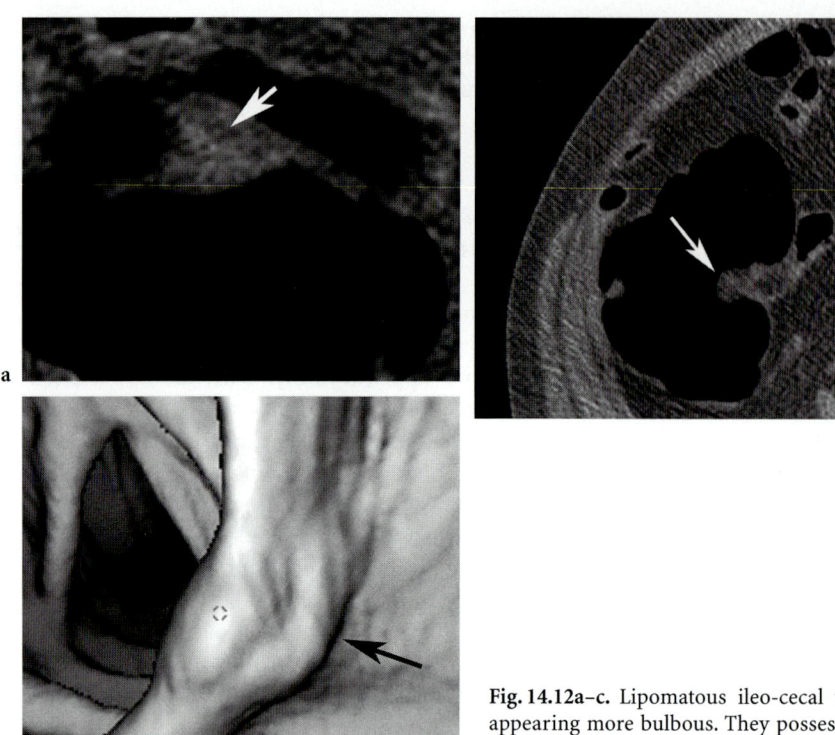

Fig. 14.12a–c. Lipomatous ileo-cecal valves retain benign features, only appearing more bulbous. They possess homogenous fatty internal attenuation and appear smoothly marginated without focal lesions on 3D endoluminal views

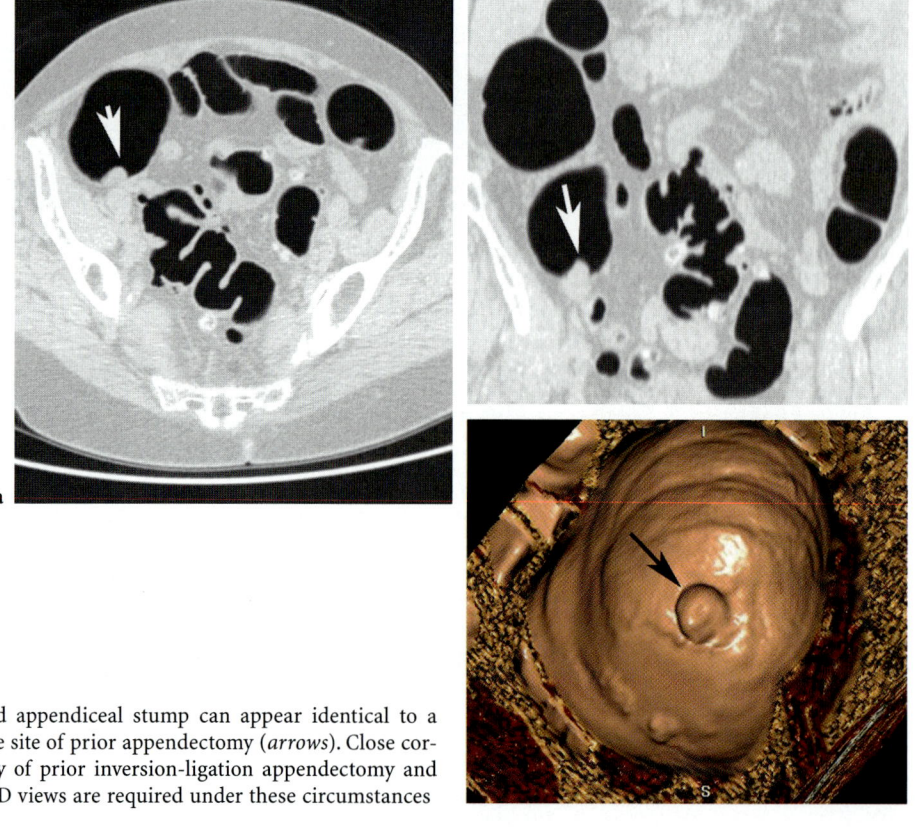

Fig. 14.13a–c. An inverted appendiceal stump can appear identical to a polyp and is located at the site of prior appendectomy (*arrows*). Close correlation to patient history of prior inversion-ligation appendectomy and absence of appendix on 2D views are required under these circumstances

ally not the case, and such filling defects require further endoscopic or fluoroscopic evaluation.

14.3
Benign Findings

14.3.1
Lipomas

Lipomas are the most common submucosal tumors of the colon and are visualized frequently. Large lipomas may bleed, and heterogeneity within a lipoma is thought to correlate with internal hemorrhage. Lipomas are smoothly marginated filling defects within the colon with internal fatty attenuation (Fig. 14.14).

14.3.2
Diverticulitis

Diverticulitis may mimic an annular constricting neoplasm when the majority of inflammation is intramural, rather than extending into the pericolonic tissues. We have infrequently encountered this occurrence. Close correlation with clinical history and clinical follow up and re-imaging or endoscopy after the episode has past is prudent. In our limited experience with this entity, contrast-enhancement may be helpful by demonstrating mural stratification and diverticula within the lesion (Fig. 14.15).

14.4
Intracolonic and Extracolonic Processes Mimicking Disease

14.4.1
Stool

Stool is the most frequent cause of false positive findings at CT colonography (FLETCHER et al. 2000). There are several imaging characteristics, which usually aid in the identification of stool. Stool has a heterogeneous internal attenuation, often with internal air (Fig. 14.16). Additionally, stool particles usually lie along the dependent colonic wall and change location with changes in patient positioning (Fig. 14.17). On 3D normal endoluminal images,

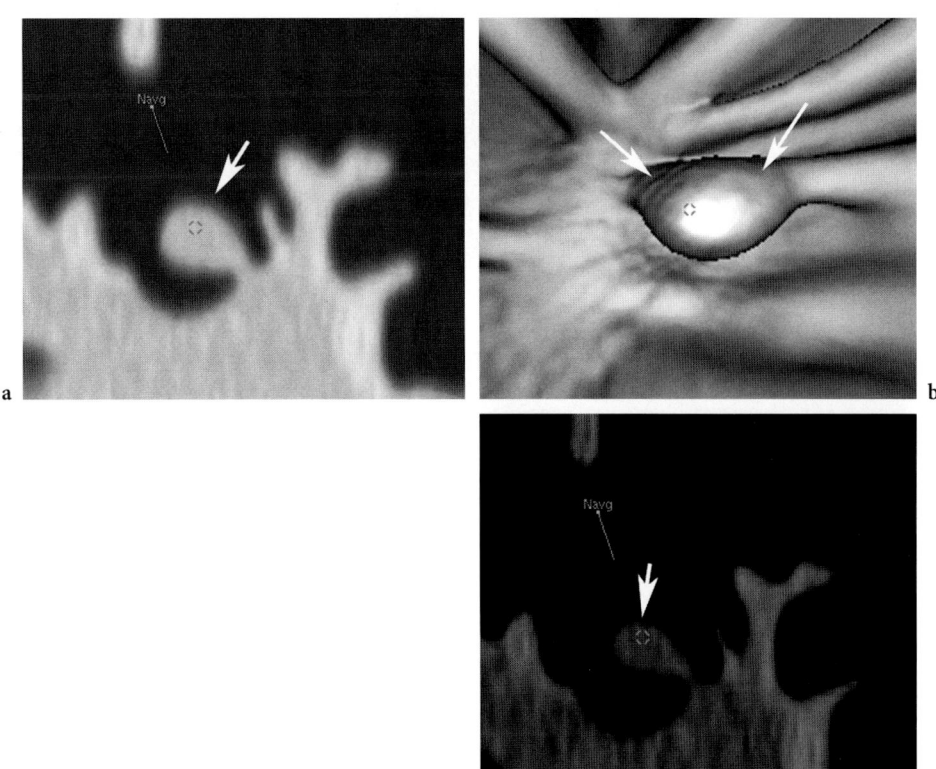

Fig. 14.14a–c. Lipoma. Note the smoothly marginated polypoid filling defect (**a,b,** *arrows*) with internal fatty attenuation (**c,** *arrow*)

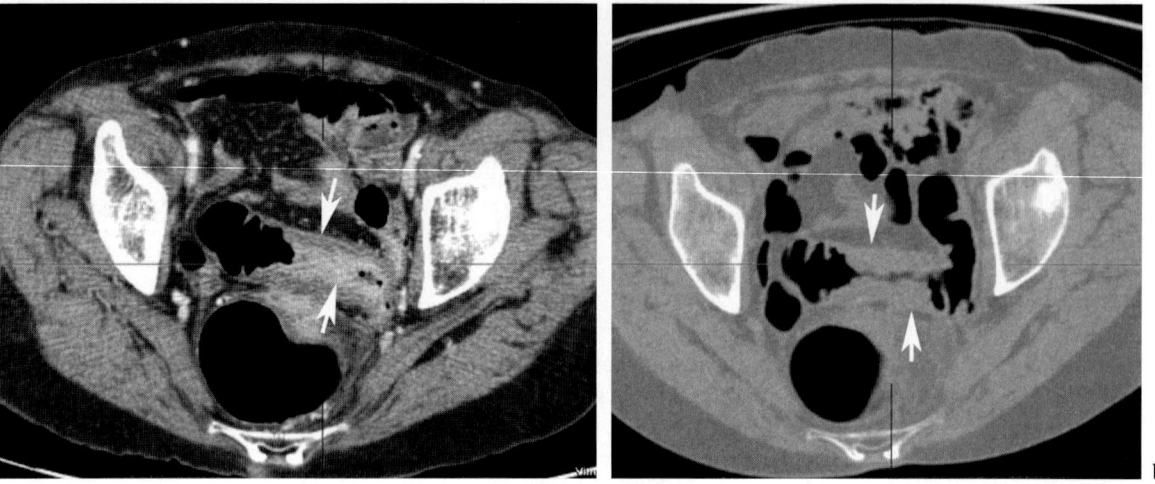

Fig. 14.15a,b. Diverticulitis may mimic an annular constricting neoplasm when the majority of inflammation is intramural, rather than extending into the pericolonic tissues (**a,b**). Contrast enhancement demonstrates mural stratification (**a**, *arrow*)

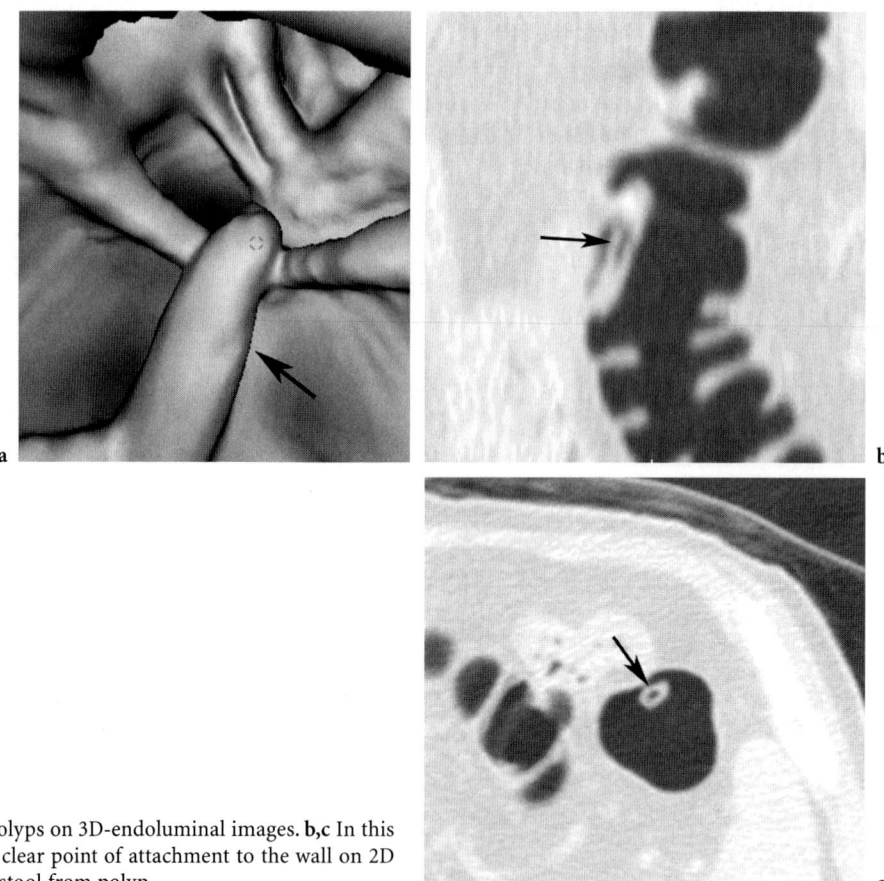

Fig. 14.16.a Stool may mimic polyps on 3D-endoluminal images. **b,c** In this case, internal air and lack of a clear point of attachment to the wall on 2D images (*arrows*) distinguishes stool from polyp

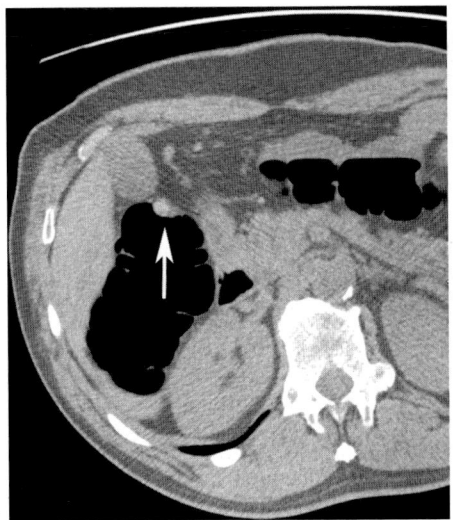 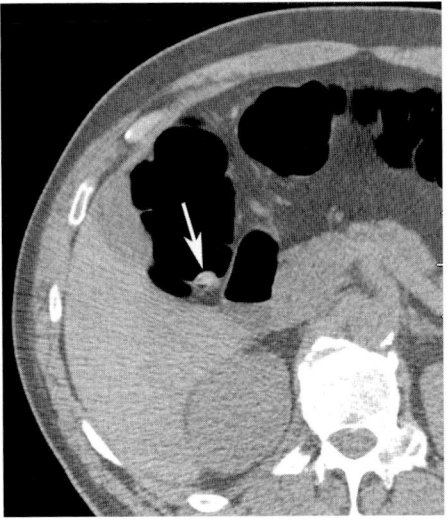

Fig. 14.17a,b. Stool particles generally change location with changes in patient positioning. Stool is usually located along the dependent wall (*arrows*)

stool often demonstrates sharp intraluminal projections (Fig. 14.18). Stool particles will demonstrate a lack of enhancement when intravenous contrast is given.

14.4.2
Fluid

Fluid redistributes between prone and supine imaging (Fig. 14.19). Polyethylene glycol electrolyte solution bowel preparation typically results in more retained colonic fluid, compared to other bowel preparation regimens, but leaves less particulate stool matter in the colon. Fluid can also be seen in 3D endoluminal images (Fig. 14.20). When there is excessive fluid, intravenous contrast can be used to enhance submerged lesions.

14.4.3
Extrinsic Compression

Extrinsic compression on the colon can result from multiple structures such as the iliac vessels, liver, renal masses, and stomach (MACARI and MEGIBOW 2001). Compression by one of the iliac arteries is a relatively common finding, and results in a linear extrinsic compression on the sigmoid colon (Fig. 14.21).

14.4.4
Technical Artifacts

Technical artifacts are easy to recognize. Breath-hold and motion artifacts are usually best seen with sagittal or coronal oblique planes which better display the motion along the z-axis (Fig. 14.22). Metallic artifacts cause beam-hardening artifacts, and can obscure the colon lumen. Stairstep artifacts are usually not seen with thin slice thickness, but with thicker slice thicknesses (such as 5 mm), and are seen on 3D endoluminal images and 2D MPR images, most commonly within the rectum and cecum, where there are great changes in the luminal diameter along the z-axis.

14.5
Colonic Neoplasia at CT Colonography

14.5.1
Polyps

Polyps maybe sessile, pedunculated, or flat (i.e., with the base measuring more than twice that of the height). Sessile polyps will possess polypoid morphology on axial, 2D multiplanar reformatted, and 3D endoluminal views (Fig. 14.23). When sessile polyps are of sufficient size (generally consid-

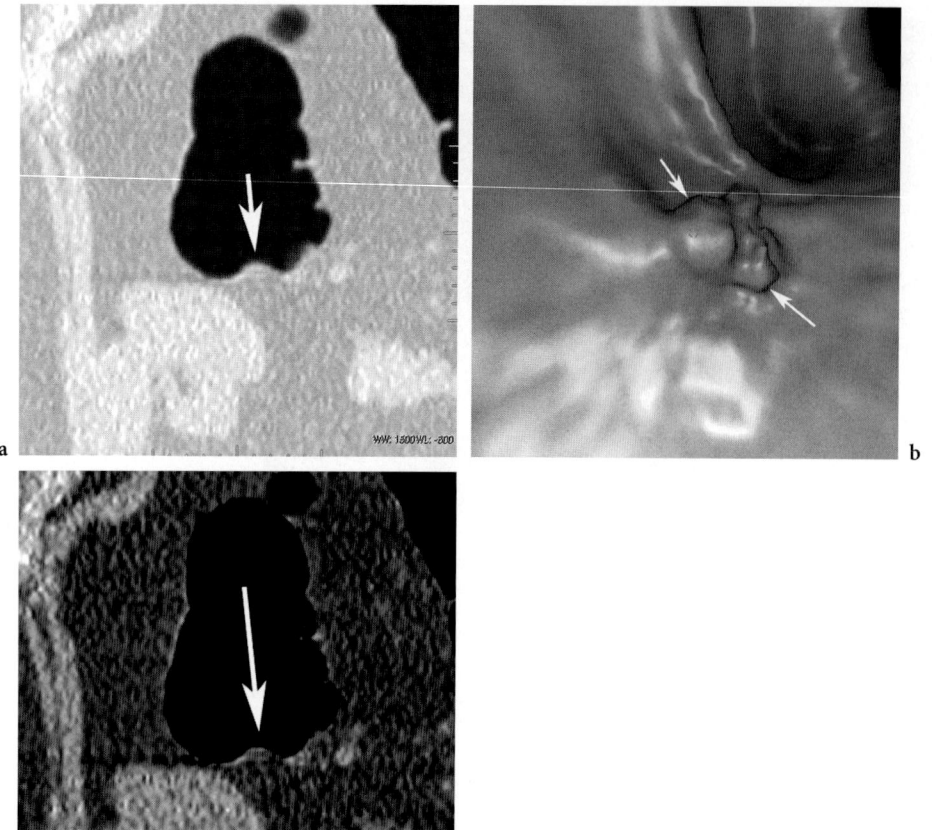

Fig. 14.18a–c. A suspicious filling defect on 2D images (**a**, arrow) demonstrates sharp intraluminal projections on 3D endoluminal images (**b**) and is not of soft tissue attenuation (**c**). These features indicate the lesion represents stool

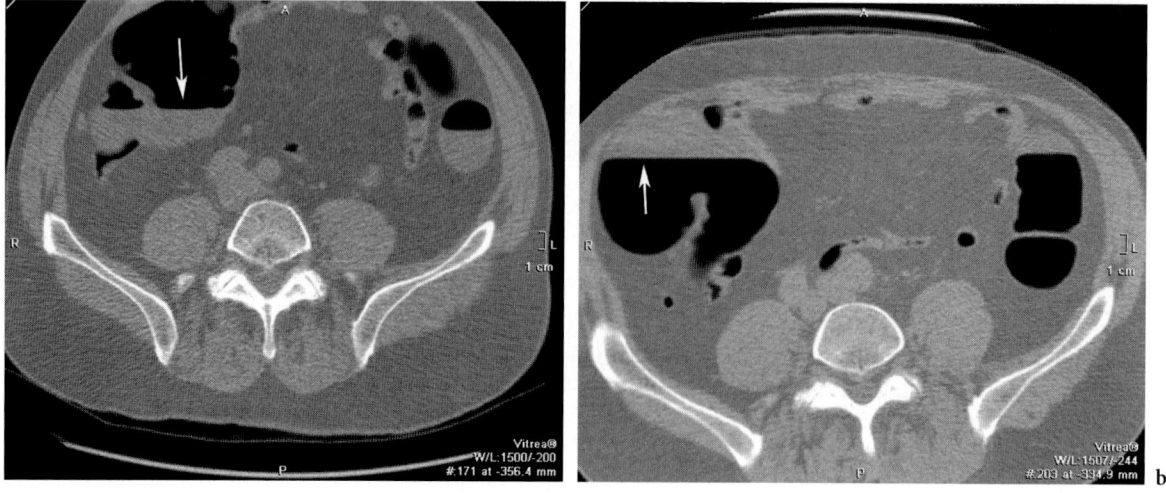

Fig. 14.19a,b. Cecal fluid redistributes between supine (**a**) and prone (**b**) imaging (*arrows*). When there is excessive fluid, intravenous contrast can be used to enhance submerged lesions. Note the dependent position of the fluid

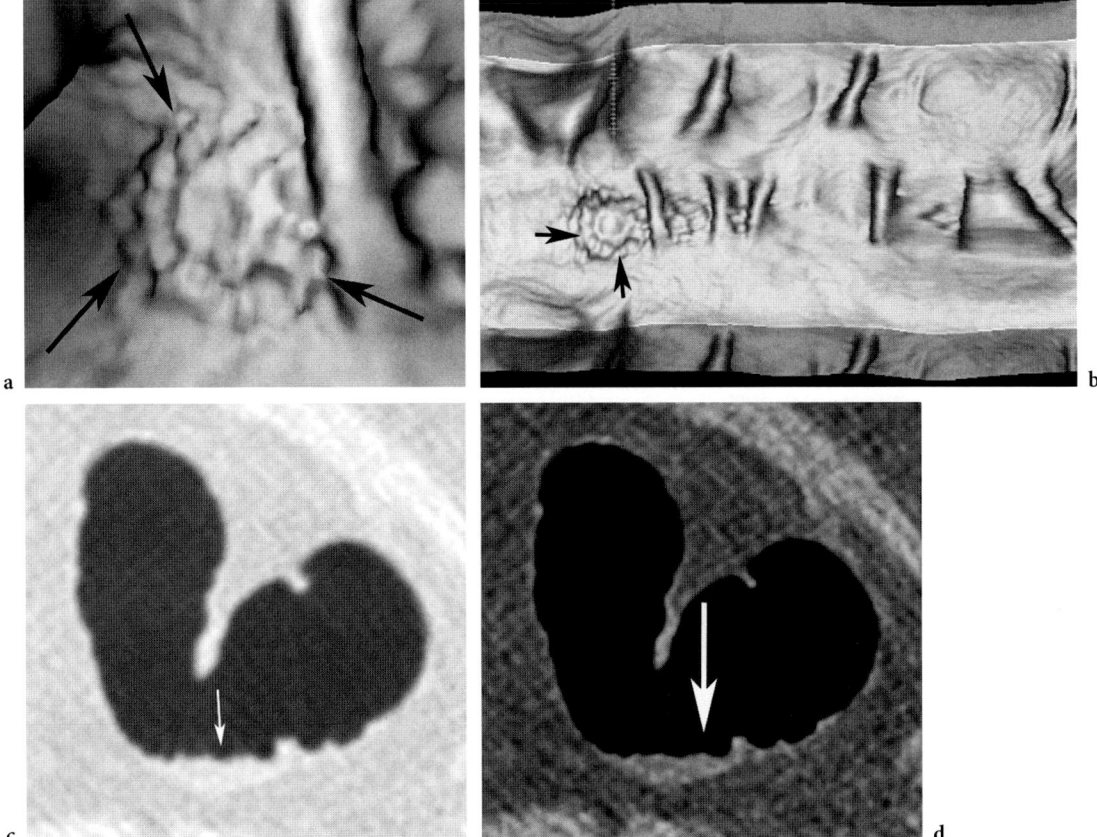

Fig. 14.20a–d. Fluid can be seen on 3D endoluminal images (a, *arrow*) and on virtual pathology (b, *arrow*) as filling defects, Axial 2D image demonstrates an air-fluid level (c, *arrow*) and soft tissue setting shows that the filling defects not have soft tissue attenuation (d, *arrow*)

ered to be three times the slice thickness), they will also possess internal soft tissue attenuation. Sessile polyps are generally seen on both supine and prone views, but about 10–15% of medium-sized polyps will be seen only in one view, due to suboptimal distention, stool or fluid in the same colonic segment in the complementary position. Lesions that appear as sessile polyps in one position should not be disregarded unless the same segment is optimally seen in the corresponding position.

Pedunculated polyps possess a stalk and a head. They are best seen on 2D axial and images (Fig. 14.24). Using 3D endoluminal renderings, the stalk of a pedunculated polyp is often inseparable from the colonic wall. Polyps with long stalks maybe missed at CT colonography, as the larger filling defect representing the head of the polyp may appear to move between colonic segments (FENLON et al. 1999). Careful interrogation of suspicious filling defects for a stalk connecting them to the colonic wall is imperative in diagnosing pedunculated polyps. In our experience, pedunculated polyps can be found with a high degree of accuracy.

Flat lesions can be difficult to visualize both endoscopically and radiographically. On CT, flat lesions appear as focal regions of colonic wall thickening with soft tissue attenuation. Flat lesions are often cigar-shaped, and are best seen on 2D axial and MPR images with narrow window settings (such as bone window settings) (FIDLER et al. 2002). Perturbation in the colonic wall can be visualized when surveying the colon with 2D images using lung windows, and when these perturbations are discovered, interrogation of soft tissue window settings is imperative (Fig. 14.25). Similar perturbations can often be seen on 3D endoluminal views, but can be occult. Like other polyps, flat lesions are usually seen in both the supine and prone views, unless the segment in which the lesion is located is suboptimally visualized in one of the views. Intravenous contrast can be useful in characterizing flat lesions. Flat lesions should not

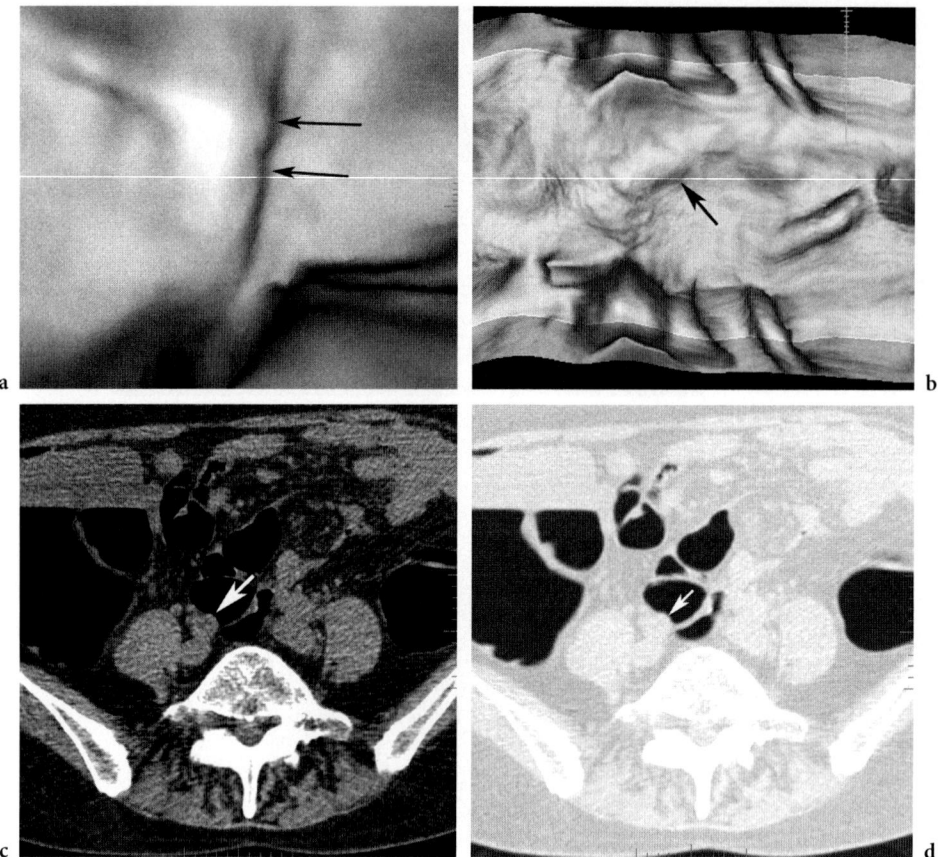

Fig. 14.21a–d. Compression by one of the iliac arteries in this case has resulted in a linear extrinsic compression on the sigmoid colon that is well demonstrated on 3 D endoluminal view (**a**, *arrows*) and virtual pathology (**b**, *arrow*). 2D axial images demonstrates the extrinsic nature of these lesions (**c,d**, *arrows*)

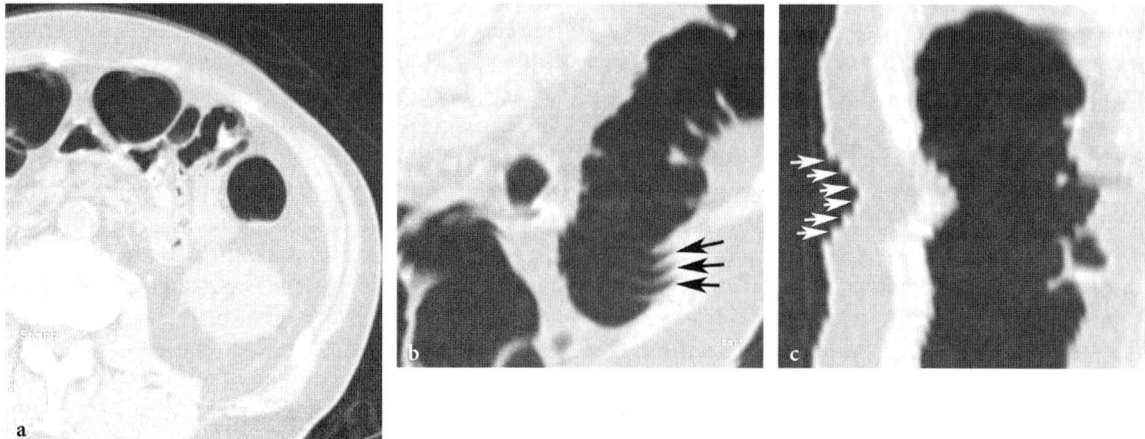

Fig. 14.22a–c. Motion artifacts cause image blur on axial images (**a**), but are best appreciated using 2D oblique coronal or sagittal images, which show luminal incongruity along Z-axis of the colon, (**b,c**, *arrows*)

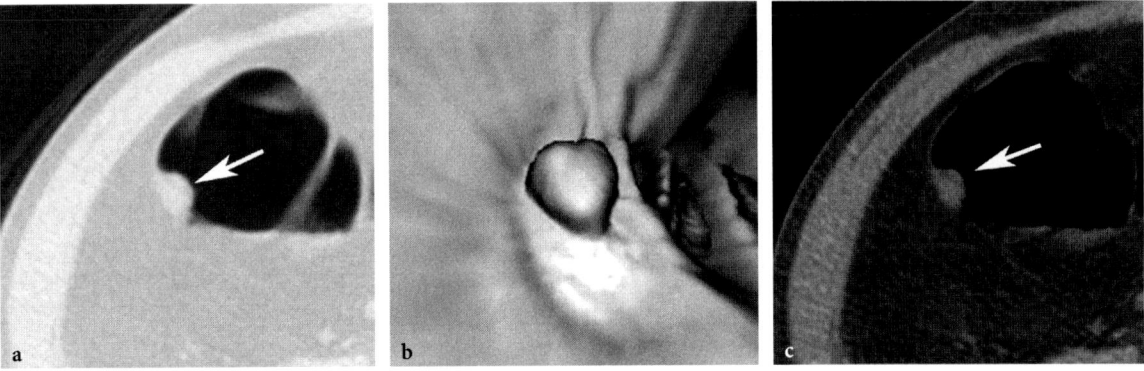

Fig. 14.23a–c. Sessile polyp: a supine 2D axial image and; b 3-D endoluminal view demonstrate a polypoid filling defect in the ascending colon; c after changing to soft tissue window setting, the homogenous soft tissue attenuation of the lesion is demonstrated. Colonoscopy demonstrated a 1.5 tubulovillous adenoma

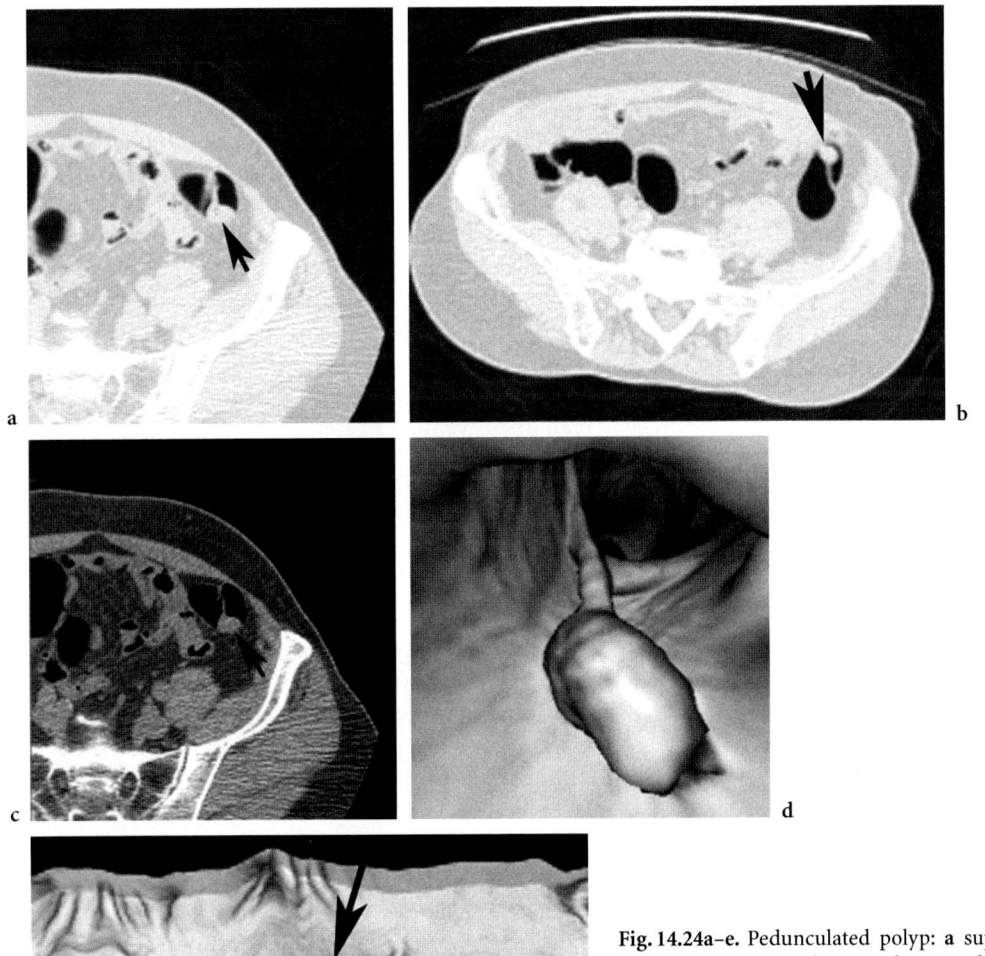

Fig. 14.24a–e. Pedunculated polyp: a supine 2D axial image and; b prone 2D axial image show a polyp in the descending colon associated with a stalk (*arrowhead*); c soft tissue window setting shows the head of the polyp to be of soft tissue attenuation. Note that the lesion changes position to the dependent position due to its long stalk; d,e endoluminal appearances of the pedunculated polyp

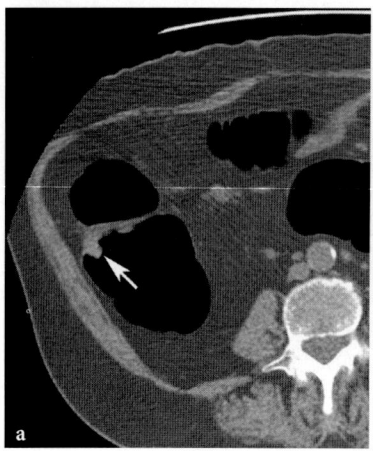 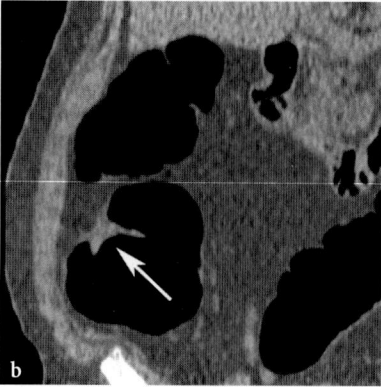 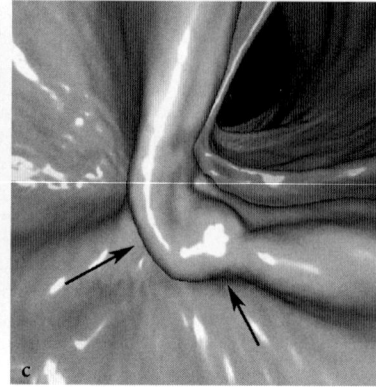

Fig. 14.25a–c. Flat cancer prone view: **a** 2D axial image and: **b** multiplanar reformatted image show a focal region of soft tissue thickening along the lateral aspect of the ascending colon lying along a haustral fold. Soft tissue window settings show the soft tissue attenuation of the lesion (*arrows*); **c** on 3-D views the lesion appears as a focal thickening along a haustral fold (*arrow*)

be confused with luminal collapse. The colonic wall does thicken as it collapses. The thickened colonic wall can be distinguished from the true flat lesion in that it is not well defined, should be distended in the corresponding position, and smoothly taper to a normal thickness in adjacent areas of appropriate distention (Fig. 14.7). The term "flat lesion" can represent a variety of pathologies, from flat adenomas to hyperplastic lesions to tubulovillous adenomas and flat carcinomas. In general, flat lesions tend to be more advanced lesions.

14.5.2
Carcinomas

Carcinomas can assume a variety of shapes. Smaller cancers may be identical to large polyps and flat lesions, while semi-annular and annular, and scirrhous cancers have a unique CT appearance. Semi-annular and annular cancers are seen as a focal, segmental regions of luminal narrowing, accompanied by focal wall thickening, usually with proximal and distal shouldering (Fig. 14.26). The intraluminal margins of the mass are irregular. Extension of soft tissue into the pericolonic fat signals invasion, as does regional lymphadenopathy or hepatic metastases. Annular cancers are best seen at 2D and 3D MPR images using soft tissue window settings.

Scirrhous cancers can constrict the lumen and are the most common type of cancer in our experience that are missed by radiologists learning colonography (FIDLER et al. 2004). Scirrhous cancers are annular lesions that constrict the colonic lumen, and may be confused with luminal collapse, usually because adjacent collapse may obscure the shouldering of the carcinoma (Fig. 14.27). Focal wall thickening of soft tissue attenuation and irregular intraluminal margins clearly separate these lesions from collapse, however. Segmental regions of luminal narrowing seen in one position or seen in both positions should be considered as potential scirrhous cancers, until repositioning and reinflation can disprove their presence.

14.6
Conclusion

CT colonography interpretation requires radiologists to create interactively two- and three-dimensional images of the colonic lumen, use a variety of window and level settings, and compare supine and prone three-dimensional datasets. Colonic datasets are interrogated systematically to screen for potential colorectal lesions, employing well-established problem-solving techniques at the computer workstation to distinguish true neoplasms from benign and normal structures. A visual understanding of the normal appearance of colorectal structures, benign lesions, disease mimics and colorectal neoplasia is necessary in utilizing the capabilities of modern CT colonography computer workstations to accurately diagnose disease.

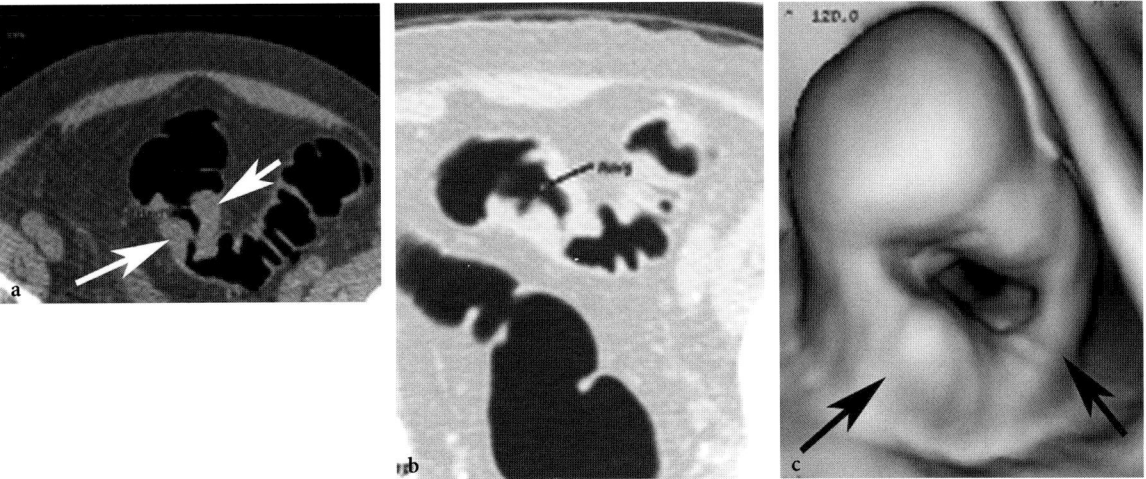

Fig. 14.26a–c. Annular cancer: **a,b** 2D axial images demonstrate focal circumferential wall thickening of soft tissue attenuation with proximal and distal shouldering (*arrows*); **c** note the shouldering of the distal edge of the lesion is visible on 3-D endoluminal view (*arrow*)

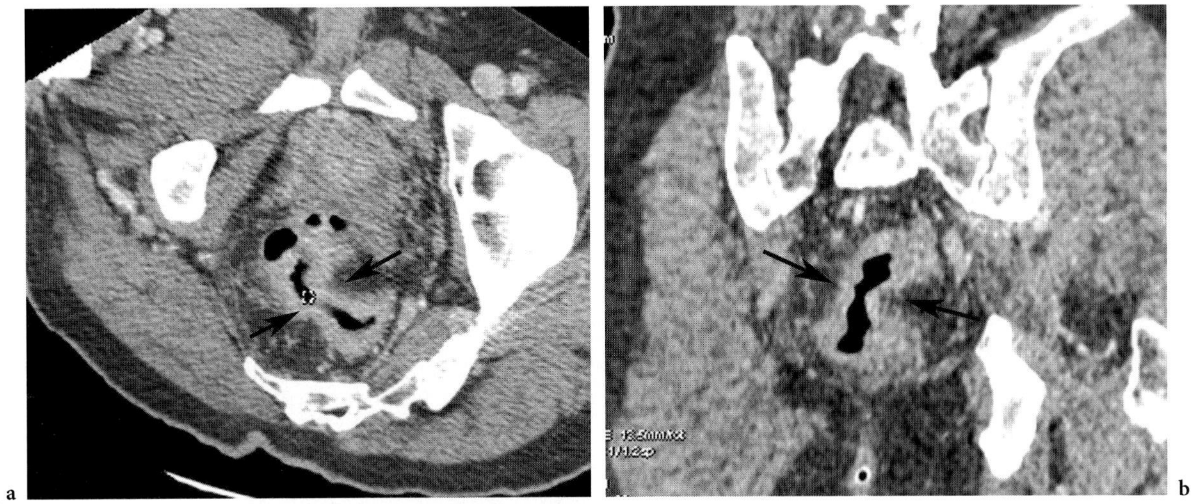

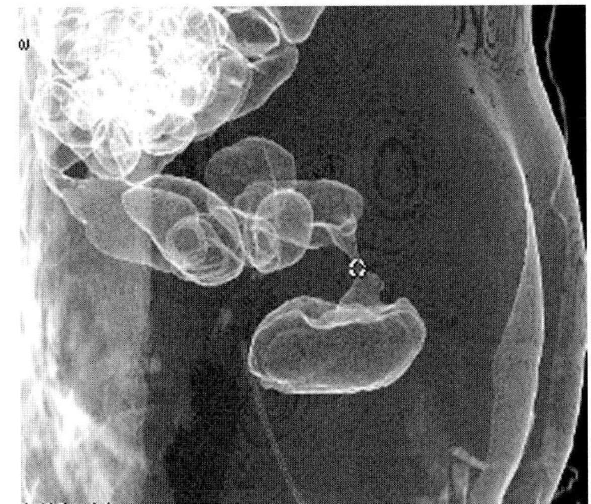

Fig. 14.27a–c. Scirrhous cancer demonstrates luminal constriction, irregularity and wall thickening in the mid-rectum: **a,b** 2D MPR images; **c** the luminal constriction best highlighted on the virtual barium enema rendering

References

Chen S, Lu D, Hecht J et al. (1999) CT colonography: value of scanning in both the supine and prone positions. Am J Roentgenol 172:595–59

Dachman A, Kuniyoshi J, Boyle C et al. (1998) CT colonography with three-dimensional problem solving for detection of colonic polyps. AJR 171:989–995

Fenlon H, Nunes D, Schroy PI et al. (1999) A comparison of virtual and conventional colonoscopy for the detection of colorectal polyps. N Engl J Med 341(20):1496–1503

Fidler JL, Johnson CD, MacCarty RL et al. (2002) Detection of flat lesions in the colon with CT colonography. Abdom Imaging 27(3):292–300

Fidler J, Fletcher JG, Johnson CD, Huprich JE, Barlow JM, Earnest F IV, Bartholmai BJ (2004) Understanding interpretive errors in radiologists learning computed tomography colonography. Acad Radiol 11:750–756

Fletcher JG, Johnson CD, MacCarty RL et al. (1999) CT colonography: potential pitfalls and problem-solving techniques. Am J Roentgenol 172(5):1271–1278

Fletcher J, Johnson C, Welch T et al. (2000) Optimization of CT colonography technique: a prospective trial in 180 patients. Radiology 216:704–711

Fletcher J, Johnson C, Reed J et al. (2001) Feasibility of planar virtual pathology: a new paradigm in volume-rendered CT colonography. J Comput Assist Tomogr 25:864–869

Hara AK, Johnson CD, Reed JE (1997) Colorectal lesions: evaluation with CT colography. Radiographics 17(5):1157–1167; discussion 1167–1168

Macari M, Megibow A (2001) Pitfalls of using three-dimensional CT colonography with two-dimensional imaging correlation. Am J Roentgenol 176:137–143

Macari M, Milano A, Lavelle M et al. (2000) Comparison of time-efficient CT colonography with two- and three-dimensional colonic evaluation for detecting colorectal polyps. Am J Roentgenol 174(6):1543–1549

Macari M, Bini EJ, Jacobs SL et al. (2003) Filling defects at CT colonography: pseudo- and diminutive lesions (the good), polyps (the bad), flat lesions, masses, and carcinomas (the ugly). Radiographics 23(5):1073–1091

Macari M, Bini EJ, Jacobs SL et al. (2004) Colorectal polyps and cancers in asymptomatic average-risk patients: evaluation with CT colonography. Radiology 230(3):629–636

Morrin M, Farrell R, Kruskal J et al. (2000) Utility of intravenously administered contrast material at CT colonography. Radiology 217(3):765–771

Pickhardt PJ, Hwang I, Butler JA, Puckett ML, Hildebrandt HA, Wong RK, Nugent PA, Mysliwiec PA, Schindler WR (2003) Computed tomographic virtual colonoscopy to screen for colorectal neoplasia in asymptomatic adults. N Engl J Med 349:2191–2200

Yee J, Akerkar G, Hung R et al. (2001) Colorectal neoplasia: performance characteristics of CT colonography for detection in 300 patients. Radiology 219:685–692

Yee J, Hung RK, Akerkar GA, Kumar PR, Wall SD (2003) Comparison of supine and prone scanning separately and in combination at CT colonography. Radiology 226(3):653–661

Subject Index

A

Accuracy   123–124
– CAD   142
ACRIN   4, 10
Adenocarcinoma, see Carcinoma
Adenoma, see Polyp
Adenoma-carcinoma sequence, see Carcinoma
Adrenal gland   129, 131
Advanced adenoma, see Polyp
Air, see Room air
Aneurysm   85, 129, 132, 135
Annular mass, see Carcinoma
Antegrade viewing   75, 89, 91, 94, 118, 120, 126
Appendix   107, 181
Apple core, see Cancer, Annular
Archiving   8
Artefact
– Blurring   63, 64
– Breathing   7, 56, 66, 101, 104, 185
– Metallic   19, 185
– Motion   143, 185, 188
– Rippling   64
– 3D   147
– Stairstep   65, 185
Artifact   see Artefact
Attenuation   120
– CAD   139
– Cefficient   117
Automatic dose delivery   67, 69
Average risk   2–5, 14–17, 153, 158

B

Balloon catheter, see Catheter
Barium
– Faecal tagging   37–48
– Fluid tagging   45
Barium enema   15–19
– Appendiceal intussusception   181
– Distension   26
– Glucagon   31
– Perforation   58
– Radiation dose   66-67
– Sodium phosphate   26
Benign mass
– Extracolonic findings   129–135
– Imaging   183
– Report   85, 156

Bisacodyl   26, 27, 37, 47, 100, 154
Blurring, see Artefact
Breathing artefacts, see Artefact
Buscopan, see Hyoscin butylbromide

C

CAD, Computer Aided Detection   11, 127, 137–151
– Carcinoma   143
– Definition   137
– False negative   142, 143–145
– Faecal tagging   146
– False positive   139–141
– Flat adenoma   143
– FROC   141
– Fuzzy merging method   145
– Performance   140–142
– Pitfalls   142
– Statistical classifier   140
– Workstation   137
Cancer, see Carcinoma, Screening
Candidate, see CAD
Cap   139
Carbon dioxide, see Distention
Carcinoma   82, 96, 167, 190
– Adenocarcinoma   157, 167
– Adenoma-carcinoma sequence   2, 14, 38, 76
– Annular   27, 96–98, 145, 156, 168, 178, 183, 190
– CAD   143, 145
– Crohn's disease   166
– Electronic cleansing   147
– Morphology   167, 190
– Obstructing   18, 29, 52
– Ovarian   158
– Report   156
– Scirrhous   178, 190
– Screening, see Screening
– Synchronous   167
– Ulcerative colitis   165
Cathartic, see Preparation
Catheter
– Balloon-tipped   8, 31, 56, 58, 90
– Foley   27, 56
– Rectal   8, 52–56, 59
Clear liquid diet, see Preparation
Collapse   23–31, 43, 53, 75, 81–83, 118, 143, 154, 178, 190
Collimation   62–67, 69, 76, 101, 154
– Prepatient   70

Colonoscopy
- Conventional   2, 15–16
- - Contra-indications   19–20
- - Diagnostic   16
- - Distension   28
- - Faecal tagging   38
- - Gold standard   2, 15, 140, 157
- - Incomplete   18, 19, 26, 38, 133, 161, 167, 171
- - Inflammatory bowel disease   19
- - Lesion morphology   157
- - Lesion size   155
- - Perforation   58
- - Polyethylene glycol   26
- - Polyp simulating mucosal prolapse syndrome   113
- - Preoperative   18
- - Postoperative   18
- - Risk   15
- - Screening   16
- - Segmental unblinding   4, 157
- - Surveillance   18
- - v Virtual colonoscopy   123
Colorectal cancer, see Carcinoma, Screening
Compliance   1–2, 26–27, 36, 54, 59, 88, 100, 123, 138
- Instruction folder   37
Computer Aided Diagnosis, see CAD
Contra-indications   20
Cone angle   69, 70
Contrast   18, 20
- Iodinated   16
- - Faecal tagging, see Preparation
- Intra-venous   1, 16, 18, 20, 38, 59, 69, 77, 167, 185
- - Extra-colonic findings   130–135
Conventional colonoscopy, see Colonoscopy
Conspicuity, see Polyp
Cost   2–4, 12, 12, 27, 85, 129, 134, 148, 155
C-RADS   11, 73, 79, 82–85, 159
Crohn's disease   19, 164–167
CTDIvol   65, 67, 69
CT dose index (CTDI)   65, 69
Cup   139

D

Depressed lesion, see Polyp
Diminutive, see Lesion, Polyp
Distension   12, 27, 38, 51–60, 66, 154, 169, 178
- Automated insufflator   54–55, 59
- Carbon dioxide   8, 29, 53–56, 59
- - Contra-indication   20
- Distension   54, 55
- Dual positioning, see Dual Positioning
- Insufflation, see Insufflation
- Multidetector row scanners   7, 56
- Perforation   55, 56, 58, 162, 164
- Rectal catheter   56
- Room air, see Room air
- Scout view, see Scout view
- Sigmoid   54
- Spasmolytics   57, 89 see also Spasmolytic
- Suboptimal   9, 23, 51, 90
Diverticulosis (diverticular disease)   90, 110, 161–163, 176
- Diverticular fecalith   110, 177
- Diverticulitis   17, 20, 162, 183
- Diverticulum   110, 156, 162
- Inverted diverticulum   111, 162
- Impacted diverticulum   162
- Muscular hypertrophy   76, 79
- Polyp-simulating mucosal prolapse syndrome   112
- Prediverticulosis   161
- Spasmolytics   57, 89
Diverticulum see Diverticulosis
Dose length product   69
Double contrast barium enema, see Barium enema
Dry preparation, see Prepation
Dual positioning   9, 31, 41, 43, 45, 51, 57, 90, 98
- Left lateral decubitus positioning   57
- Radiation exposure   65
DVD   8
Dysplasia, see Polyp

E

Effective dose   21, 65–67
Effective section thickness   64, 69, 70
Electronic cleansing   16, 21, 88, 123, 147
Endoscopist, see Gastroenterologist
Experience   9-11, 123, 138, 142, 145, 147, 178
Extracolonic findings   9, 85, 129–136
- Definitions   129
- Economical impact   134
- Ethical impact   135
- False positives   134
- Frequency   130
- IV contrast   134
- Nature   132
- Patient population   132
Extraction, see Segmentation
Extrinsic impression   106, 185

F

Faecal material, see Fluid, Stool
Faecal tagging, see Preparation
False negative   23, 36, 43, 51, 87-99, 134–135, 155
- CAD, 142-143
False positive   9, 23, 36, 63, 67, 76, 99–116, 123–125, 155, 157, 183
- CAD   143-145
- Extra-colonic findings   134–135
Familial adenomatous polyposis   14, 17, 179
Faecal occult blood test   2, 15, 18
Faecal tagging, see preparation
Fat
- Attenuation   68, 155
- Carcinoma   168
- Fibrofatty proliferation   164
- Fold   178
- Hernia   129
- Inverted diverticulum   112, 162, 178
- Ileo-cecal valve   104, 181
Fecal, see Faecal
Fecal tagging, see Preparation, Faecal tagging
Filling defect   39, 43, 90, 171, 175–178, 181, 183, 187

Subject Index

Flat, *see* Lesion, Polyp
Fluid
- Residual   23–27, 36, 57, 74, 88, 89, 99, 118, 123, 143, 146, 153–156, 185
- Tagging   35–37, 43, 45, 48

Foam   45
Fold
- Complex   10, 79, 89, 94, 96, 106, 144, 155
- Distension   51
- Diverticulosis   90, 162
- Normal   23, 118, 121, 139, 178
- Tagging   40, 43
- Thickened   67, 74, 79, 81, 89, 106, 139

Foley, *see* Catheter
FROC   141
Fuzzy merging method   145

G

Gastroenterologist   4, 11, 76, 85, 87, 112, 153, 155–157, 176
Glucagon   30-33, 57–60, 88, 154, 169, 178
Gold standard   2, 15, 140, 157, *see also* Colonoscopy

H

Haustral, *see* Fold
Heart failure   26, 37, 47
Hemorrhoid (varices)   107, 176
Hyoscin butylbromide   31, 38, 57–59, 88, 104, 154, 169
Hyperplane   69
Hyperplastic lesion, *see* Polyp

I

Ileo-cecal valve   104, 181
- Imaging   90-98, 104, 144, 181
- Competent   54
- Crohn's disease   19
- Incompetent   17, 19-21, 154

Impacted diverticulum, *see* Diverticulosis
Incomplete colonoscopy, *see* Colonoscopy
Inflammatory bowel disease   19, 58, 164–167, 170
Instruction, *see* Compliance
Insufflation   8, 27–30, 51–59, 85, 154, 166
- Contra-indication   20, 164

Insufflator, see Distension, Insufflation
Intra-venous, *see* Contrast
Inverted diverticulum, *see* Diverticulosis
Iodinated, see Contrast
Isocenter   69, 70
Interpretation   9, 59, 73–85, 119, 138, 148, 154, 175, *see also* Reading
- Tagging   39–46
- Time   120, 125, 148

L

Laxative-free, *see* Preparation
Learning curve   9, 47, 55, 87

Lesion, *see also* Carcinoma, Polyp
- Diminutive   157
- Flat   80, 94, 96, 157
- Focal polypoid v stool   76
- Location   85, 155
- Morphology   157
- Mural   80
- Pedunculated   79, 99
- Sessile   79
- Surveillance   85, *see also* Surveillance

Liver   18, 67, 78, 106, 132, 185
Lipoma   17, 74, 85, 106, 175, 183
Location correspondence   145
Longitudinal resolution   70
Low dose,   21, 38, 65–68, 132–135
Low residue diet   37, 47
Lung   3, 11, 14, 137
Lymphoma   161, 166, 170, 172, 173

M

Magnesium citrate   25, 27, 37, 88, 100, 154
Mammography   4, 11, 135, 139, 148, 158
Measurement   4, 10, 79, 84, 155–156
Meta-analysis   27, 142, 153
Metachronous, *see* Polyp
Metallic artefact, *see* Artefact
Motion artefact, *see* Artefact
Mucosal reconstruction   147
Mucous filaments   45
Multidetector CT (MDCT)   7, 56, 61–70
Muscular hypertrophy   76, 79, 80, 82, 176

N

Negative predictive value   4, 158
Network   7, 8
- Neural   140, 141, 149

Noise   61–70, 117, 127, 134

O

Obstructing mass, *see* Carcinoma
Occlusive, *see* Carcinoma
Ovarian carcinoma, *see* Carcinoma

P

PACS   8
Panoramic endoscopy   119
Parameters   7–10, 13, 61–71, 154
Partial volume effect   62, 64, 76, 143, 147, 175
Patient information   11, 37, 52, 58
Patient tolerance   29–31, 54–56, 59
Pedunculated, *see* Lesion, Polyp
Perforation
- Conventional colonoscopy   15, 58
- CT colonography   20, 55, 56, 58, 164
- Diverticulosis   162
- Inflammatory bowel disease   164

Phosphosoda, *see* Sodium phosphate
Pitch   64–71, 101, 115, 140, 154
Pitfal   9–10, 12, 87-116, 138, 142-145, 169
Polyethylene glycol, 25-27, 37, 38, 88, 154, 185
Polyp
- Adenoma, Adenomatous   2, 3, 5, 14-18, 21–22, 25, 62, 124, 131, 156, 157, 159, 170
- Adenoma-carcinoma sequence   2, 14, 38
- Advanced   2, 3, 16, 156
- Candidate   127, 139, 146
- Conspicuity   35, 39, 41, 65, 94, 96, 103, 139, 156
- Depressed   14, 62, 96
- Diminutive   3, 143, 156, 157
- Dysplasia   14, 157
- Faecal tagging   39–41, 100
- False negative   36, 87–99, *see also* False negative
- False positive   36, 76, 99-116, *see also* False positive
- Flat   14, 62, 76, 79-81, 85, 94, 96, 107, 110, 127, 143, 157, 186, 187, 190
- Hyperplastic   3, 14, 96, 99, 157, 190
- Measurement   4, 10, 79, 84, 155–156
- Metachronous   18, 22, 171, 173
- Pedunculated (stalk)   45, 64, 76, 77, 79-84, 96, 99, 155, 156, 185, 187
- Polypectomy   2-3, 5, 14–16, 19, 21, 22, 107, 143
- Pseudopolyp   36, 40, 41, 111, 112, 162–166
- Screening, *see* Screening
- Sensitivity   1, 16, 18, 47, 63, 66, 81, 87, 119, 123–127, 138, 140-142, 146
- Sessile   64, 76, 79, 81,82, 94, 96, 99, 155, 170, 185, 187
- Size   2–4, 8-11, 14–16, 62, 82, 94, 155–157
- Stalk, *see* Pedunculated
- Synchronous   18, 158, 167
- Villous   3, 14, 157, 190
Polypectomy, *see* Polyp
Polyp-simulating mucosal prolapse syndrome, *see* Diverticulosis
Post-surgery   171
Prediverticulosis, *see* Diverticulosis
Preparation   23-33, 35–49, 153
- Cathartics   25, 88
- - Reduced cathartic cleansing   36, 100, 147
- Clear liquid diet   24, 47
- Dry   27, 88, 114, 149, 154
- Faecal tagging   16, 21, 35–49, 73, 79, 96, 123, 154
- - CAD   138, 146-149
- - Electronic cleansing   16, 21, 88, 123, 147
- - False positive   100
- - Fluid tagging   35, 88
- - Imaging findings   39
- - Incomplete colonoscopy   38
- - Indications   38
- - Non-tagged stool   41
- - Obstructing tumor   38
- - Optical colonoscopy   38
- - Rationale   36
- - Reading   39
- - Results   47
- - Stool tagging   35, 100
- - Tagged stool   39
- Fluid, see fluid
- Laxative-free   4, 21, 48, 88, 99
- Magnesium citrate   25, 27, 88, 100, 154
- Mild cathartic cleansing   37
- Phosphosoda, see Sodium phosphate
- Polyethylene glycol   25-27, 37, 38, 88, 154, 185
- Regular preparation   24–27
- Sodium phosphate   4, 25–27, 37, 47–49, 88, 100, 154
- Wet   26, 88
Pregnancy   20
Prepless   21, see also Preparation
Primary 2D read   13, 51, 73, 117, 120, 123–127
- Faecal tagging   39
Primary 3D read   4, 13, 48, 51, 73, 91, 94, 123–127
- Faecal tagging   39
Problem solving   175, 190
Prolapsing mucosa   110
Pseudopolyp, *see* Polyp

Q

Quality assurance   12, 59, 85

R

Radiation dose   9, 20, 57, 61, 65–68
- Effective patient dose   69
- Noise   127
- Recommendations   69
- Weighted dose index   69
RADLEX   85
Reading, 9-11, *see also* Interpretation
- Fatigue   10, 158
- Time   125
Rectal catheter, *see* Catheter
Rectal examination   15, 52, 56
Reflux, ileo-cecal   55, 154
Reimbursement   1, 12, 21
Renal failure (insufficiency)   26, 37, 47
Renal mass   85, 131–136, 185
Report   4, 5, 9–11, 16, 82, 153–159
- C-RADS C-RADS   11, 73, 79, 82–85, 159
- Extra-colonic findings   85, 129–136
- Measurement   84
Residual stool, *see* Stool
Retrograde viewing   75, 89, 91, 94, 118, 120, 126
Ridge   139
Rippling artefact, *see* Artefact
Room air   8, 29, 53, 55–56
- Contra-indication   20

S

Scanning parameters, *see* Parameters
Scirrhous, *see* Carcinoma
Scout view   29, 31, 51, 54, 55, 59
Screening   1-5, 153
- CT colonography   13, 14
- Colorectal cancer   14–16
- Conventional colonoscopy   2
- Double contrast barium enema   2, 17–19
- Faecal occult blood test   2
- Polypectomy   2–3

Subject Index

– Rationale   2
– Sigmoidoscopy   2
Second reader   11, 127, 137, 148
Segment, colon   155
Segmental unblinding   4, 157
Segmentation (extraction)   74, 139, 149, 150
Sensitivity, *see* Polyp
Sessile see Lesion, Polyp
Shape index   139
Shoulder formation   98, 162, 165, 168, 169, 176, 190
Sigmoidoscopy   2, 4, 14, 15, 158
Size, *see* Polyp
Slice sensitivity profile   64, 70
Sodium phosphate (Phosphosoda)   4, 25–27, 37, 47, 77, 88, 100, 154
Soft tissue (abdominal) settings   17, 41, 42, 75, 82, 96
Spasm   30, 53, 88, 89, 96, 104, 110, 154, 169, 178
Spasmolytic   30–32, 57–59, 88, 154
Sphincter   52, 53, 104, 110
Spleen   106
Stairstep artefact, *see* Artefact
Stalk see, Lesion, Polyp
Statistical classifier   140
Stomach   185
Stool
– Residual   24, 36, 39, 41, 67, 74, 76–79, 96, 99, 110, 118, 120, 122, 144, 154, 162, 176, 183
– Tagging   35, 36, 39, 41
Surface rendering   117, 154
Surveillance   3, 17, 18, 19, 21, 82, 85, 156, 171
Synchronous lesion, *see* Carcinoma, Polyp

T

Tagging, see Preparation
Technician   9
Three-dimensional (3D)   117–127, 175
– Antegrade and retrograde viewing   75, 89, 91, 94, 118, 120, 126
– Artefact, *see* artefact
– 2D v 3D   123-125
– Display

– – Alternative   119
– – Conventional   118
– Flattening method   119
– Fly-through   73, 75, 117
– Measurement   84
– Panoramic endoscopy   119
– Problem-solving   74
– Surface area visualisation   75
– Transparency view   76
– Unfolded cube   120
– Virtual colon dissection   119
Training   4, 5, 9–12, 76
Transfer, data   8
Tube current   65–68, 70, 140
Tube potential   67, 70
Two-dimensional (2D)   175
– 2D v 3D   123–125
– MPR   73
– Primary   74, 120

U

Ulcerative colitis   19, 58, 164, 165

V

Variability
– Reader   9, 137–139, 142
Viewing angle   91, 118
Villous, see Polyp
Volume-rendering technique   70, 117, 140, 154, 162, 175
Voxel   70, 117, 139

W

Weighted dose index   69
Weighted hyperplane reconstruction   61, 66, 70,

Z

Z axis   64
Z filter reconstruction   70

List of Contributors

FARGOL BOOYA, MD
Department of Radiology
Mayo Clinic Rochester
Mayo Building East 2-B
200 First Street SW
Rochester, MN 55905
USA

DAVID BURLING, MD
Intestinal Imaging Unit
Level 4V
St. Mark's Hospital
Watford Road
Harrow, HA1 3UJ
Middlesex
UK

ABRAHAM H. DACHMAN, MD, FACR
Professor, Department of Radiology, MC 2026
The University of Chicago
5841 S. Maryland Avenue
Chicago, IL, 60645
USA

AYSO H. DE VRIES, MD
Department of Radiology
Academic Medical Center
University of Amsterdam
Meibergdreef 9
1105 AZ G1-226 Amsterdam
The Netherlands

HELEN FENLON, MD
Department of Radiology
Mater Misericordiae University Hospital
Eccles Street
Dublin 7
Ireland

JOSEPH T. FERRUCCI, MD
Chair Emeritus and Professor of Radiology
Boston University School of Medicine
Boston Medical Center
88 East Newton Street
Boston, MA 02118
USA

J. G. FLETCHER, MD
Department of Radiology
Mayo Clinic Rochester
Mayo Building East 2-B
200 First Street SW
Rochester, MN 55905
USA

STEFAAN GRYSPEERDT, MD
Stedelijk Ziekenhuis
Department of Radiology
Bruggesteenweg 90
8800 Roeselare
Belgium

STEVE HALLIGAN, MD
Intestinal Imaging Unit
Level 4V
St Mark's Hospital
Watford Road
Harrow, HA1 3UJ
Middlesex
UK

ANDREA LAGHI, MD
Department of Radiological Sciences
University of Rome "La Sapienza"
Polo Didattico Pontino
I.C.O.T.
Via Franco Faggiana 34
04100 Latina
Italy

PHILIPPE LEFERE, MD
Stedelijk Ziekenhuis
Department of Radiology
Bruggesteenweg 90
8800 Roeselare
Belgium

ANDREA MAIER, MD
Assistant Professor, Department of Radiology
Medical University of Vienna
Waehringer Guertel 18–20
1090 Vienna
Austria

THOMAS MANG, MD
Department of Radiology
Medical University of Vienna
Waehringer Guertel 18–20
1090 Vienna
Austria

BETH G. MCFARLAND, MD
Diagnostic Imaging Associates
Center for Diagnostic Imaging
St. Luke's Hospital
232 S. Woods Mill Road
Chesterfield, MO 63017

and

Adjunct Professor
Washington University School of Medicine
Mallinckrodt Institute of Radiology
510 S. Kingshighway Boulevard
St. Louis, MO 63110
USA

KOENRAAD J. MORTELÉ, MD
Assistant Professor of Radiology
Harvard Medical School
Director, Abdominal and Pelvic MRI
Associate Director, Division of Abdominal Imaging
and Intervention
Department of Radiology
Brigham and Women's Hospital
75 Francis Street
Boston, MA 02115
USA

AYODALE S. ODULATE, MD
Resident in Radiology
Department of Radiology
Brigham and Women's Hospital
75 Francis Street
Boston, MA 02115
USA

ALAN O'HARE, MD
Department of Radiology
Mater Misericordiae University Hospital
Eccles Street
Dublin 7
Ireland

PASQUALE PAOLANTONIO, MD
Department of Radiological Sciences
University of Rome "La Sapienza"
Polo Didattico Pontino
I.C.O.T.
Via Franco Faggiana 34
04100 Latina
Italy

PETER POKIESER, MD
Professor, Department of Radiology
Medical University of Vienna
Waehringer Guertel 18–20
1090 Vienna
Austria

WOLFGANG SCHIMA, MD
Department of Radiology
Medical University of Vienna
Waehringer Guertel 18–20
1090 Vienna
Austria

JAAP STOKER, MD
Professor of Radiology, Department of Radiology
Academic Medical Center
University of Amsterdam
Meibergdreef 9
1105 AZ G1-226 Amsterdam
The Netherlands

STUART TAYLOR, MD
Intestinal Imaging Unit, Level 4V
St Mark's Hospital
Watford Road
Harrow, HA1 3UJ
Middlesex
UK

ROGIER E. VAN GELDER, MD
Department of Radiology
Academic Medical Center
University of Amsterdam
Meibergdreef 9
1105 AZ G1-226 Amsterdam
The Netherlands

JUDY YEE, MD
Associate Professor and Vice Chair of Radiology,
UCSF
Chief of Radiology, SFVAMC
4150 Clement Street
San Francisco, CA 94121
USA

HIROYUKI YOSHIDA, PhD
Associate Professor, Department of Radiology
Massachusetts General Hospital and
Harvard Medical School
75 Blossom Court, Suite 220
Boston, MA 02114
USA

MICHAEL E. ZALIS, MD
Department of Radiology (White 270)
Massachusetts General Hospital
55 Fruit Street
Boston MA, 02114
USA

MEDICAL RADIOLOGY   Diagnostic Imaging and Radiation Oncology
Titles in the series already published

DIAGNOSTIC IMAGING

Innovations in Diagnostic Imaging
Edited by J. H. Anderson

Radiology of the Upper Urinary Tract
Edited by E. K. Lang

The Thymus - Diagnostic Imaging, Functions, and Pathologic Anatomy
Edited by E. Walter, E. Willich, and W. R. Webb

Interventional Neuroradiology
Edited by A. Valavanis

Radiology of the Pancreas
Edited by A. L. Baert,
co-edited by G. Delorme

Radiology of the Lower Urinary Tract
Edited by E. K. Lang

Magnetic Resonance Angiography
Edited by I. P. Arlart, G. M. Bongartz, and G. Marchal

Contrast-Enhanced MRI of the Breast
S. Heywang-Köbrunner and R. Beck

Spiral CT of the Chest
Edited by M. Rémy-Jardin and J. Rémy

Radiological Diagnosis of Breast Diseases
Edited by M. Friedrich
and E.A. Sickles

Radiology of the Trauma
Edited by M. Heller and A. Fink

Biliary Tract Radiology
Edited by P. Rossi,
co-edited by M. Brezi

Radiological Imaging of Sports Injuries
Edited by C. Masciocchi

Modern Imaging of the Alimentary Tube
Edited by A. R. Margulis

Diagnosis and Therapy of Spinal Tumors
Edited by P. R. Algra, J. Valk, and J. J. Heimans

Interventional Magnetic Resonance Imaging
Edited by J.F. Debatin and G. Adam

Abdominal and Pelvic MRI
Edited by A. Heuck and M. Reiser

Orthopedic Imaging
Techniques and Applications
Edited by A. M. Davies
and H. Pettersson

Radiology of the Female Pelvic Organs
Edited by E. K.Lang

Magnetic Resonance of the Heart and Great Vessels
Clinical Applications
Edited by J. Bogaert, A.J. Duerinckx, and F. E. Rademakers

Modern Head and Neck Imaging
Edited by S. K. Mukherji
and J. A. Castelijns

Radiological Imaging of Endocrine Diseases
Edited by J. N. Bruneton
in collaboration with B. Padovani and M.-Y. Mourou

Trends in Contrast Media
Edited by H. S. Thomsen,
R. N. Muller, and R. F. Mattrey

Functional MRI
Edited by C. T. W. Moonen
and P. A. Bandettini

Radiology of the Pancreas
2nd Revised Edition
Edited by A. L. Baert
Co-edited by G. Delorme
and L. Van Hoe

Emergency Pediatric Radiology
Edited by H. Carty

Spiral CT of the Abdomen
Edited by F. Terrier, M. Grossholz, and C. D. Becker

Liver Malignancies
Diagnostic and Interventional Radiology
Edited by C. Bartolozzi
and R. Lencioni

Medical Imaging of the Spleen
Edited by A. M. De Schepper
and F. Vanhoenacker

Radiology of Peripheral Vascular Diseases
Edited by E. Zeitler

Diagnostic Nuclear Medicine
Edited by C. Schiepers

Radiology of Blunt Trauma of the Chest
P. Schnyder and M. Wintermark

Portal Hypertension
Diagnostic Imaging-Guided Therapy
Edited by P. Rossi
Co-edited by P. Ricci and L. Broglia

Recent Advances in Diagnostic Neuroradiology
Edited by Ph. Demaerel

Virtual Endoscopy and Related 3D Techniques
Edited by P. Rogalla, J. Terwissscha Van Scheltinga, and B. Hamm

Multislice CT
Edited by M. F. Reiser, M. Takahashi, M. Modic, and R. Bruening

Pediatric Uroradiology
Edited by R. Fotter

Transfontanellar Doppler Imaging in Neonates
A. Couture and C. Veyrac

Radiology of AIDS
A Practical Approach
Edited by J.W.A.J. Reeders
and P.C. Goodman

CT of the Peritoneum
Armando Rossi and Giorgio Rossi

Magnetic Resonance Angiography
2nd Revised Edition
Edited by I. P. Arlart,
G. M. Bongratz, and G. Marchal

Pediatric Chest Imaging
Edited by Javier Lucaya
and Janet L. Strife

Applications of Sonography in Head and Neck Pathology
Edited by J. N. Bruneton
in collaboration with C. Raffaelli and O. Dassonville

Imaging of the Larynx
Edited by R. Hermans

3D Image Processing
Techniques and Clinical Applications
Edited by D. Caramella
and C. Bartolozzi

Imaging of Orbital and Visual Pathway Pathology
Edited by W. S. Müller-Forell

MEDICAL RADIOLOGY Diagnostic Imaging and Radiation Oncology
Titles in the series already published

Pediatric ENT Radiology
Edited by S. J. King
and A. E. Boothroyd

**Radiological Imaging
of the Small Intestine**
Edited by N. C. Gourtsoyiannis

Imaging of the Knee
Techniques and Applications
Edited by A. M. Davies
and V. N. Cassar-Pullicino

Perinatal Imaging
From Ultrasound to MR Imaging
Edited by Fred E. Avni

Radiological Imaging of the Neonatal Chest
Edited by V. Donoghue

**Diagnostic and Interventional
Radiology in Liver Transplantation**
Edited by E. Bücheler, V. Nicolas,
C. E. Broelsch, X. Rogiers,
and G. Krupski

Radiology of Osteoporosis
Edited by S. Grampp

Imaging Pelvic Floor Disorders
Edited by C. I. Bartram
and J. O. L. DeLancey
Associate Editors: S. Halligan,
F. M. Kelvin, and J. Stoker

Imaging of the Pancreas
Cystic and Rare Tumors
Edited by C. Procacci
and A. J. Megibow

**High Resolution Sonography
of the Peripheral Nervous System**
Edited by S. Peer and G. Bodner

Imaging of the Foot and Ankle
Techniques and Applications
Edited by A. M. Davies,
R. W. Whitehouse,
and J. P. R. Jenkins

Radiology Imaging of the Ureter
Edited by F. Joffre, Ph. Otal,
and M. Soulie

Imaging of the Shoulder
Techniques and Applications
Edited by A. M. Davies and J. Hodler

Radiology of the Petrous Bone
Edited by M. Lemmerling
and S. S. Kollias

Interventional Radiology in Cancer
Edited by A. Adam, R. F. Dondelinger,
and P. R. Mueller

**Duplex and Color Doppler Imaging
of the Venous System**
Edited by G. H. Mostbeck

Multidetector-Row CT of the Thorax
Edited by U. J. Schoepf

Functional Imaging of the Chest
Edited by H.-U. Kauczor

**Radiology of the Pharynx
and the Esophagus**
Edited by O. Ekberg

**Radiological Imaging
in Hematological Malignancies**
Edited by A. Guermazi

**Imaging and Intervention in
Abdominal Trauma**
Edited by R. F. Dondelinger

Multislice CT
2nd Revised Edition
Edited by M. F. Reiser, M. Takahashi,
M. Modic, and C. R. Becker

**Intracranial Vascular Malformations
and Aneurysms**
From Diagnostic Work-Up
to Endovascular Therapy
Edited by M. Forsting

Radiology and Imaing of the Colon
Edited by A. H. Chapman

Coronary Radiology
Edited by M. Oudkerk

Dynamic Contrast-Enhanced Magnetic Resonance Imaging in Oncology
Edited by A. Jackson, D. L. Buckley,
and G. J. M. Parker

**Imaging in Treatment Planning
for Sinonasal Diseases**
Edited by R. Maroldi and P. Nicolai

Clinical Cardiac MRI
With Interactive CD-ROM
Edited by J. Bogaert,
S. Dymarkowski, and A. M. Taylor

Focal Liver Lesions
Detection, Characterization,
Ablation
Edited by R. Lencioni, D. Cioni,
and C. Bartolozzi

Multidetector-Row CT Angiography
Edited by C. Catalano
and R. Passariello

Paediatric Musculoskeletal Diseases
With an Emphasis on Ultrasound
Edited by D. Wilson

Contrast Media in Ultrasonography
Basic Principles and Clinical Applications
Edited by Emilio Quaia

**MR Imaging in White Matter Diseases of the
Brain and Spinal Cord**
Edited by M. Filippi, N. De Stefano,
V. Dousset, and J. C. McGowan

Diagnostic Nuclear Medicine
2nd Revised Edition
Edited by C. Schiepers

Imaging of the Kidney Cancer
Edited by A. Guermazi

**Magnetic Resonance Imaging in
Ischemic Stroke**
Edited by R. von Kummer and T. Back

Imaging of the Hip & Bony Pelvis
Techniques and Applications
Edited by A. M. Davies, K. J. Johnson,
and R. W. Whitehouse

**Imaging of Occupational and
Environmental Disorders of the Chest**
Edited by P. A. Gevenois and
P. De Vuyst

Contrast Media
Safety Issues and ESUR Guidelines
Edited by H. S. Thomsen

Virtual Colonoscopy
A Practical Guide
Edited by P. Lefere and S. Gryspeerdt

Vascular Embolotherapy
A Comprehensive Approach
Volume 1
Edited by J. Golzarian. Co-edited by
S. Sun and M. J. Sharafuddin

Vascular Embolotherapy
A Comprehensive Approach
Volume 2
Edited by J. Golzarian. Co-edited by
S. Sun and M. J. Sharafuddin

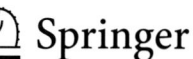

MEDICAL RADIOLOGY Diagnostic Imaging and Radiation Oncology

Titles in the series already published

RADIATION ONCOLOGY

Lung Cancer
Edited by C.W. Scarantino

Innovations in Radiation Oncology
Edited by H. R. Withers
and L. J. Peters

**Radiation Therapy
of Head and Neck Cancer**
Edited by G. E. Laramore

**Gastrointestinal Cancer –
Radiation Therapy**
Edited by R.R. Dobelbower, Jr.

**Radiation Exposure
and Occupational Risks**
Edited by E. Scherer, C. Streffer,
and K.-R. Trott

**Radiation Therapy of Benign Diseases
A Clinical Guide**
S. E. Order and S. S. Donaldson

**Interventional Radiation
Therapy Techniques – Brachytherapy**
Edited by R. Sauer

Radiopathology of Organs and Tissues
Edited by E. Scherer, C. Streffer,
and K.-R. Trott

**Concomitant Continuous Infusion
Chemotherapy and Radiation**
Edited by M. Rotman
and C. J. Rosenthal

**Intraoperative Radiotherapy –
Clinical Experiences and Results**
Edited by F. A. Calvo, M. Santos,
and L.W. Brady

**Radiotherapy of Intraocular
and Orbital Tumors**
Edited by W. E. Alberti and
R. H. Sagerman

**Interstitial and Intracavitary
Thermoradiotherapy**
Edited by M. H. Seegenschmiedt
and R. Sauer

**Non-Disseminated Breast Cancer
Controversial Issues in Management**
Edited by G. H. Fletcher and
S.H. Levitt

**Current Topics in
Clinical Radiobiology of Tumors**
Edited by H.-P. Beck-Bornholdt

**Practical Approaches to
Cancer Invasion and Metastases
A Compendium of Radiation
Oncologists' Responses to 40 Histories**
Edited by A. R. Kagan with the
Assistance of R. J. Steckel

Radiation Therapy in Pediatric Oncology
Edited by J. R. Cassady

Radiation Therapy Physics
Edited by A. R. Smith

Late Sequelae in Oncology
Edited by J. Dunst and R. Sauer

Mediastinal Tumors. Update 1995
Edited by D. E. Wood
and C. R. Thomas, Jr.

**Thermoradiotherapy
and Thermochemotherapy**
Volume 1:
Biology, Physiology, and Physics
Volume 2:
Clinical Applications
Edited by M.H. Seegenschmiedt,
P. Fessenden, and C.C. Vernon

**Carcinoma of the Prostate
Innovations in Management**
Edited by Z. Petrovich, L. Baert,
and L.W. Brady

**Radiation Oncology
of Gynecological Cancers**
Edited by H.W. Vahrson

**Carcinoma of the Bladder
Innovations in Management**
Edited by Z. Petrovich, L. Baert,
and L.W. Brady

**Blood Perfusion and
Microenvironment of Human Tumors
Implications for
Clinical Radiooncology**
Edited by M. Molls and P. Vaupel

**Radiation Therapy of Benign Diseases
A Clinical Guide
2nd Revised Edition**
S. E. Order and S. S. Donaldson

**Carcinoma of the Kidney and Testis,
and Rare Urologic Malignancies
Innovations in Management**
Edited by Z. Petrovich, L. Baert,
and L.W. Brady

**Progress and Perspectives in the
Treatment of Lung Cancer**
Edited by P. Van Houtte,
J. Klastersky, and P. Rocmans

**Combined Modality Therapy of
Central Nervous System Tumors**
Edited by Z. Petrovich, L. W. Brady,
M. L. Apuzzo, and M. Bamberg

**Age-Related Macular Degeneration
Current Treatment Concepts**
Edited by W. A. Alberti, G. Richard,
and R. H. Sagerman

**Radiotherapy of Intraocular
and Orbital Tumors
2nd Revised Edition**
Edited by R. H. Sagerman,
and W. E. Alberti

**Modification of Radiation Response
Cytokines, Growth Factors,
and Other Biolgical Targets**
Edited by C. Nieder, L. Milas,
and K. K. Ang

Radiation Oncology for Cure and Palliation
R. G. Parker, N. A. Janjan,
and M. T. Selch

**Clinical Target Volumes in Conformal and
Intensity Modulated Radiation Therapy
A Clinical Guide to Cancer Treatment**
Edited by V. Grégoire, P. Scalliet,
and K. K. Ang

**Advances in Radiation Oncology
in Lung Cancer**
Edited by Branislav Jeremić

New Technologies in Radiation Oncology
Edited by W. Schlegel, T. Bortfeld,
and A.-L. Grosu

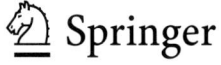

Printing and Binding: Stürtz GmbH, Würzburg

RC
804
.T65
V57

DATE DUE

SOUTH UNIVERSITY
709 MALL BLVD.
SAVANNAH, GA 31406